.95

369 0289745

ISSUES IN HEALTH AND HEALTH CARE RELATED TO RACE/ETHNICITY, IMMIGRATION, SES AND GENDER

RESEARCH IN THE SOCIOLOGY OF HEALTH CARE

Series Editor: Jennie Jacobs Kronenfeld

RESEARCH IN THE SOCIOLOGY OF HEALTH CARE
VOLUME 30

ISSUES IN HEALTH AND HEALTH CARE RELATED TO RACE/ETHNICITY, IMMIGRATION, SES AND GENDER

EDITED BY

JENNIE JACOBS KRONENFELD
Department of Sociology, Arizona State University, USA

United Kingdom – North America – Japan
India – Malaysia – China

Emerald Group Publishing Limited
Howard House, Wagon Lane, Bingley BD16 1WA, UK

First edition 2012

Copyright © 2012 Emerald Group Publishing Limited

British Library Cataloguing in Publication Data
A catalogue record for this book is available from the British Library

ISBN: 978-1-78190-124-3
ISSN: 0275-4959 (Series)

ISOQAR certified
Management Systems,
awarded to Emerald for
adherence to Quality
and Environmental
standards ISO 9001:2008
and 14001:2004,
respectively

Certificate Number 1985
ISO 9001
ISO 14001

INVESTOR IN PEOPLE

CONTENTS

SECTION IV: POLICY ISSUES AND RACE/ETHNICITY

LIST OF CONTRIBUTORS

Kathryn Freeman Anderson	Department of Sociology, University of Arizona, Tucson, AZ, USA
Jennifer Arney	Department of Sociology, University of Houston-Clear Lake, Houston, TX, USA; Department of Medicine, Section on Health Services Research, Baylor College of Medicine, Houston, TX, USA
Marriam Ewaida	Graduate School of Education, College of Education and Human Development, George Mason University, Fairfax, VA, USA
Angélica Forero-Quintana	Department of Emergency Medicine, Texas Tech University Health Sciences Center at El Paso, El Paso, TX, USA
Elena Frank	Women and Gender Studies, Arizona State University, Tempe, AZ, USA
Christopher J. Fries	Department of Sociology, University of Manitoba, Winnipeg, Manitoba, Canada
Andrew S. Fullerton	Department of Sociology, Oklahoma State University, Stillwater, OK, USA
Jean Giles-Sims	Department of Sociology, Texas Christian University, Fort Worth, TX, USA
Joanne Connor Green	Department of Political Science,Texas Christian University, Fort Worth, TX, USA

Sara E. Grineski   Environment Core of the Hispanic Health
                            Disparities Research Center, Department
                            of Sociology and Anthropology, University
                            of Texas at El Paso, El Paso, TX, USA

Atsuko Kawakami   School of Social and Family Dynamics,
                            Arizona State University, Tempe, AZ, USA

Katina B. Kearney   Graduate School of Education, College of
                            Education and Human Development,
                            George Mason University, Fairfax, VA,
                            USA

Jennie Jacobs   School of Social and Family Dynamics,
Kronenfeld   Arizona State University, Tempe, AZ, USA

Charles Lockhart   Department of Political Science,Texas
                            Christian University, Fort Worth, TX, USA

Melinda S. Markham   School of Family Studies and Human
                            Services, Kansas State University at Salina,
                            Salina, KS, USA

Eileen J. Porter   School of Nursing, University of Wisconsin-
                            Madison, Madison, WI, USA

Kim Price-Glynn   Department of Sociology & Urban and
                            Community Studies Program, University of
                            Connecticut, West Hartford, CT, USA

Carter Rakovski   Department of Sociology, California State
                            University, Fullerton, CA, USA

Igor Ryabov   Department of Sociology, The University of
                            Texas-Pan American, Edinburg, TX, USA

Colleen K. Vesely   Graduate School of Education, College of
                            Education and Human Development,
                            George Mason University, Fairfax, VA,
                            USA

Rose Weitz   School of Social Transformation, Arizona
                            State University, Tempe, AZ, USA

SECTION I
RACE/ETHNICITY, IMMIGRATION, SES AND GENDER, AS FACTORS IN HEALTH AND HEALTH CARE

HEALTH CARE SYSTEM ISSUES AND RACE/ETHNICITY, IMMIGRATION, SES AND GENDER AS SOCIOLOGICAL ISSUES LINKING TO HEALTH AND HEALTH CARE

Jennie Jacobs Kronenfeld

ABSTRACT

This chapter will initially review some health care system issues with a focus on the US health care system. It will then review some of the sociological literature about race/ethnicity, immigration, socioeconomic status (SES) and gender and how these factors link to health and health care. In addition, the chapter will serve as an introduction to the volume and will briefly review the contents of the other sections and chapters in this volume.

Keywords: Review; USA; health; health care; health care system; race; ethnicity; immigration; SES; gender

Issues in Health and Health Care Related to Race/Ethnicity, Immigration, SES and Gender
Research in the Sociology of Health Care, Volume 30, 3–18
Copyright © 2012 by Emerald Group Publishing Limited
All rights of reproduction in any form reserved
ISSN: 0275-4959/doi:10.1108/S0275-4959(2012)0000030003

This chapter provides an introduction to Volume 30 of the *Research in the Sociology of Health Care* series. This volume is entitled *Issues in Health and Health Care Related to Race, Ethnicity, Immigration, SES, and Gender*. The overall volume is divided into four sections. The first section is this introductory chapter. The second section includes chapters related to race, ethnicity, immigration, and SES and is the largest section in the volume. The third section includes chapters linked to gender. The last section includes chapters linked to policy issues and race/ethnicity.

HEALTH CARE SYSTEMS AND HEALTH CARE USE

While most of the chapters in the section focus on the impact of sociological factors such as race/ethnicity, immigration, SES, and gender on health and health care, at least for those articles that use data linked to health and health care issues in the United States, issues of the health care system in which these actions occur is important. Currently in the United States there is a major ongoing debate about the need to reform aspects of the health care delivery system. Certain aspects of the major legislation passed in the United States in March 2010 as part of the Patient Protection and Affordable Care Act of 2010 health insurance reform, are currently being debated in the United States Supreme Court while this volume is being prepared. While this introductory chapter cannot predict how that challenge to aspects of the law will be resolved, it is important to understand a few basic facts about health care in the United States as an underpinning for many of the chapters in this volume. This first part of the chapter will review some current material on health care insurance and health care in the United States, followed by sections on important social factors and health and health care and a last section summarizing the chapters included in this volume.

Compared to many other countries, health care debates in the United States have become volatile conversations and, more so in recent years. In some ways, these debates have become flashpoints to ideological conflict (Starr, 2011). This is not because there have not been controversies in the past about the passage of major new health programs. At the time of the passage of Medicare in the United States, there was major debate between the political parties. In addition, there were debates with health related organizations such as the American Medical Association and many health insurance organizations, especially about Medicare. Some of these same issues resurfaced during the debates over the failed Clinton health care reforms. Once the Medicare program was first passed and then implemented, it became clear that costs for the program were going to be higher than the initial estimates, leading to new controversies (Kronenfeld, 2011). As programs such as Medicare for the elderly and Medicaid for the poor became more accepted parts of the American approach to health care services, more of the discussion about health care often focused on who had access to care, what to do about some groups who were not being covered, whether costs were becoming too high, and whether the quality of health care being delivered was appropriate. Often, the public discussion became part of a debate over whether there was a "crisis" in health care. Certainly, this was true of the discussion in public at the time of the proposing of the Clinton health care plan, which eventually failed (Kronenfeld, 1997). During that time frame, any major push on health care reform ceased, and what became the major accomplishment of the Clinton administration in health care policy was the passage of the state child health insurance program (SCHIP) that expanded coverage for health care services to the children of the working poor.

In the 2000 election, George W. Bush won the presidency in an extremely close election that ended up with final decisions on the outcome of the election by the Supreme Court due to issues about the appropriateness of the ballot and contested results in certain states, especially issues with ballots in the state of Florida. This meant that for the first time in over 100 years, the United States elected a person as president (George W. Bush) who had lost the popular vote. Bush had not focused much in his campaign on health care, in contrast to his opponent, Al Gore who proposed extensions to SCHIP and to Medicare. When health care became part of the campaign in September 2000, Bush did propose a plan to convert Medicare into a system of competing private health insurance plans that would include prescription drugs in their benefits, an important deficit in the original Medicare program. The initial Bush focus was on a tax cut, which he accomplished. After that Bush became interested in accomplishing one part of what had been mentioned during the campaign, a prescription drug option for Medicare, rather than any type of comprehensive health care reform. In 2004, the Medicare Prescription Drug, Improvement and Modernization Act, generally known as the Medicare Modernization Act, was passed. This act had three separate parts, the prescription drug addition to Medicare, new provisions for private insurance coverage in Medicare, and tax incentives for health savings accounts. The part most anticipated by the public, the prescription drug addition to Medicare, did not begin until January 1, 2006. Prior to that, there was a distribution of drug discount cards to the low-income elderly in mid-2004 so that they would obtain some financial relief from high drug costs. Once the complete plan began, many of the elderly were initially confused by the amount and complexity of some of the details of the program, since people had to pick among different private plans with different sets of drugs included. Some experts even think that confusion among the public about aspects of this plan may have played a role in the Republicans' loss of Congress in November 2006.

One thing that did happen by early 2000 was that rising health care costs returned to the United States. During the 1990s, the rise in costs had slowed some, and there were some people who hoped that the marketplace was playing a role in this effort to keep health care costs from rising as rapidly as it had in some previous decades. As an example, from 2000 to 2006, average annual premiums for employer-sponsored family coverage rose by 87 percent, going from 6,348 dollars in 2000 to 11,480 dollars in 2006. As part of these rising costs, fewer employers decided to continue offering health insurance to their workers, and from 2001 to 2006, the number of firms providing health insurance declined from 69 to 61 percent (Starr, 2011). Even though in this same time period there were some increases in coverage by Medicaid, the proportion of people who had a high financial burden from health care costs, defined as more than 10 percent of pretax income on insurance premiums and out-of-pocket expenses, rose one percentage point each year, up to 19 percent by 2006. Absolute numbers of people uninsured at any one time rose from 40 to 45 million, or about 15.3 percent of the population (Starr, 2011). Other indicators of how Americans were increasingly viewing health care as a concern were that in a Kaiser Family Foundation Survey in 2004, health costs ranked among Americans' major worries about the future (Commonwealth Fund, 2007).

Quality also became a focus of concern and of attention by some major health policy and health research groups during a similar time frame. As compared to the cost area, one difficulty in accessing quality is that measurement is less clear and the US health care system is less easily amenable to evaluation than systems in some other countries, because it is not one unified system with an available database to use to understand quality issues. Quality is often defined as the degree of excellence or conformation to high standards, and it cannot be assessed without a clear understanding of the standards of excellence (Kronenfeld, 2002).

Two important reports from the Institute of Medicine have dealt with quality concerns in the United States. The first was a 1999 report, *To Err Is Human*, which argued that while physicians, nurses, and other health professionals were doing their best to provide quality care, the current system did not reward innovation and communication (Institute of Medicine, 1999). This report documented that more people die each year in the United States from medical mistakes than from highway deaths, breast cancer, and AIDS. A second report focused on quality issues was published in 2001, entitled *Crossing the Quality Chasm* (Institute of Medicine, 2001). This report argued that the current U.S. health care system is a tangled, highly fragmented web that often wastes resources with unnecessary services and duplicated efforts. Possible solutions would include revamping the system to deal not only with the needs and values of patients, but also to develop greater teamwork among health professionals and greater use of information technology. Some suggested technological solutions that are also included in the new health reform legislation are better medical information systems and use computers for the maintenance of medical records.

By the time of the election of President Obama in 2008, these problems with the availability of health care insurance, the overall rising costs of health care, and quality concerns again made health care an important campaign issue. Discussion about how to reform the health care delivery system in the United States was particularly a part of the Democratic primary debates, with Obama and Clinton having somewhat different proposals. By the time of the general election campaign, Obama had made more comprehensive health reform a major promise in his election discussions. Once elected, accomplishing some of his goals in the area of health care reform became an important push, even though both the President and his advisers were all aware of the ways in which the failure of health care reform in the Clinton administration had been an important failure in Clinton's first term as President. Thus, with great difficulty and many compromises in the specifics of the plan, the Affordable Health Care Act of 2010 was eventually passed. In reality, many of the provisions of this plan take place in different years, and some of the most important will not be put into place until 2014. This includes the creation of health exchanges to help make health insurance more available for people who do not have work-based health insurance available (some of these people include those who are unemployed). It also includes the mandate that employers must offer health insurance and people must purchase it, or pay penalties, provisions that are currently under consideration as to the determination of their legality by the Supreme Court.

RACE/ETHNICITY, IMMIGRATION, AND HEALTH AND HEALTH CARE

In the early years of sociology within the United States, there was a major focus on social class differences, to the extent that data was available.

As differences in recent years have become redefined as disparities with the growth of federal government efforts in health, there has been more focus on race/ethnicity. Partially, this was due to greater data availability and partially a belief, especially in the United States, that a policy focus necessitated more attention to race/ethnicity than to class. In the past few years, there is now a growing consensus whether in the United States or Great Britain that looking only at data on race/ethnicity without a consideration of social class differences is problematic (Adler & Rehkopf, 2008; Davey Smith, 2000; Kawachi, Daniels, & Robinson, 2005). One important issue is variability in the distribution of racial/ethnic groups across levels of income, wealth, education, and occupation. If studies look only at race/ethnicity and ignore social class issues, it is too easy to conclude that differences are linked either specifically to race/ethnicity or even to biological differences that may be linked to race and ethnicity (Issacs & Schroeder, 2004).

Recent studies tend to examine issues in a more complex way, although this complexity can make interpretations of results more difficult and also make it more difficult to arrive at clear policy-oriented conclusions. Two recent articles published in the *Journal of Health and Social Behavior* in a section entitled "Unraveling Racial and Ethnic Health Disparities" looked at race/ethnicity in combination with other factors and illustrated these complexities. They also build upon some important recent trends in the United States as well as in many parts of Europe, the growth in immigration. Walton (2009) examined racial and ethnic minorities in the United States and the impact of racial segregation on birth weights. The second article perceived ethnic discrimination as contrasted with acculturation stress as factors that influence substance use among Latino youth in the southwest (Kulis, Marsiglia, & Nieri, 2009). More than half of the sample of fifth grade students from the southwestern United States perceived some discrimination and almost half reported some acculturation stress. Spanish dominant and bilingual youth perceived more discrimination than English dominant youth. Youth in the United States for less time (five or fewer years) perceived more discrimination than youth who had been in the United States longer. The most acculturation stress was reported by Spanish dominant youth or more recent arrivals. Because some of these results (such as that youth with less time in the United States perceived more discrimination) are inconsistent with research on Latino adults and because linguistic acculturation and time in the United States did not moderate the effects of perceived discrimination or acculturation stress, the chapter ends up discussing the need for longitudinal data and a much better understanding of the context of determining adaptation processes among immigrants.

Issues of immigration complicate considerations of race/ethnicity as well as socioeconomic status (SES). SES is covered in the next section in this chapter. Immigration and race/ethnicity issues as linked to health and health services are growing in importance in many countries. In a commentary article in the *American Journal of Public Health* about the role of acculturation research in advancing science and practice to reduce health care disparities among Latinos in the United States, Zambrana and Carter-Pokras (2010) argue that despite an impressive body of public health knowledge accumulated over the past decade on health care disparities among Latinos, inconclusive and conflicting results on predictors of health care disparities remain. If forced to make conclusions, they argue that social and economic determinants are more important predictors than culture in understanding health care disparities. Not all researchers agree with that type of conclusion. In a review article, Takeuchi, Walton, and Leung (2010) argue that there is an important role played by segregation as a social process. It contributes to differential exposure to many particular environments and contexts and these different opportunity structures and community structures may influence health by shaping social processes. Similarly, a recent review article about the Hispanic paradox by Dubowitz, Bates, and Acevado-Garcia (2010) points out how the sociopolitical context and patterns of migration contribute to health and to the paradox that Hispanics/Latinas have higher life expectancies than would be expected based on their higher representation among the poor.

These varying articles illustrate that the more factors researchers consider in trying to understand the complexity between health differences, immigration, race/ethnicity, and SES, the more confusing and conflicting results researchers may find. One hope for this volume is that some of the studies will add to the complexity of this confusing literature, even given the reality that any one chapter will not be able to be the definitive chapter on these complex topics.

An issue that connects research on race/ethnicity and social class relates to measurement concerns. In a report from the Institute of Medicine (2009), there is a recommendation that researchers develop more detailed categories for race, ethnicity, and English language proficiency. The Institute of Medicine began to work on this topic in early 2009, at the request of the Agency for Healthcare Research and Quality. A subcommittee on Standardized Collection of Race/Ethnicity Data for Healthcare Quality Improvement was formed and this group recommended collection of the existing Office of Management and Budget (OMB) race and Hispanic ethnicity categories as well as more fine-grained categories of ethnicity and language need. In addition to these national standards, the committee also recommended that locally relevant categories of granular ethnicity and languages be made available and that individuals should be given the opportunity to self-identify their ethnicity or language when it is not listed on local data collection instruments. An important aspect of the recommendations from the Institute of Medicine is that it will become more likely that hospitals, health plans, and physician practices may actually modify categories they currently use and this would then make these applied sources of data more useful for research in the future.

SES AND HEALTH AND HEALTH CARE

Similar concerns about how information is gathered and disparate results depending on the exact ways data are gathered apply to the issue of SES and health disparities. Three traditional ways of measuring SES are occupation, income, and education. Each of these have somewhat different associations with health outcomes (Adler & Rehkopf, 2008; Kitigawa & Hauser, 1978; Kliss & Scheuren, 1978). In addition, another way to consider SES is social capital (Kawachi, 2010). In the United States, most studies now use income and education more often than occupation, because those questions are much simpler to ask and to code. In addition, in the United States, weaker associations have been found with measures of occupation as compared with income and education, perhaps because of the difficulty of having more standardized measures across studies (Adler & Rehkopf, 2008; Braveman et al., 2005). Some authors argue that education is the key to socioeconomic differentials in health (Ross & Mirowsky, 2010). A slightly different way to look at SES and its relationship to health disparities is the fundamental cause argument (Link & Phelan, 2010).

Braveman et al. (2005) argue that SES is often implicitly or explicitly equated with income, especially in the United States. There are many issues with this approach. Even though researchers all recognize how important it is to obtain income information, many practitioners and some researchers consider income information to be too difficult or too sensitive to collect. Instead, information about education (typically measured as years completed or credentials of formal schooling) is more easily obtained and thus is often treated as a proxy for income (or for SES overall). In addition, income itself is a limited measure, and it is better to include measures of wealth as well as income. There is evidence that wealth measures are even more widely varied when racial/ethnic information is examined as linked to SES. Beyond the basic collection of information, in many studies when both income and education are obtained, researchers have methodological concerns about the inclusion of both in analytic models due to colinearity. According to Braveman et al. (2005), both evidence from literature and new analyses indicates that while standard measures of education and income are correlated, these correlations are generally not usually strong enough to justify education as a proxy for income (or vice versa). Earnings do vary at similar educational levels, and this is even truer if researchers also take into account different social (e.g., racial/ethnic, sex, age) groups.

The fundamental cause approach is no longer a new approach in medical sociology. It first emerged in the 1990s and was developed in response to the emphasis in public health on risk factor approaches, an approach that dominated medicine and epidemiology then (House, 2002; Link & Phelan, 1995). In its essence, the fundamental cause argument is that the unequal distribution of socioeconomic resources leads to health inequalities as those with more resources are then able to use those resources to acquire and act upon the new and better information, such as in the areas of diet, exercise, and hazards, to both protect and improve their health. Given this, interventions that aim at proximal causes of health disparities will never close the gap. The authors of this theory are now clear that they view it as a middle range theory as is social stress theory or theories of health selection (Link & Phelan, 2010).

Kawachi (2010) has focused recently on social capital and has used this concept to shift the focus from individuals to communities. He views the application of resources as a group level construct. Advantages can flow across social networks, and become an additional resource to create social inequalities in health.

While the earlier discussion on measurement of SES stressed the greater simplicity and perhaps accuracy of collection of education data, Ross and Mirowsky (2010) argue that there are advantages to the use of education as the one measure of SES that go beyond simplicity and accuracy. They argue that education can operate as both human capital and a commodity and is the key to socioeconomic differentials in health.

GENDER AND HEALTH AND HEALTH CARE

Gender is an important social factor that has received greater attention in sociology overall and in medical sociology in the last 20 years. As most research has now documented, women live longer than men, although they may actually report poorer health status and especially more disabilities as they age. The sex/gender difference in life expectancy in the United States is now well known, with women living on average 5.2 years longer than men do (Rieker, Bird, & Lang, 2010). Women also generally are higher utilizers of the health care system (Anspach, 2010). Previous research on gender and health and health care utilization also points out that gender differences may also vary by categories considered in the previous sections, such as race/ethnicity and SES.

Recent specific studies, whether looking at broader health indicators such as self-rated health (Zheng, 2009) or more specific issues, sometimes in specific age groups such as among adolescents and sometime with specific health outcomes such as smoking cessation (Castro et al., 2009) or adolescence and obesity (Clark, O'Malley, Schulenberg, & Lantz, 2009), find complexities in examining issues of gender and health and health care disparities. The more general studies point to the need to consider social factors beyond gender to understand health disparities. In a study looking at rising United States income inequality and gender and self-rated health, Zheng (2009) finds that most previous research on the effect of income inequality on health has been based on sectional data and often finds mixed results. Using data from 1972 through 2004, Zheng finds that increases in income inequality increase the odds of worse self-reported health by 9.4 percent, but that overall income inequality and gender specific income inequality harm men's, but not women's, self-rated health. Lack of attention to gender composition may be an important factor in discrepant findings in earlier studies. In a study looking at many indicators of health and health care utilization among adolescents, Mulye et al. argue that young adulthood is a particularly important period of life to examine when interested in health disparities (Mulye et al., 2009). They find large differences on many different outcomes, after examining such areas as mortality, health-related behaviors, and health care access and utilization. They particularly point out that large disparities persist in many areas by race/ethnicity and gender, pointing out the importance of looking at gender but also looking at in along with other social factors such as race/ethnicity.

Recent studies that focus mainly on one or a few health outcomes but include gender as an important social factor in disparities in health and health care use also tend to argue that studies need to look at gender in relationship to other social factors. Rieker et al. (2010) in their recent review article in the newest edition of the *Handbook of Medical Sociology* point out that in the past binary approaches to gender often treated men and women as distinct homogenous groups, whereas most scholars today would emphasize the importance of understanding gender as a factor along with other important social factors such as age, race/ethnicity, and SES. In particular, these researchers stress an approach they call constrained choices. This approach emphasizes how structural constraints narrow the opportunities and choices that are available for individuals. In addition, choices that people make may play an important part in creating health and health care utilization outcomes. Differences in work and family roles, in different workplaces and in communities all may impact differences in health and health care utilization between men and women. There are linkages between this approach and the fundamental cause approach, and all of this points out how interrelated important social factors such as gender, SES, race/ethnicity, and immigration become, especially when researchers relate those to health and health care outcomes and differentials in such outcomes.

ORGANIZATION OF THIS VOLUME

This volume is divided into four sections. The first section is this chapter that represents an introduction to the rest of the volume, and both reviews briefly each of the other chapters in this section, as well as reviewing the basic concepts all chapters deal with in this volume as the first part of this chapter.

The second section is the largest section of the volume, and includes six chapters dealing with different aspects of race/ethnicity, immigration, and SES, as linked to health and health care services. The first three chapters each deal with specific racial/ethnic groups, with two focusing on Mexican-Americans and border issues and one on Japanese immigrants to the United States. The other three chapters focus on issues more broadly related to race/ethnicity, immigration, and SES as linked to health and health care. The first chapter is titled "Obesity in Mexican-American Adults: Interplay of Immigrant Generation, Gender and Socioeconomic Status" by Igor Ryabov. Using the data from a unique sample of Mexican-American adults from the U.S.–Mexico border area, this chapter offers explanations for Mexican-American obesity, with a special focus on immigrant generation status, income, and gender. This chapter applies nutrition transition theory to the study of immigrant assimilation in a regional context. Age of arrival is found to be a stronger predictor of obesity than country of birth. As Mexican-American immigrants' length of residence increases, so does their Body Mass Index (BMI) that reflects the adoption of less diverse diet and sedentary lifestyles. The second chapter also deals with issues along the

U.S.–Mexico border region and focuses on delayed diagnosis of tuberculosis in that area using a health narratives approach. This chapter by Angélica Forero-Quintana and Sara Grineski finds that 14 of the 15 patients experienced delayed diagnosis. Important themes were provider's lack of awareness, including repeated misdiagnosis and TB test errors, and patient disadvantage, including fear of U.S. immigration authorities and few economic resources for care. The chapter concludes that prompt diagnosis of TB could be achieved if providers were more cognizant of TB and its symptoms and public health policies increased access to health care regardless of immigration status or SES. The third chapter focuses on the views of Japanese immigrant women as they age as linked to needed care and is by Atsuko Kawakami and Jennie Jacobs Kronenfeld.

Although other research on Japanese in their homeland has pointed out how people in Japan feel ashamed when elderly members of the family are cared for by formal services such as day care or government/commercial-based nursing homes due to cultural norms of the consciousness of social appearance, this was not found in this study of elderly Japanese immigrant women's preference for utilization of formal care services in the United States. Instead, these women felt that receiving family-based care could be a burden on their middle-aged children (or grandchildren) and preferred to purchase formal long-term care services. These immigrant women held rather positive views on formal care in the United States, including nursing homes.

The last three chapters in this section are more diverse in terms of ethnic groups that are studied. The next chapter by Colleen K. Vesely, Marriam Ewaida, and Katina B. Kearney is entitled "Two Sides of the Potomac: A Qualitative Exploration of Immigrant Families' Health Care Experiences in Virginia and Washington, DC." This chapter examined how micro- and macro-level issues including access to child-only or family public health insurance helps to shape low-income immigrant families' health care experiences, looking at first-generation, low-income immigrant Latin American and African mothers. Pregnancy was the entry for most into the U.S. health care system. The fifth chapter in this section explores a very different issue, the use of accepted and rejected complementary and alternative medical therapies, not in the United States, but in Canada. In this chapter, Christopher J. Fries compares Whites with Asians, South Asians, Blacks, Latin Americans, Aboriginals, and Others and reports that whites and North American born immigrants had higher odds of using "accepted" therapies whereas immigrant visible minorities and those with Asian ethnic identities were more likely to use "rejected" therapies. The last chapter in this section by Kathryn

Freeman Anderson and Andrew S. Fullerton looks at racial residential segregation and access to health care coverage. Both this chapter and the fifth chapter in this section use quantitative analytical approaches to study their topics. The Anderson and Fullerton's chapter utilizes multilevel binary logit models based on individual-level health data from the 2008 Behavioral Risk Factor Surveillance System linked to metropolitan-area level data to examine the association between Black/White segregation in 136 metropolitan statistical areas in the United States and health care coverage. They find an increase in Black/White segregation is related to a decrease in the likelihood of having health insurance for Black residents and an increase in the Black-White gap in health care coverage. These effects are substantial even when controlling for the effects of educational, social and economic factors.

The third section focused on articles linked to gender and includes three different chapters. The first chapter is "Gendering Affective Disorders in Direct-to-Consumer Advertisements" by Jennifer Arney and Rose Weitz. This chapter explores how direct-to-consumer advertisements (DTCA) for major depression and anxiety disorders use contemporary gender scripts to sell medications and disease definitions to consumers, and in the process reflect and reinforce those scripts for both men and women. Between 1997 and 2006, antidepressant DTCA in popular magazines overwhelmingly depicted depression as a (white) female disorder, as did anti-anxiety DTCA. DTCA suggested that medication would yield benefits for women primarily in their close relationships and for men primarily in their work lives, thus reinforcing the binary sex divisions implicit in hegemonic masculinity and emphasized femininity. The second chapter is entitled "'More than Boobs and Ovaries': BRCA Positive Young Women and the Negotiation of Medicalization in an Online Message Board" by Elena Frank. The discovery of the BRCA1 and BRCA2 genes has facilitated the construction of a new group of women referred to as "previvors" – individuals who are survivors of a predisposition to cancer but who are not presently ill. These "previvors" are the first generation of women faced with the option to make preventative health choices based on this kind of genetic information. This research examines how young BRCA positive women negotiate the medicalization of their bodies based on their new "potentially ill" status. The majority share an "anything's better than cancer" mantra, suggesting that fear of death largely outweighs all other fears or concerns. The women appear to believe that they must undergo prophylactic surgery and disassociate from their bodies in order to save their lives. The third chapter deals with "Close-Calls That Older Homebound Women Handled Without

Help While Alone at Home" by Eileen J. Porter and Melinda S. Markham. This chapter points out that competence to live alone is typically associated with measures of activities of daily living, but such measures fail to capture problematic situations that older people face in daily life, especially how older homebound women handle potentially harmful incidents. In a descriptive phenomenological study of the experience of reaching help quickly (RHQ) with 40 older homebound women, 33 women spontaneously reported 139 incidents (falls, "tight spots," near-falls, health problems, and unwanted visitors) that they managed alone. The purpose of this secondary phenomenological analysis of RHQ project data was to describe the experience of those women with handling "close-calls." Data yielded a typology of close-call incidents and developed five components of the phenomenon.

The fourth section includes two chapters that have a stronger policy orientation, as linked to issues of race/ethnicity, gender, and health. The first chapter in the section is on "Countervailing Influences of Black and Women Legislators on State Age Friendliness" by Jean Giles-Sims, Joanne Green, and Charles Lockhart. The chapter examines the influences of African-American and female legislators on the supportiveness of states toward elders, using a cross-sectional data set for the 50 American states around the year 2000. They find that, controlling for the most prominent alternative factors generally shaping state orientations and policies, women legislators are selectively supportive of dimensions of state elderly friendliness, but African-American legislators do not share this support. The second chapter in this section deals with "Intersectional Identities and Worker Experiences in Home Health Care: The National Home Health Aide Survey" by Carter Rakovski and Kim Price-Glynn. They look at the topic of growth of home health care, as important topic as the population ages in the United States. Small, regional, qualitative studies have indicated both satisfaction and exploitation in home health care work. This study broadens the scope of current research by addressing issues facing home health care workers using large scale, nationwide data available as part of the National Home Health Aide Survey. The prevalence and sources of discrimination and working conditions are examined according to workers' intersectional gender, race, ethnicity, and class identities. Satisfaction was highest for those who were extremely satisfied with challenging work, learning new skills, and were most supported in their caring labor. Salary was an area with frequent dissatisfaction. Black women and men reported the highest levels of discrimination followed by Hispanic women and men and the largest source of discrimination was from patients.

REFERENCES

Adler, N. E., & Rehkopf, D. H. (2008). U.S. disparities in health: Descriptions, causes and mechanisms. *Annual Review of Public Health, 29*, 235–252.

Anspach, R. R. (2010). Gender and health care. In C. E. Bird, P. Conrad, A. M. Fremont & S. Timmermans (Eds.), *Handbook of medical sociology* (5th ed.). Nashville, TN: Vanderbilt University Press.

Braveman, P. A., Cubbin, C., Egerter, S., Chideya, S., Marchi, K. S., Metzler, M., & Posner, S. (2005). Socioeconomic stats in health research – One size does not fit all. *Journal of the American Medical Association, 294*, 2879–2888.

Castro, Y., Reitzel, L. R., Businelle, M. S., Kendzor, D. E., Mazas, C. A., Li, Y., ... Wetter, D. W. (2009). Acculturation differentially predicts smoking cessation among Latino men and women. *Cancer Epidemiology, Biomarkers and Prevention, 18*(12), 3468–3475.

Clark, P. J., O'Malley, P. M., Schulenberg, J. E., & Lantz, P. (2009). Differential treatment in weight-related health behaviors among American young adults by gender, race/ethnicity and socioeconomic status, 1984–2006. *American Journal of Public Health, 99*, 1893–1901.

Commonwealth Fund. (2007). Americans spend more out-of-pocket on health care expenses. In *Health system performance in selected nations: A chartpack*. Washington, DC: Commonwealth Fund.

Davey Smith, G. (2000). Learning to live with complexity: Ethnicity, socioeconomic position and health in Britain and the United States. *American Journal of Public Health, 90*, 1694–1698.

Dubowitz, T., Bates, L. M., & Acevado-Garcia, D. (2010). The Latino health paradox: Looking at the intersectionality of sociology and health. In C. E. Bird, P. Conrad, A. M. Fremont & S. Timmermans (Eds.), *Handbook of medical sociology* (5th ed.). Nashville, TN: Vanderbilt University Press.

House, J. S. (2002). Understanding social factors and inequalities in health: 20th century progress and 21st century prospects. *Journal of Health and Social Behavior, 43*, 124–142.

Institute of Medicine. (1999). *To err is human*. Washington, DC: National Academy of Sciences.

Institute of Medicine. (2001). *Crossing the quality chasm: A new health system for the 21st century*. Washington, DC: National Academy of Sciences.

Institute of Medicine. (2009). *Race, ethnicity, and language data: Standardization for health care quality improvement*. Washington, DC: Institute of Medicine.

Issacs, S. L., & Schroeder, S. A. (2004). Class – The ignored determinant of the nation's health. *New England Journal of Medicine, 351*(11), 1137–1142.

Kawachi, I. (2010). Social capital and health. In C. E. Bird, P. Conrad, A. M. Fremont & S. Timmermans (Eds.), *Handbook of medical sociology* (5th ed.). Nashville, TN: Vanderbilt University Press.

Kawachi, I., Daniels, N., & Robinson, D. E. (2005). Health disparities by race and class: Why both matter. *Health Affairs, 24*, 343–352.

Kitigawa, E., & Hauser, P. (1978). *Differential mortality in the United States*. Cambridge, MA: Harvard University Press.

Kliss, B., & Scheuren, F. J. (1978). The 1973 CPS-IRS-SSA exact match study. *Social Security Bulletin, 42*, 14–22.

Kronenfeld, J. J. (1997). *The changing federal role in U.S. health care policy*. Westport, CT: Praeger Press.

Kronenfeld, J. J. (2002). *Health care policy: Issues and trends*. Westport, CT: Praeger Press.

Kronenfeld, J. J. (2011). *Medicare*. Santa Barbara, CA: Greenwood Press (an imprint of ABC-Clio).

Kulis, S., Marsiglia, F. F., & Nieri, T. (2009). Perceived ethnic discrimination versus acculturation stress: Influences on substance use among Latino Youth in the Southwest. *Journal of Health and Social Behavior, 50*(4), 443–459.

Link, B. G., & Phelan, J. C. (1995). Social conditions as fundamental causes of disease. *Journal of Health and Social Behavior* (extra issue). In C. E. Bird, P. Conrad, A. M. Fremont, & S. Timmermans (Eds), *Handbook of Medical Sociology* (5th ed., pp. 80–94). Nashville, TN: Vanderbilt University Press.

Link, B. G., & Phelan, J. C. (2010). Social conditions as fundamental causes of health inequalities. In C. E. Bird, P. Conrad, A. M. Fremont & S. Timmermans (Eds.), *Handbook of medical sociology* (5th ed.). Nashville, TN: Vanderbilt University Press.

Mulye, T. P., Park, M. J., Nelson, C. D., Adams, S. H., Irwin, C. E., & Brindes, C. D. (2009). Trends in adolescent and young health in the United States. *Journal of Adolescent Health, 45*, 8–24.

Rieker, P. P., Bird, C. E., & Lang, M. E. (2010). Understanding gender and health: Old patterns, new trends and future directions. In C. E. Bird, P. Conrad, A. M. Fremont & S. Timmermans (Eds.), *Handbook of medical sociology* (5th ed.). Nashville, TN: Vanderbilt University Press.

Ross, C. E., & Mirowsky, J. (2010). Why education is the key to socioeconomic differentials in health. In C. E. Bird, P. Conrad, A. M. Fremont & S. Timmermans (Eds.), *Handbook of medical sociology* (5th ed.). Nashville, TN: Vanderbilt University Press.

Starr, P. (2011). *Remedy and reaction: The peculiar American struggle over health care reform*. New Haven, CT: Yale University Press.

Takeuchi, D. T., Walton, E., & Leung, M. C. (2010). Race, social contexts and health: Examining geographic spaces and places. In C. E. Bird, P. Conrad, A. M. Fremont & S. Timmermans (Eds.), *Handbook of medical sociology* (5th ed). Nashville, TN: Vanderbilt University Press.

Walton, E. (2009). Residential segregation and birth weight among racial and ethnic minorities in the United States. *Journal of Health and Social Behavior, 50*(4), 427–442.

Zambrana, R. E., & Carter-Pokras, O. (2010). Role of acculturation research in advancing science and practice in reducing health care disparities among Latinos. *American Journal of Public Health, 100*(1), 18–23.

Zheng, H. (2009). Rising U.S. income inequality, gender, and individual self-rated health, 1972–2004. *Social Science and Medicine, 69*(9), 1333–1342.

SECTION II
RACE/ETHNICITY, IMMIGRATION, AND SES

OBESITY IN MEXICAN-AMERICAN ADULTS: INTERPLAY OF IMMIGRANT GENERATION, GENDER, AND SOCIOECONOMIC STATUS

Igor Ryabov

ABSTRACT

Using the data from a unique sample of Mexican-American adults from the U.S.-Mexico border area, this chapter offers explanations for Mexican-American obesity, with the special focus on immigrant generation status, income, and gender. On a theoretical plane, this study attempts to apply the nutrition transition theory to the study of immigrant assimilation in a regional context. Considered are the most important structural dimensions of immigrant assimilation – country of birth (the United States vs. Mexico) and age of arrival. Of the two aforementioned factors, age of arrival is found to be a stronger predictor of obesity that country of birth. As Mexican-American immigrants' length of residence increases, so does their Body Mass Index (BMI) that reflects the adoption of less diverse diet and sedentary lifestyles. Through the use of multilevel hierarchical modeling, I also found sizeable variation in obesity

Issues in Health and Health Care Related to Race/Ethnicity, Immigration, SES and Gender
Research in the Sociology of Health Care, Volume 30, 21–43
Copyright © 2012 by Emerald Group Publishing Limited
All rights of reproduction in any form reserved
ISSN: 0275-4959/doi:10.1108/S0275-4959(2012)0000030004

by income, gender, and family history of obesity. The analyses suggest that the interventions aimed at reducing overweight and obesity among Mexican-Americans in the U.S.-Mexico border region should be better targeted by focusing on women and low-income households.

Keywords: Obesity; Mexican-American adults; nutrition transition theory; immigrant assimilation

INTRODUCTION

At the beginning of the 21st century, obesity represents a major health problem in the United States because it greatly increases risk for almost every chronic disease (CDC, 2008). Hispanics, and especially Mexican-Americans, are at particularly high risk for obesity and the incidence rates of obesity grow faster for Hispanics than for non-Hispanic whites (CDC, 2003, 2009). In an attempt to shed light on the obesity epidemic among Mexican-American adults, this chapter adds to the literature on Hispanic paradox, assimilation, and nutrition transition by using multilevel modeling on a unique dataset (Alliance for Healthy Border, hereafter AHB) from the U.S.-Mexico border region. It builds upon prior research methodologically by expanding the notion of immigrant acculturation to include the immigrant generational status and theoretically by testing the premises of nutrition transition theory (NTT).

The NTT describes a stage-wise, historically determined global process of food consumption and physical activity (Popkin, 2001; Popkin & Gordon-Larsen, 2004). At the dawn of civilization (i.e., preindustrial societies), diets tend to consist of starchy, low fat, and high fiber foods, and work tends to be physically intensive. Obesity is generally rare and positively associated with higher socioeconomic status (SES). But with time, everyday life becomes more sedentary and the availability of sugar, fat, and processed foods increases, thus leading to higher prevalence of degenerative disease and disability. In the concluding stage of the transition, behavioral changes in diet and exercise begin to reverse the negative effects of lifestyles associated with modern life. Overall, as the nutrition transition advances through time, growth of obesity is expected to match that of economic development. At the same time, the burden of obesity will shift from the upper and middle classes to the poor. In the context of the United States, the NTT states that the diets of immigrants are shifting toward a more "Americanized" diet high in fat, sugars, and animal sourced products (Popkin, 2001; Popkin & Gordon-Larsen, 2004). Exposure to the American environment (i.e., fast food industry, readily available cheap, prepackaged foods, and reliance on cars) may lead to the "Americanization" of health-related behaviors involving diet and activity, which sequentially may lead to obesity (Barcenas et al., 2007; Blumenthal, Hendi, & Marsillo, 2002).

THEORETICAL CONSIDERATIONS

Obesity Epidemic

The globe has succumbed to the pandemic of obesity that has put a significant number of the global population at a risk of developing noncommunicable diseases (WHO, 2000). While all regions of the world have experienced significant increases in obesity during the second half of the 20th century, no other industrialized country is as heavy (per capita) as the United States (Cutler, Glaeser, & Shapiro, 2003; Wang & Beydoun, 2007). While estimates of the extent of the problem vary, there is no doubt that obesity in the United States has increased dramatically in the past three decades. Adult obesity rates have doubled since 1980, from 15% to 30%. Two-thirds of US adults are now either overweight or obese (CDC, 2003). Noteworthy is that not only is average weight increasing but also the right end of the weight distribution is expanding particularly rapidly. Here, in the United States, as elsewhere in the world, obesity has become a disease of the poor, women, racial and ethnic minorities, i.e. groups that are socially underprivileged (Cutler et al., 2003; Wang & Beydoun, 2007). Most of the increases in the right end of the weight distribution are among the aforementioned groups (Wang & Beydoun, 2007). Therefore, it is essential to look into differences in obesity by social class, race, and ethnicity, nativity/immigrant status, and gender.

Obesity and Social Class

In the United States, the incidence of acute obesity and related morbidity is much higher among the poor than among the affluent (Cutler et al., 2003; Hofferth, 2004). As a whole, literature (e.g., Blumenthal et al., 2002; Hofferth, 2004; Wang & Beydoun, 2007) suggests that people in deep poverty (e.g., homeless) may not have a stable access to food and may be underweight, whereas people with low incomes are likely to be the most obese socioeconomic strata because of their excessive exposure to fast food, limited access to affordable fresh vegetables and fruits, and lack of medical insurance. Paradoxically, obesity coexists with the pattern of persistent malnutrition among the poor (Doak, Adair, Bentley, Monteiro, & Popkin, 2005). Underweight and overweight individuals are often found within the same households, referred to by (Doak et al. 2005; Doak, Adair, Monteiro, & Popkin, 2000) as "dual burden" households. As prior research has shown (Coady et al., 2002; Perusse & Bouchard, 1994), the problem of "dual burden" households may not only rooted in persistent malnutrition but also in hereditary factors.

Obesity and Ethnicity

It is a well-established fact that racial and ethnic minorities in the United States have higher obesity incidence and prevalence rates than non-Hispanic whites and the gap is getting larger (CDC, 2009; Ogden et al., 2006). Given my focus on Mexican-Americans in this study, I do not approach the larger issue of obesity epidemic among other racial and ethnic minorities. However, it is worth mentioning that in terms of the incidence of obesity, Hispanics rank second after African-Americans and the gap between these two groups is diminishing. Although ethnic disparities in obesity and obesity-related morbidity have been examined in a number of studies, there is a relative shortage of inquiries into Mexican-American obesity. Only a few studies attempted to analyze the factors contributing to Mexican-American obesity (e.g., Abrafdo-Lanza, Dohrenwend, Ng-Mak, & Turner, 1999; Barcenas et al., 2007; Gordon-Larsen, Harris, Ward, & Popkin, 2003). These studies, which are national in scope, overwhelmingly emphasize the importance of the Hispanic health paradox. The paradox refers to the well-known fact that, Hispanics enjoy substantially better health than the average population in spite of what their aggregate socioeconomic indicators would predict (Abrafdo-Lanza et al. 1999; Palloni & Arias, 2004). The Hispanic health paradox is particularly surprising because Hispanics tend to have higher rates of poverty than non-Hispanic whites and because, in their majority, they come from countries that have lower standards of living than that in the United States.

All the explanations of the paradox that have been offered (for the detailed summary see Palloni & Arias, 2004) emphasize nativity status and the extent of cultural assimilation as the decisive factors. It has been argued that healthier individuals choose to immigrate (Abrafdo-Lanza et al., 1999), and some immigrants go back to their home country to meet their health care needs (Alba & Nee, 2003; Jasso & Rosenzweig, 1990). It is worth mentioning, though, that only limited evidence exists in support of the argument that, as a result of both in- and out-migration selections, disproportionately healthy Hispanic immigrants remain in the United States (see the summary of the empirical evidence in Palloni & Arias, 2004). The most pertinent explanation of the paradox is that Hispanics' social and cultural practices, while being partially preserved during the acculturation process, prevent a rapid adoption of unhealthy behavior and lifestyle of the native born population (Antecol & Bedard, 2006; Palloni & Arias, 2004). Thus, even over a considerable duration in the United States, Hispanic immigrants may retain partial health advantage over non-Hispanic whites. As Noh & Kaspar (2003, p. 325) put it, "The more 'they' become like 'us,' immigrants and immigrant children fail to maintain their initial health advantages ... The process is poorly understood, but may be the result of the adoption of our poor health behaviors and lifestyles, leaving behind resources (social networks, cultural practices, employment in their field of training, etc.), and ways in which the settlement process wears down hardiness and resilience." Thus, the most possible explanation of the Hispanic paradox, that is the initial health advantage, has to do with immigrant status, rather than with ethnicity. Therefore it is useful to consider the Hispanic paradox as a special case within a larger and more encompassing theoretical framework – the NTT that parallels the historical changes described by demographic and epidemiological transition theories (Bean & Stevens, 2003; Kaplan et al., 2004; Portes & Rumbaut, 2001; Portes & Rumbaut, 2006). It is worth noting that, unlike demographic and epidemiologic transition theories, the NTT is a relatively recent theoretical development by Popkin and colleagues (Gordon-Larsen et al., 2003; Popkin, 2001; Popkin & Gordon-Larsen, 2004).

Obesity and Assimilation

The demographic, epidemiological and nutrition transitions have one feature in common — all of them were triggered by modernization (Doak et al., 2000). Particularly, the nutrition transition has been defined in five broad patterns. The first pattern is that of food collection in hunting and gathering societies. In the second pattern diets became less varied and there were episodic periods in which there was extreme food shortage. This pattern of periodic famine accompanied the advent of agriculture. Popkin (2001) suggests that in this phase social stratification has become pronounced and the elites were better off nutritionally than the masses. In pattern three the recession of famine started gradually and the consumption of fruits, vegetables, and animal proteins became less important. The diet grew heavy on starches. The third pattern fits most countries in Asia with still predominantly rural population, such as India, China (rural areas), and Philippines. These are also the main immigrant sending countries to the United States (Popkin & Gordon-Larsen, 2004).

While pattern three comes into existence in the wake of or as a result of the industrial revolution, pattern four involves a major dietary shift to increased animal fat, sugar, and processed foods. Pattern four is most commonly seen among contemporary postindustrial societies. Here the majority of people are not engaged in intensive physical activity, while enjoying all "spoils" of civilization, such as mechanized transportation and labor-saving household appliances. Pattern four is characterized by problems of degenerative diseases related to diet and inactivity. The majority of immigrants to the United States come from societies that are in patter four of the transition. This includes much of Mexico (Gordon-Larsen et al., 2003; Popkin & Gordon-Larsen, 2004).

Emerging within the currently prevalent pattern four is pattern five. This newest pattern is characterized by a reduction in dietary fat and processed foods, and an increased intake of complex carbohydrates, fruits, and vegetables. Individuals focus on a reduction in body fat and leisure exercise that is designed to offset sedentary jobs. In pattern five, life expectancy continues to rise and there is a decline in cardiovascular mortality and improvement in age-specific chronic morbidity rates. This pattern is spreading within the privileged strata of postindustrial societies (Popkin, 2001; Popkin & Gordon-Larsen, 2004).

The NTT can be applied to the study of immigrant assimilation in the United States. A prevalent theoretical paradigm in immigrant studies today – segmented assimilation theory – suggests that assimilation processes vary across groups depending on norms in immigrants' countries of origin, the level of resources immigrant groups possess when they arrive in their new country, and the social and economic contexts of reception (Portes & Rumbaut, 2001; Portes & Rumbaut, 2006). The newcomers from Mexico, who are, in their majority, representatives of lower socioeconomic strata of the sending society, may experience two possible assimilation paths:

– The straight-line upward assimilation that foretells that immigrants' nutritional and behavioral norms will change across generations until they correspond to the latest (fifth) pattern of nutrition transition adopted by

the white middle- and upper-class. In this case immigrants' acculturation may go hand-in-hand with experiencing the better health conditions.
- The straight-line downward assimilation when that the first generation will have better health outcomes than higher generation immigrants owing to the protective character of ethnic cultural norms infused in them by their families and communities. In this case, immigrants' worsening health outcomes over time in the United States may result from the more sedentary lifestyles and greater reliance on convenience foods.

Obesity and Gender

It has long been recognized that gender differences in obesity rates are not only due to biological differences but also to social factors. Women are more likely to be employed in "pink-color" jobs of lower occupational prestige and demanding no or very little physical activity, while both of the aforementioned factors (i.e., occupational prestige and physical activity) are deemed to be important protective factors from obesity (Wardle, Waller, & Jarvis, 2002). Some of the aspects of everyday experience may also affect women differently from men. For example, women spend, on average, more time preparing food, while men spend little (Cutler et al., 2003). This, together with other societal factors, puts women at a greater risk of obesity. The accumulated empirical evidence points to the fact that the gender gap in obesity among Mexican-Americans has to do with the pervasiveness of traditional gender roles (Hunt, Schneider, & Comer, 2004; Wardle et al., 2002). In the Mexican-American community, the overall nonegalitarian nature of gender roles may deleteriously affect women's health.

U.S.-Mexico Border Health and the AHB study

The present study is regional in focus. It utilizes the data that were collected in the U.S.-Mexico border region, which is characterized by the U.S. government as "medically underserved area" (TACHC, 2010). The region is predominantly rural, its underlying condition is poverty and many of its residents lack private insurance. Lack of insurance or, more exactly, of insurability has been aggravated by a deficient health care infrastructure, which is itself a product of poverty. Many residents of the region take long hours waiting at the Community Health Centers for Medicare and Medicaid services, while missing school and work, or, even worse, endure until their conditions are severe and only then travel long distances for care. In view of that fact, there exists a number of health programs, both publicly and privately funded, that aim at improving health delivery system in the U.S.-Mexico border region. The data that I use were collected by one of such programs – AHB funded by Pfizer Inc. AHB is a chronic disease prevention initiative that funded nutrition and physical activity education programs at 12 federally qualified Community Health Centers located along the U.S.-Mexico border in Texas, New Mexico, Arizona and California. The Community Health Centers serve predominately rural, underprivileged Mexican-American families who commute for their health care needs. Pfizer committed $4.5 million over three years (2006–2008) to these community centers with the aim of preventing the twin epidemics of diabetes and cardiovascular disease among the Mexican-American population (AHB, 2010). In order to determine the effectiveness of the intervention, the project evaluators conducted three surveys at three data collection points (Waves 1, 2, and 3). The survey instrument was partially based on CDC's Behavioral Risk Factor Surveillance System (BRFSS) and Community Tracking Study Household Survey (see the *Methods* section for a more detailed description of the data). As a community-level intervention, the AHB program was success. By the end of the program period, the participating community centers reported statistically significant improvement in the following areas: healthy weight loss, lower cardio-risk, and lower blood sugar. These results were attributed to an increase in health literacy which, in turn, improved frequency of exercise and healthier eating habits (AHB, 2010). *The present study goes beyond the descriptive analyses and attempts to identify the groups in the AHB study for which similar interventions will be the most effective.*

The AHB survey contains information on two measures of assimilation – country of birth and the Short Acculturation Scale for Hispanics (SASH), a scale developed by Marín, Sabogal, Marín, Otero-Sabogal, and Perez-Stable (1987) to determine a degree of linguistic assimilation. I propose a different approach to measure assimilation. In the present work, I will use the concept that frequently appears in the studies of immigrant assimilation – *immigrant generational* status (Kepka, Ayala, & Cherrington, 2007; Negy & Woods, 1992; Vernez & Abrahamse, 1996). It is common among immigration scholars to distinguish at least three generations: generation 1 (immigrants themselves), generation 2 (children of immigrants) and generation "three plus" (everybody else). Further, it is increasingly more accepted to conceptualize immigrant generation as a 4-category variable (Bean & Stevens, 2003; Oropesa & Landale, 1997). *Age at arrival* is often used as the distinguishing factor to differentiate 1 and 1.5 generations. This variable captures the length of exposure to the mainstream culture which country of birth cannot. Because previous studies showed that arrival by age sixteen is associated with a markedly different health outcomes (Portes & Rumbaut, 2001; Portes & Rumbaut, 2006), I propose to use the sixteen-year threshold to distinguish 1 and 1.5 generations.

CONTRIBUTION TO THE LITERATURE

The obesity epidemic among rural Mexican-Americans has received startlingly little attention in the literature. Earlier research stemming from NTT and conducted on Hispanic populations (Barcenas et al., 2007; Gordon-Larsen et al., 2003; Wang & Beydoun, 2007) is broad and lacks regional focus: the type of residence (rural vs. urban) is not usually controlled for, while the findings are often assumed to be applicable to all locales and all Hispanic ethnic origin groups. Even with the large proportion of Hispanics among immigrants, the degree to which ethnic disparities in BMI are masked by immigrant status is seldom assessed in the literature. This study focuses on rural Mexican-Americans and thus controls the effects of ethnicity and type of residence but centers on the role immigrant generational status plays in reducing obesity among Mexican-Americans. Further, the present study differs from this literature in its empirical strategy. In most previous studies, explanations for assimilation on Hispanic obesity are mainly from the linguistic perspective that confounds the residence duration and immigrant/nativity status. The present study expands the notion of immigrant acculturation to include both aspects of the immigrant generational status – age at arrival and country of birth. Finally, the present study is longitudinal in design. This point is worth emphasizing since thee effectiveness of a multi-year, culturally-sensitive intervention program like the AHB cannot be assessed by a cross-sectional analysis.

HYPOTHESES

The main hypothesis of the study is that immigrant generational status is positively associated with BMI. Because of the way immigrant generational status is conceptualized in this study (i.e., as an asymmetrical interaction of *country of birth* and *age at arrival*), this hypothesis should be further subdivided into two parts: (1) persons born in the United States will have higher BMI than those born in Mexico, and (2) the greater length of residence in the United States is likely to be associated with higher BMI (measured at the baseline and at the program end).

The secondary hypothesis concerns SES and it is derived from numerous studies indicating that people with lower incomes, lower educational attainment and unemployed are more likely to be obese than those with higher incomes, higher educational attainment and employed in paid labor force (Cutler et al., 2003; Wang & Beydoun, 2007). Hence, I hypothesize that: (1) lower-income Mexican-American adults will have higher BMI than their middle-income counterparts; (2) higher educational attainment is negatively associated with obesity; and (3) people actively employed in paid labor force will have lower BMI than those who are not (e.g., homemakers, retirees, and students).

Building on the previous research (Hunt et al., 2004; Pérez-Escamilla & Putnik, 2007; Wardle et al., 2002) that noted significant gender differences in the way gender influences obesity, I will test the tertiary hypothesis stating that females are more likely to be obese than males. This hypothesis is based on research that attributes higher prevalence of obesity among females to lower exposure to physical activity, which, in turn, is determined by the character of jobs demanding more (for males) or less (for females) physical activity.

DATA AND METHOD

Sample

The present study included a random unstratified sample of adults who were recruited from several community settings in the Southwestern United States. Because respondents were selected from regular patients of community health care centers, the representativeness of the sample is limited. The survey was administered in three waves: Wave 1 (the baseline) was administered in 2006, Wave 2 in 2008, and Wave 3 in 2009 (six months after the program end). An important consideration is the retention of respondents: given that the post-program-end survey (Wave 3) was modified to include a qualitative component and did not target all respondents, its sample size was only 55% of the baseline (Wave 1).

Because of the completeness of information on the variables on interest, I use Waves 1 and 2 of the AHB survey ($N = 2,782$) for the current analyses. Except for BMI the information on which is obtained from Waves 1 and 2, all study variables analyzed hereto were measured in Wave 1. These cases were not excluded from the further analyses but their values were imputed using the Markov Chain Monte Carlo technique (the SAS' *proc mi*), with the efficiency of the resulting estimates within 95% confidence interval (for more information on the Markov Chain Monte Carlo imputation see Rubin, 1987, 1996). The Markov chain Monte Carlo yields a successive simulation of the distribution of missing values, conditioned on both observed data and assuming that the data are missing at random. This imputation was carried out via a procedure (Proc MI) in the SAS software. It requires that missing data are imputed in m data sets ($m =$ number of imputations required by the procedure) and that data analyses are run for those m data sets. In order to compute m, I used the formula provided by Rubin (1987, p. 114):

$$CI = \left(1 + \frac{\gamma}{m}\right)^{-1}$$

where *CI* is the efficiency of estimate (in our case, confidence interval = 95) and γ is the rate of missing information for the quantity being estimated. It should be noted that the majority of variables in the AHB dataset have a comparatively low rate of missing information (less than 15%). Putting this information into the aforementioned equation and knowing that the efficiency of the estimate that need to be achieved (95% CI), I obtained the number of datasets to be imputed, which equals 3. Subsequently, parameter estimates from the analyses run on those data sets were averaged to obtain single parameter estimates. The covariance diagnostic test confirmed that the covariance matrix had not undergone any significant changes as a result of imputations.

Since this study focuses on Mexican-Americans, I use a subsample of the AHB survey that includes only Mexican-Americans who represent 79% of the sample (final $N = 2,179$). The reason for limiting sample to Mexican-Americans, instead of including categorical variables for ethnicity (e.g., Anglo and other Hispanic) is that mechanisms linking acculturation and obesity, as it is know from literature (Barcenas et al., 2007; Gordon-Larsen et al., 2003; Wang & Beydoun, 2007), vary among ethnic groups, including those within "Hispanic" mega-ethnicity.

MEASURES

Dependent Variables

The dependent variable of this study is Body Mass Index (BMI). The indicator of BMI is called from the Wave 1 and 2 surveys, which helps to address concerns about causal ordering. BMI is intended to measure how heavy a particular person is relative to their height. As a convention, it is calculated as a ration of body weight in kilograms to the height in meters squared. Table 1 shows that the average BMI in the sample was 32.0, with the standard deviation of 8.4.

Independent Variables

Immigrant generational status is the key independent variable in the study. I divided all respondents into three categories: first-, 1.5-, and second- and higher-immigrant generations. Because of the theoretical importance of age of migration (Bean & Stevens, 2003; Oropesa & Landale, 1997; Portes & Rumbaut, 2001; Portes & Rumbaut, 2006), I subdivided foreign-born adults into those who moved to the United States before age sixteen (generation 1.5) and those who moved to the United States at sixteen or older ages (generation 1). Hence, two immigrant generations will be compared – "first generation" and "first-and-half generation" – while simultaneously controlling for the effect of age at arrival. For all of my analyses, the "second-plus" immigrant generation is the reference group. Respondents included in this category have parents or grandparents who were immigrants, but because the immigration experience is much further removed from the social context of their everyday life, this category is considered the native population and the fundamental comparison group for generations 1 and 1.5. In my sample, the majority of respondents (64%) were 1.5 generation and fewer (18% and 18%) were, respectfully, first- and second-plus generations (see Table 1).

Arguably, the most important predictor of obesity is SES. It is also of one of the key independent variables in the NTT. I consider three dimensions of SES—family income, educational attainment and employment status. It important for the purposes of the present study to measure and analyze these variables separately, because some immigrant groups, especially Mexican-Americans, report very low levels of educational attainment, and in part because the jobs (and therefore income) available to immigrants often do not correspond to their educational attainment. It is also worth

Table 1. Descriptive Statistics of Study Variables ($N = 2,782$).

	Weighted Mean	SD	Minimum	Maximum
Dependent variable				
BMI (Wave 2)	31.6	8.4	15.7	52.3
Independent variables				
Family-level indicators				
No family obese[a]	0.54	0.43	0	1
Individual-level indicators				
Generational status				
Immigrant generation 1.0	0.18	0.26	0	1
Immigrant generation 1.5	0.64	0.44	0	1
Immigrant generation 2+	0.18	0.40	0	1
Socioeconomic status				
Some college education[b]	0.15	0.35	0	1
Primary or secondary school[c]	0.86	0.45	0	1
Homemaker or retired	0.37	0.48	0	1
Employed or other[d]	0.63	0.47	0	1
Annual income $< = \$10,000$	0.42	0.50	0	1
Annual income $> \$10,000$	0.58	0.47	0	1
Gender				
Male	0.24	0.42	0	1
Female	0.77	0.43	0	1
Control variables				
BMI (Wave 1)	32.4	6.9	14.8	62.3
Single (Not married)	0.32	0.47	0	1
Married	0.68	0.48	0	1
Age	50.23	14.17	18	91

[a]Respondents reporting neither of parents being obese.
[b]Educational attainment above high school diploma or GED.
[c]Educational attainment at the level of high school diploma/GED or below.
[d]Employed, self-employed or student.

mentioning that the scale that the AHB survey uses to measure income is not particularly sensitive to the lowest end of SES, as 42% of Mexican-American respondents in the baseline survey fall into the lowest income category, that is, less than $10,000 annually (see Table 1). Similarly, the majority of respondents never went to college (87%) and are employed for wages, self-employed, and/or students (63%). I dichotomized the three aforementioned variables (annual incomes less than $10,000 vs. incomes equal or more than $10,000; no college education vs. some college education; homemakers and/or retired vs. employed, self-employed and/or student) because exploratory cluster analyses (not shown for parsimony) indicated that the aforementioned thresholds marked significantly different health outcome (i.e., BMI).

In order to test my third research hypothesis I include gender. The data allowed controlling for the influence of other factors that have been documented to impact BMI. With respect to individual characteristics, these include marital status (married vs. single) and age. Because, as it is a well-known fact, obesity is determined by the hereditary factors (Coady et al., 2002; Perusse & Bouchard, 1994), I control for family history of obesity. Specifically, I compare respondents who has/had obese parents/grandparents (reference category) with those who has/had not. Unlike all other variables, this is a family-level variable. Luckily, the AHB data contain a family identifier that justifies multilevel modeling, an analytical technique described in the following section.

ANALYTIC STRATEGY

Considering the fact that family history of obesity is a family-level trait (i.e., the one that all family members share) while all other variables are measured at the individual level, I use multilevel modeling for multivariate analyses. Specifically, I treat families as level-1 units (the multiple observations for each respondent within their family) and the individual respondents as level-2 units (for more information on multilevel modeling see Bryk & Raudenbush, 1992). This technique will be possible using the SAS *proc mixed*.

The regression analyses presented below are performed using HLM. If I denote i as the ith individual (level-1) and j as the jth family (level-2), the individual-level (level-1) model can be presented as follows:

$$BMI = \beta_{0j} + \beta_{1j}X_{1ij} + \beta_{2j}X_{2ij} + \cdots + \beta_{nj}X_{nij} + \rho_{ij}$$

where $\beta_{(0-n)j}$ are regression coefficients of individual-level factors $X_{(0-n)ij}$ and ρ_{ij} is normal error with mean 0 and variance σ^2.

The generalized formula of the family-level (level-2) intercept is

$$\beta_{0j} = \gamma_0 + \gamma_1 Y_{1j} + \omega_{0j}$$

where $\gamma_{(1)}$ are regression coefficient of family-level factor Y_{1j} (there is only one in my model – family history of obesity) and ω_j is the family-level error.

Table 2. Weighted Means and Standard Deviations of All Variables by Immigrant Generational Status $(N = 2,782)^a$.

	Immigrant Generation Status					
	1		1.5		2+	
$N = 2,782$	511		1,785		486	
	Mean	SD.	Mean	SD	Mean	SD
Dependent variable						
BMI	30.0^d	6.7	32.3^e	9.5	$33.7^{d,e}$	7.1
Independent variables						
Family-level indicators						
No family obese^a	0.59	0.41	0.53	0.56	0.51	0.44
Individual-level indicators						
Socioeconomic status						
Some college Education^b	0.14^d	0.36	$0.10^{c,e}$	0.31	$0.23^{d,e}$	0.43
Homemaker or retired	0.34^d	0.42	0.37^e	0.49	$0.24^{d,e}$	0.45
Annual income $<\$10,000$	0.38	0.47	0.45	0.51	0.39	0.48
Gender (male)	0.20^d	0.42	0.22^e	0.41	$0.29^{d,e}$	0.45
Individual-level controls						
Single (not married)	0.32^d	0.45	0.29^e	0.44	$0.42^{d,e}$	0.49
Age	45.18^c	14.03	$52.25^{c,e}$	13.20	49.38^e	16.53

^{a}Respondents reporting neither of parents being obese.
^{b}Educational attainment above high school diploma or GED.
^{c}The difference in the means between 1 and 1.5 generations.
^{d}The difference in the means between 1 and 2 generations.
^{e}The difference in the means between 1.5 and 2 generations.

UNIVARIATE RESULTS

Means and standard deviations of the study variables across generational status groups are shown in Table 2. The Bonferroni method of comparing multiple means was used in the analysis. It is evident that the largest difference in BMI (measured at Waves 1 and 2) is found between generations 1 and 2, with generation 1 having the lowest BMI and generation 2 having the highest. The post-hoc tests comparing means across generational groups by time of measurement (not shown for the sake of parsimony) demonstrate that,

Table 3. Regression Coefficients of Predictors of BMI, Wave 1 ($N = 2{,}782$).

	Models						
	1		2		3		4
	b	p-value	B	p-value	B	p-value	B	p-value
Family-level indicators								
No Family Obese	-5.97	0.000	-5.10	0.000	-2.73	0.000	-2.56	0.000
Individual-level indicators								
Generational status								
Immigrant generation[a] 1.0	-4.33	0.000	-3.16	0.000	-3.25	0.000	-3.31	0.000
Immigrant generation[a] 2+	1.65	0.000	1.19	0.000	1.35	0.039	0.96	0.083
Socioeconomic status								
Some college education[b]			-0.16	0.910	0.11	0.251	0.23	0.152
Homemaker or retired[c]			0.48	0.055	0.36	0.134	0.70	0.111
Annual income $\leq$ \$10,000[d]			1.56	0.000	1.32	0.009	1.12	0.016
Gender (male)[e]					-1.51	0.000	-1.35	0.003
Individual-level controls								
Single (not married)[f]							-1.02	0.035
Age							0.67	0.135
Constant	36.78	0.000	35.81	0.000	37.11	0.000	35.79	0.000
Model comparison test			1,095	0.000	661	0.000	287	0.025

[a]Generation 1.5.
[b]Educational attainment at the level of high school diploma/GED or below.
[c]Employed, self-employed or student.
[d]Annual income > \$10,000.
[e]Female.
[f]Married.

Table 4. Regression Coefficients of Predictors of BMI, Wave 2 ($N = 2{,}782$).

	Models							
	1		2		3		4	
	b	p-value	B	p-value	B	p-value	b	p-value
Family-level indicators								
No Family Obese	-4.84	0.000	-3.44	0.000	-3.20	0.000	-1.78	0.019
Individual-level indicators								
Generational status								
Immigrant generation[a] 1.0	-1.39	0.065	-1.50	0.067	-1.12	0.093	-0.56	0.103
Immigrant generation[a] 2+	0.83	0.000	0.47	0.001	0.56	0.025	0.40	0.154
Socioeconomic status								
Some college education[b]			-0.18	0.177	-0.16	0.219	-0.04	0.315
Homemaker or retired[c]			0.24	0.093	0.20	0.134	0.15	0.107
Annual income $\leq$ $10,000[d]			1.40	0.012	1.27	0.035	0.86	0.125
Gender (male)[e]					-1.56	0.000	-0.63	0.076
Individual-level controls								
BMI (Wave 1)							4.73	0.000
Single (Not married)[f]							-0.41	0.135
Age							0.14	0.282
Constant	35.90	0.000	35.79	0.000	36.57	0.000	32.51	0.000
Model comparison test			842	0.000	524	0.000	750	0.000

[a]Generation 1.5.
[b]Educational attainment at the level of high school diploma/GED or below.
[c]Employed, self-employed or student.
[d]Annual income > $10,000.
[e]Female.
[f]Married.

although the reduction in BMI between Waves 1 and 2 is significant for all
generations, generation 1 made the most significant stride toward reducing
obesity ($p < 0.001$). Also noteworthy is that the difference in BMI between
generations 1.5 and 2, while being significant at Wave 1, disappears at Wave 2.
The differences in BMI between immigrant generations highlight necessity for
examining the generational status effects further using regression analyses.
Tables 3 and 4 also shed light on some of the similarities/differences in
independent variables across immigrant status groups. All independent
variables, except family history of obesity and annual income, vary significantly among generations.

In the case of educational level, employment and marital statuses, the
major difference is found between 1.5 and 2 generations. The largest share of
adults with college education is among generation 2, while the lowest is
among generation 1.5. The opposite is true about the share of homemakers
and retirees, which is the largest among generation 1.5 and the lowest among
generation 2. The analyses also reveal that the distribution of single adults
across generational status groups match the distribution of adults with
college education. With respect to gender, the general pattern of change
across immigrant generation emulates that of BMI and suggests that more
recent arrivals have higher share of females than later immigrant waves,
with generation 1 having the highest proportion of females and generation
2 having the lowest. The straight-line pattern of change across immigrant
generations, observable in case of BMI and gender, is not characteristic for
age. Generation 1.5 is the "oldest" among immigrant generational status
groups, while generation 1 is the "youngest".

MULTILEVEL REGRESSION RESULTS

Table 3 shows results of multilevel regression coefficients and their significance of individual- and family-level predictors on BMI measured in Wave
1. Because all variables come from Wave 1 data, the results presented in
Table 3 are cross-sectional in character. Model 1 documents the effects of
the core subset of independent variables – immigrant generational status,
while controlling for family history of obesity. It demonstrates that all of
these measures were significant in the predicted directions. First, family
history of obesity has a strong effect on BMI. Particularly, those having no
obese parents or grandparents are less likely to be obese than those who do.
This effect is robust and remains significant in all subsequent models that
include control variables. Second, the effect of immigrant generation 1 is

negative (generation 1.5 is reference group). This implies that those adults who immigrated at age sixteen or older are more likely to be obese than those persons who arrived at younger ages. Third, the coefficient for generation 2 is positive, thus indicating an "obesity advantage" of the immigrants over the natives. All these findings are largely consistent with the expectations derived from the NTT.

Model 2 adds SES measures – educational attainment, employment status and income. Among these there is only one significant effect – that of income ($p < 0.001$). Persons falling into the lowest income category (less than $10,000 annually) have higher chances of being obese than the rest of respondents. This finding partially supports my second research hypothesis, suggesting an inverse relationship between income and obesity. However, no association between obesity and educational attainment and employment status was observed. The effects of variables introduced in model 1 retained their significance, indicating that SES is unlikely to mediate relationship between immigrant generation and BMI.

Gender (male; female is reference) is added in model 3. The negative and significant effect for male is not a surprisingly finding because the literature (Wang & Beydoun, 2007; Wardle et al., 2002) confirms a "weight gap" in favor of men, owing to higher frequency and intensity of physical activity among men than women. Hence, the results lend support to my hypothesis that Mexican-American women are at a grater risk of obesity epidemic than Mexican-American men. Incorporating gender in model 3 alters baseline coefficients for family history of obesity, which decreases in magnitude but retains significance, and for generation 1, which loses in significance (from $p < 0.001$ to $p < 0.05$). This implies that gender explains some of the differences in BMI among immigrant generations.

Two variables are introduced in model 4 – age and marital status (single; married is control category). Age does not seem to matter in predicting obesity outcome, but marital status does. Singlehood has a significant ($p < 0.05$) and negative effect on BMI. Hence, married Mexican-American adults in the AHB sample are more prone to obesity than their single counterparts. As evidenced in model 4 of Tables 3, the drop in the significance level of the coefficient for generation 2 accompanies the introduction of the aforementioned control variables. Consequently, the difference between generations 1.5 and 2 is not statistically significant, when marital status and age are controlled.

Table 4 repeats the above exercise using BMI at Wave 3 as the dependent variable and controlling for BMI at Wave 1. The models of Table 3 and 4 are identical, except for model 4 that includes BMI at Wave 1 in addition to the other control variables. With few exceptions, the results are almost identical to those presented in Table 3. The main difference is that the few significant effects present in Table 3 lose their significance in Table 4. As expected from the descriptive analyses shown in Table 2, the difference between generations 1 and 1.5 becomes insignificant. However, the effect of generation 2 is robust and persists in all Table 4 models ($p < 0.05$), with an exception of model 4 that controls for BMI at baseline. Generally, because the effect of BMI at Wave 1 is, by far, the most important predictor of BMI at Wave 2, only one effect is significant in model 4 (complete model) – that of family history of obesity. Observe that the two predictors that were significant in prior models, the effects of being poor and female, lose their significance in a complete model. This is quite an anticipated finding as it is usually prior history of obesity that is known to define future risks of obesity.

DISCUSSION

Using a sample of Mexican-American adults residing along the U.S.-Mexico border, I analyzed variations in BMI across immigrant generational status groups, while controlling for family history of obesity, SES, marital status, age and gender. The main purpose of the study was to apply the NTT, which describes the graduate change in health status of immigrant groups on the United States through the process of nutritional transition, to the context of Mexican immigrant assimilation. I approached the multidimensional phenomena of assimilation by focusing on immigrant generation to show that combinations of two main components of the assimilation process (country of birth and age at arrival) have a differential impact on various individual- and family-level characteristics (presented in Table 2), including BMI.

The multilevel regression results indicated that immigrant generational status can be utilized as a measure of assimilation when predicting BMI as well as its change over time. However, my main research hypothesis that the further immigrant experience is removed from the present-day, the higher the odds of becoming overweight or obese, was only partially supported by the regression analyses. Age at arrival has been found to be a strong predictor of obesity, but the effect of country of origin was not significant in the full model that controlled for age and marital status. Whether controlling for individual- and family-level variables or not, the multilevel results showed that generation 1 turns out to have the lowest BMI in all regression models. When approaching the question of whether or not immigrant generation matters in reducing BMI as a desired outcome of the AHB intervention program, it should be noted that generation 1 was the one that made the most significant improvement toward declining BMI. Yet, the average BMIs of generations 1.5 (foreign-born arrived before the age of 18) and 2 (U.S.-born) do not differ significantly from each other at the AHB program end. Thus, the "immigrant advantage" in the case of generation 1 (that follows from the way this generation was defined in this study) seems to be a cumulative effect of being an immigrant parents and arriving in this country after the school age. Hence, as seen through the lens of assimilation theory, obesity is affected by both factors that define immigrant generation in this study: age at arrival and country of birth. Finally, these finding are fairly consistent with the expectations of the NTT about the process of assimilation whereby immigrants are posited to adopt the host community's practices with respect to diet and physical activity.

Another important observation is that, among the SES measures analyzed in this study, only annual income has a strong and negative effect on BMI. No significant differences were found between employment status groups and educational attainment, on the one hand, and BMI, on the other. Likewise, no relationship was found between marital status and obesity. Consequently, the findings of this study suggest that obesity is a problem primarily among Mexican-American women and those falling into the lowest income segment of population. It is among these population segments that the interventions, such as the AHB, can be the most effective.

It is possible that the absence of significant effects is influenced by the limitations of this study, such as small sample size and selection bias (e.g., the majority of the participants in the present study were women and were below the poverty level). The sampling method of selecting the participants attending community health care centers that cater primarily to medically indigent populations might have contributed to having a higher number of low-income and female participants than expected. Although the sample may be representative of the Mexican-American population of the Southwest, it is uncertain whether and to what extent the findings of the present study can be generalized to all Mexican-Americans. Further research with larger samples and better controls is warranted.

REFERENCES

Abrafdo-Lanza, A., Dohrenwend, B. P., Ng-Mak, D. S., & Turner, J. B. (1999). The Latino mortality paradox: A test of the "salmon bias" and healthy migrant hypotheses. *American Journal of Public Health, 89*(10), 1543–1548.

AHB (Alliance for a Healthy Border). (2010). *Alliance for a Healthy Border, Study description.* Retrieved from: http://www.pfizer.com/responsibility/global_health/alliance_healthy_border.jsp. Accessed on October 29, 2010.

Alba, R. D., & Nee, V. (2003). *Remaking the American mainstream: Assimilation and contemporary immigration.* Cambridge, MA: Harvard University Press.

Antecol, H., & Bedard, K. (2006). Unhealthy assimilation: Do immigrants converge to American weights? *Demography, 43*(2), 337–360.

Barcenas, C. H., Wilkinson, A. V., Strom, S. S., Cao, Y., Saunders, K. C., Mahabir, S., ... Bondy, M. L. (2007). Birthplace, years of residence in the United States, and obesity among Mexican-American adults. *Obesity, 15*(4), 1043–1052.

Bean, F. D., & Stevens, G. (2003). *America's newcomers and the dynamics of diversity.* New York, NY: Russell Sage Foundation.

Blumenthal, S. J., Hendi, J. M., & Marsillo, L. (2002). A public health approach to decreasing obesity. *The Journal of American Medical Association, 288*(17), 2178.

Bryk, A., & Raudenbush, S. W. (1992). *Hierarchical linear models for social and behavioral research: Applications and data analysis methods.* Newbury Park, CA: Sage Publications.

CDC (Center for Disease Control and Prevention). (2003). *National health and nutrition examination survey.* Retrieved from: http://www.cdc.gov/nchs/nhanes.htm. Accessed on November 15, 2010,

CDC (Center for Disease Control and Prevention). (2008). *Overweight and obesity – Introduction.* Retrieved from http://www.cdc.gov/nccdphp/dnpa/obesity/index.htm. Accessed on November 4, 2010.

CDC (Center for Disease Control and Prevention). (Center for Disease Control and Prevention). Differences in prevalence of obesity among black, white, and Hispanic adults – United States, 2006–2008. *Morbidity and Mortality Weekly Report, 58*(27), 740–744.

Coady, S. A., Jaquish, C. E., Fabsitz, R. R., Larson, M. G., Cupples, L. A., & Myers, R. H. (2002). Genetic variability of adult body mass index: A longitudinal assessment in Framingham families. *Obesity, 10*, 675–681.

Cutler, D. M., Glaeser, E. L., & Shapiro, J. M. (2003). Why have Americans become more obese? *Journal of Economic Perspectives, 17*(3), 93–118.

Doak, C. M., Adair, L. S., Bentley, M., Monteiro, C., & Popkin, B. M. (2005). The dual burden household and the nutrition transition paradox. *International Journal of Obesity, 29*, 129–136.

Doak, C. M., Adair, L. S., Monteiro, C., & Popkin, B. M. (2000). Overweight and underweight co-Exist in Brazil, China, and Russia. *Journal of Nutrition, 130*, 2965–2980.

Gordon-Larsen, P., Harris, K. M., Ward, D. S., & Popkin, B. M. (2003). Acculturation and overweight related behaviors among Hispanic immigrants to the US: The National Longitudinal Study of Adolescent Health. *Social Science and Medicine, 57*, 2023–2034.

Hofferth, S. L. (2004). *Persistence and change in the food security of families with children, 1997-99.* Washington, DC: U.S. Department of Agriculture.

Hunt, L. M., Schneider, S., & Comer, B. (2004). Should 'acculturation' be a variable in health research? A critical review of research on U.S. Hispanics. *Social Science and Medicine, 59*, 973–986.

Jasso, G., & Rosenzweig, M. (1990). *The new chosen people: Immigrants in the United State.* New York, NY: Russell Sage Foundation.

Kaplan, M. S., et al. (2004). *American Journal Preventive Medicine, 27*, 323–326.

Kepka, D., Ayala, G. X., & Cherrington, A. (2007). Do Latino immigrants link self-rated health with BMI and health behaviors? *American Journal of Health Behavior, 31*(5), 535–544.

Marín, G., Sabogal, F., Marín, B., Otero-Sabogal, R., & Perez-Stable, E. J. (1987). Development of a short acculturation scale for Hispanics. *Hispanic Journal of Behavioral Science, 9,* 183–205.

Negy, C., & Woods, D. J. (1992). The importance of acculturation in understanding research with Hispanic-Americans. *Hispanic Journal of Behavioral Science, 14*(2), 224–247.

Noh, S., & Kaspar, V. (2003). Diversity and immigrant health. In P. Anisef & M. Lanphier (Eds.), *The world in a city* (pp. 316–353). Toronto: Toronto University Press.

Ogden, C., Carroll, M. D., Curtin, L. R., McDowell, M. A., Tabak, C. J., & Flegal, K. M. (2006). Prevalence of overweight and obesity in the United States, 1999–2004. *The Journal of American Medical Association, 295,* 1549–1555.

Oropesa, R. S., & Landale, N. (1997). Immigrant legacies: Ethnicity, generation, and children's familial and economic lives. *Social Science Quarterly, 78,* 399–416.

Palloni, A., & Arias, E. (2004). Paradox lost: Explaining the Hispanic adult mortality advantage. *Demography, 41*(3), 385–415.

Pérez-Escamilla, R., & Putnik, P. (2007). The role of acculturation in nutrition, lifestyle, and incidence of type 2 diabetes among Latinos. *Journal of Nutrition, 137,* 860–870.

Perusse, L., & Bouchard, C. (1994). Genetics of energy intake and food preferences. In C. Bouchard (Ed.), *The Genetics of Obesity.* Boca Raton, FL: CRC Press.

Popkin, B. M. (2001). The nutrition transition and obesity in the developing world. *Journal of Nutrition, 131,* 871S–873S.

Popkin, B. M., & Gordon-Larsen, P. (2004). The nutrition transition: Worldwide obesity dynamics and their determinants. *International Journal of Obesity, 28,* S2–S9.

Portes, A., & Rumbaut, R. G. (2001). *Legacies: The story of the immigrant second generation.* Berkeley, CA: University of California Press.

Portes, A., & Rumbaut, R. G. (2006). *Immigrant America: A portrait* (3rd ed.). Berkeley, CA: University of California Press.

Rubin, D. B. (1987). *Multiple imputation for nonresponse in survey.* New York, NY: John Wiley & Sons.

Rubin, D. B. (1996). Multiple imputation after 18 + years. *Journal of the American Statistical Association, 91,* 473–489.

TACHC (The Texas Association of Community Health Centers). (2010). *The Texas Association of Community Health Centers.* Retrieved from http://www.tachc.org/Home.asp. Accessed on October 21, 2010.

Vernez, G., & Abrahamse, A. (1996). *How immigrants fare in U.S. Education.* Santa Monica, CA: RAND.

Wang, Y., & Beydoun, M. A. (2007). The obesity epidemic in the United States – gender, age, socioeconomic, racial/ethnic, and geographic characteristics: A systematic review and meta-regression analysis. *Epidemiologic Reviews, 229,* 6–28.

Wardle, J., Waller, J., & Jarvis, M. J. (2002). Sex differences in the association of socioeconomic status with Obesity. *American Journal of Public Health, 92,* 1299–1304.

WHO (World Health Organization). (2000). Obesity: Preventing and managing the global epidemic. *WHO Technical Report No. 894,* Geneva, Switzerland: WHO Press.

DELAYED DIAGNOSIS OF TUBERCULOSIS IN THE U.S.-MEXICO BORDER REGION: A HEALTH NARRATIVES APPROACH

Angélica Forero-Quintana and Sara E. Grineski

ABSTRACT

Purpose – *One-third of the world's population is infected with tuberculosis (TB) and there are two million TB-related deaths worldwide every year. Along the U.S.-Mexico border, migration patterns, and reduced access to health care contribute to high rates of TB. Delayed diagnosis of TB, the focus of this chapter, increases the likelihood that a patient will progress to more advanced stages of the disease and heightens the risk of TB transmission to others as patients are contagious for longer periods of time.*

Approach – *Despite the seriousness of these consequences, few socio-logical studies have examined delayed diagnosis of TB and why people affected by TB symptoms delay care. Because of this, we take a health narratives approach to understanding the experiences of 15 TB patients of*

Issues in Health and Health Care Related to Race/Ethnicity, Immigration, SES and Gender
Research in the Sociology of Health Care, Volume 30, 45–65
Copyright © 2012 by Emerald Group Publishing Limited
All rights of reproduction in any form reserved
ISSN: 0275-4959/doi:10.1108/S0275-4959(2012)0000030005

Mexican descent in a high-risk border community (e.g., El Paso, Texas) in order to discover why delayed diagnoses happen and how they impact patients.

Findings – *Fourteen of the fifteen patients experienced delayed diagnosis. Analysis of these fourteen narratives revealed two broad themes: (1) provider lack of awareness, including repeated misdiagnosis and TB test errors, and (2) patient disadvantage, including fear of U.S. immigration authorities and few economic resources for care.*

Implications – *Findings from this study suggest that prompt diagnosis of TB could be achieved if providers were more cognizant of TB and its symptoms and public health policies increased access to health care regardless of immigration status or socioeconomic status.*

Keywords: Tuberculosis; delayed diagnosis; U.S-Mexico border; health narratives; immigration; access to health care

INTRODUCTION AND LITERATURE REVIEW

Delayed diagnosis of tuberculosis (TB) has serious implications for patients and society as a whole. Delayed diagnosis increases the likelihood that a patient will progress to more advanced stages of the disease (Deiss et al., 2011; Gaviria, Henao, Martinez, & Bernal, 2010; Moya & Lusk, 2009; Tsai, Hung, Chen, Chew, & Lee, 2008; Wallace et al., 2009) and transmit the bacteria to others as the patient stays in active disease (and contagious) longer (Gaviria et al., 2010). By delayed diagnosis, we mean when a symptomatic patient does not receive diagnosis and treatment within 60 days from the onset of initial symptoms (Asch, Leake, Anderson, & Gelberg, 1998). Despite the seriousness of the consequences for patients and society, little is known about why and how people affected by TB symptoms suffer, often for many months (Gaviria et al., 2010), without being treated for TB. Because of this, we take a qualitative approach to exploring TB patients' experiences with delayed diagnoses in order to better understand why delayed diagnosis happens and their impacts on patients in El Paso, Texas, which is located on the U.S. side of the border with Mexico.

To begin, TB is a disease caused by *Mycobacterium tuberculosis*. The bacterium usually attacks the lungs, but it can attack any part of the body such as the kidneys, spine, and brain (CDC, 2008). TB is spread through the air from person to person, but not everyone infected with TB becomes sick. Those who do not get sick are said to have latent TB infection (LTBI) (the majority of those infected with TB), and those that do get sick have active TB disease and can spread the disease to others. People with LTBI do not present any symptoms; the only sign of TB infection is a positive reaction to a tuberculin skin test or a TB blood test (CDC, 2008). People with active TB disease often spread it to people they often spend time with, such as family members, coworkers, and friends. Some people develop TB disease soon after becoming infected (within weeks), before their immune system can fight the TB bacteria. Other people may get sick years later, when their immune system becomes weak for another reason (e.g., stress and HIV infection) (CDC, 2008).

Literature on Delayed Diagnosis

Literature suggests that a lack of health-care provider knowledge/awareness and patient disadvantage contribute to delayed diagnosis of active TB disease. Nationally in the United States, there has been an increase in the number of active pulmonary TB cases relative to the number of latent pulmonary TB cases (Wallace et al., 2009). These active pulmonary TB cases were found in areas with low prevalence rates and among subgroups less "at risk" (e.g., whites, the employed, U.S.-born persons, and those who do not abuse alcohol). This likely reflects, as explained by Wallace et al. (2009), the fact that TB has become a relatively uncommon disease, which has led to delayed diagnoses, especially for these groups, because providers were less cognizant of its existence. In addition to delayed diagnosis, provider lack of awareness may also be related to initial misdiagnosis of TB symptoms as another lung disease. For example, in Taiwan, of patients that experienced a delayed diagnosis of TB, 68% were first diagnosed incorrectly with pneumonia (Tsai et al., 2008). Provider lack of awareness can have serious consequences for patient care. In Medellín, Colombia, Gaviria et al. (2010) found that the lack of knowledge and patient stereotyping by doctors and nurses were the leading causes of their misinterpretation of patients' TB symptoms. This misinformation and inappropriate treatment led patients to experience discriminatory practices in the clinic/hospital setting (Gaviria et al., 2010).

In addition to the health-care provider issues, patient disadvantage (e.g., immigration status and low incomes) would seem to contribute to a delayed diagnosis, although the TB literature has not investigated this as directly as the barriers to care literature. Immigrants may have delayed diagnoses because of not seeking care when experiencing symptoms due to fear of immigration authorities. This theme has been commonly identified in the barriers to care literature (e.g., Berk & Schur, 2001; Derose, Escarse, & Lurie, 2007; Heyman, Nunez, & Talavera, 2009). In El Paso, Texas, the site of this study, undocumented immigrants have reported: being afraid of authorities, obstacles to movement due to the presence of immigration law enforcement, and hierarchical social interactions in health-care settings, which negatively influenced their access to health care. While seeking health care, these immigrants felt at-risk of being arrested and deported, so many were not willing to seek health care in formal settings (Heyman et al., 2009). It logically follows that these challenges would likely make immigrants less likely to seek care for TB symptoms.

Another reason that people delay care that has been highlighted in the health-care barriers literature is they possess insufficient economic resources to do so. In one of the few studies to examine delayed TB diagnosis directly, Asch et al. (1998) surveyed 248 patients in treatment for TB in Los Angeles, California who self-reported a delay in seeking care (20% delayed care for more than 60 days). In terms of their reasons for doing so, 25% worried about the cost of care because they were unemployed; similar percentages of respondents did not know where to go for care (28%) and believed they could treat themselves (26%). Since 1998, health-care costs have risen and the U.S. government has enacted additional provisions that make it more difficult for adult immigrants to access public benefits; this makes economic concerns likely a bigger problem for immigrants today than in 1998.

Few studies have examined the process of delayed diagnosis to uncover reasons behind the delays and even fewer the direct experiences of people involved, as we do here. One case study of TB does provide a detailed example of one El Paso woman who suffered for four years without being diagnosed with TB (Moya & Lusk, 2009). The dearth of focus on experiences is in part because the majority of studies related to delayed diagnosis and TB have been quantitative (Asch et al., 1998; Gaviria et al., 2010; Tsai et al., 2008; Wallace et al., 2009). As such, we take a health narratives approach to this topic in a U.S.-Mexican border city (i.e., El Paso, Texas).

Health narratives are an effective method to describe the impacts of TB on residents of El Paso, Texas undergoing treatment. The health narratives approach involves soliciting people's stories about their illness, including how the person and members of their family understand illness and how they live with the illness, respond to symptoms of disability, and cope with the illness (Bell, 2000). TB is not the most common illness studied from this perspective (see only Araujo Paz & Moita Sa, 2009; McEwen, 2003, 2005). Unlike these studies, our study included people with active disease (unlike McEwen, 2003, 2005) and had a broader focus than explanatory models for TB (the focus of McEwen, 2003, 2005) and treatment delivery (the focus of Araujo Paz & Moita Sa, 2009). Because little is known about the experiences of people seeking treatment for TB in U.S.-Mexico border communities, these narratives are important to report.

CONTEXT AND METHODS

Study Context

This study was conducted in El Paso Texas, which has a population of approximately 800,000. El Paso County has a population whose majority is an ethnic minority, with 82% being Latino/a; in addition, 4% are African American and 13% are non-Latino white. The city is generally working class, with a median household income of $36,000 (US Bureau of the Census, 2012). Forty percent of adults do not have health insurance (Rivera, Ortiz, & Cardenas, 2009), meaning the County has one of the highest rates of uninsured residents in the state of Texas, the state with the highest rate in the United States.

TB is a serious health concern in El Paso, and its Mexican sister city Ciudad Juárez. For 2008 and 2009, the TB rates in El Paso were 5.4 and 8.9 per 100,000, and in Ciudad Juárez, 13.5 and 13.3 per 100,000. The number of new TB cases in 2008 and 2009 for El Paso were 40 and 67 cases and for Ciudad Juárez, they were 311 and 306 cases (Moya, 2010). A possible reason for these changes in rates is that many residents of Ciudad Juárez have fled the city to escape the drug-related violence that has claimed nearly 10,000 lives since 2008 (Molloy, 2012), and these include migrants with TB. Important risk factors (for the infected population ages 18 years and up in 2009 in El Paso) were: 76% were foreign-born; 36% had a history of alcohol use; 15% had diabetes; 12% had HIV/AIDS; 3% were or had been homeless; and 12% had an incarceration history (Moya, 2010).

The dynamics of TB infections in El Paso reflects conditions along the rest of the U.S.-Mexico border, where TB is one of the top ten diseases that account for high rates of mortality and morbidity (Pan American Health Organization, 2007). Immigration, which is prevalent along the border, has changed the epidemiology of TB in the United States as the number of TB cases in the native-born population has declined and as the number of cases in the foreign-born population has increased (Deiss et al., 2009; De Heer, Moya, Lacson, & Sheldin, 2009; Quitugua et al., 2002). The higher incidence of TB within the northern Mexican border area and the continuous cyclical migration of Mexican nationals to and from the United States contribute to the transmission of TB across the border (Quitugua et al., 2002). In addition, the large number of periodic return visits of persons to Mexico from the United States increases the chances for infections in the United States. In Mexico, "the TB rate is estimated to be fivefold than that of the US, [which] increases the risk for exposure to TB and thus ultimate transmission of TB within the US" (Wells et al., 1999, p. 837).

Despite its prevalence in the border region, TB remains a stigmatized health issue (De Heer et al., 2009; Moya, 2010). Delayed diagnosis is also a problem on the border. In a sample of 167 Hispanic border residents, the median duration of symptoms was four months prior to receiving a diagnosis and that one-third of all patients had been symptomatic for six months or longer (Wells et al., 1999).

Data Collection

We interviewed people of Mexican descent (immigrants and native born) under treatment for tuberculosis at the public TB clinic in El Paso, Texas. The TB clinic, funded by the Department of Health and Human Services of Texas, was selected because it treats all TB patients in El Paso. Interviews were conducted, by the first author, in a private and secure space at the clinic. All protocols were approved by the University of Texas Institutional Review Board and by the Texas Department of Health (i.e., TB clinic).

Participants were recruited with the assistance of the TB clinic staff. First, potential participants were given a study flyer by the nurses. Then, if they were interested in participating, they provided their phone number on a form included in the flyer. TB clinic staff then contacted the first author with each patient's phone number. All potential participants were contacted within a 48 hour period to schedule an interview. The total number of people we contacted by phone was 14, and all 14 were interviewed (the primary interviewees were these 14 individuals, but three daughters also participated in the interviews with their respective parent) between June and August of 2010. The majority of the participants were at the end of their treatment: five participants were two to three weeks away from completing treatment, two participants completed treatment the day of the interview, and five participants were three months away from completing treatment; only one participant still had six months to go to complete treatment. The respondents were provided with $25 to thank them for their participation.

In addition to the fourteen interviews, a pilot interview took place before the clinic-based interviews at the university office of the first author. All fifteen interviews were used in the analysis. All but one of the interviews was conducted in Spanish and all interviews were digitally recorded, with the respondent's consent, and averaged 60 minutes in length. The interviews were transcribed in the language in which they were conducted and analyzed using N*VIVO qualitative analysis software. Characteristics of each participant are presented, by pseudonym, in Table 1.

During the interview, a variety of themes were discussed. Related to this chapter were questions about the participant's story with TB, which included sections about his/her initial symptoms, length of time with symptoms, time spent waiting to seek health care, sources of infection, and other health conditions. In addition, the participant was asked about the process of being diagnosed and seeking treatment and if he/she sought care in Mexico, in addition to the United States. Also discussed, but less relevant to this chapter, were: the impact of TB on the participants' life, feelings about medications, side effects of medications, infecting others with TB, process of finding the TB clinic, experience of receiving treatment at the TB clinic, and resources offered to the participant by the TB clinic (contact authors for a copy of the interview schedule).

Data Analysis

The first authored created a node for "Delayed Diagnosis" as it emerged from a series of questions based on the participants' experiences with TB, and we then subcoded it into four emergent subnodes that can be broadly grouped into two themes. These are (1) repeated misdiagnosis and (2) TB test errors, which fall under the general theme of provider lack of awareness and (3) fear of U.S. immigration authorities and (4) few economic resources for care, which relate more generally to patient disadvantage.

RESULTS

Residents living in El Paso, Texas with TB had different experiences during their diagnosis process. While not a selection criteria for participation in

Table 1. Participants' Demographic Information.

Pseudonym	Age	Country/Place of Birth	# Of Years in El Paso	English Speaker	Type of Health Insurance	Annual Income (2010 US $)	Level of Education/ Country	Referred to TB Clinic by
Jorge	24	MX/Cd. Juarez	14	No	None	5,000–10,000	Elementary/MX	Health-care provider
Ivan	66	MX/Durango	4	No	Medicare/Edna	5,000–10,000	Elementary/MX	Lung specialist
Esteban	80	MX/Durango	19	No	Medicare/Medicaid	5,000–10,000	None	Health-care provider/ Providence
Dianna	19	U.S./El Paso	19	Yes	None	Less <5,000	Some College/US	Health-care provider
Mercedes	52	MX/Durango	34	Yes	Tricare/Military	5,000–10,000	Part of High School/MX	Health-care provider
Fernando	75	MX/Chihuahua	3	No	None	Less <5,000	Elementary/MX	Health-care provider/ Texas-Tech
Samuel	63	MX/Cd. Juarez	18	No	None	Less <5,000	High School Degree/MX	Family/Daughter
Beatriz	83	MX/Zacatecas	20	No	Medicare/Medicaid	5,000–10,000	Elementary/MX	Health-care provider
Julieta	70	MX/Durango	24	No	Medicare/Medicaid	10,000–14,000	Elementary/MX	Health-care provider
Daniel	72	MX/Chihuahua	40	No	Medicare/Medicaid	Less <5,000	Part of High School/MX	Health-care provider
Marcela	47	U.S./El Paso	.33	No	Medicaid	Less <5,000	Some High School/MX	Health-care provider
Sebastian	24	MX/Cd. Juarez	6	Yes	None	10,000–14,000	Some College/US	ICE agents
Alexandra	23	MX/Durango	12	Yes	None	15,000–19,999	Some College/US	Health-care provider
Mia	24	MX/Cd. Juarez	13	Yes	None	10,000–14,000	B.A./US	Health-care provider
Esperanza	42	MX/Unknown	39	Yes	None	Less <5,000	B.A./US	Health-care provider

this study, fourteen of the fifteen participants had experienced a delayed diagnosis (i.e., when a symptomatic patient does not receive diagnosis and treatment within 60 days from the onset of initial symptoms). The fifteenth patient (Sebastian) may also have had a delayed diagnosis, but he did not indicate for how many months he had been coughing before being diagnosed while in detention for narco-trafficking. Because of our focus on health narratives, we will highlight one person in detail in each of the four subthemes related to delayed diagnosis. We will provide information about the sample first, to illustrate how this person's story compares to the group as a whole. This strategy of selecting one story was chosen because it allows us to provide detailed information that emphasizes the richness of the health narratives approach.

Provider Lack of Awareness: Repeated Misdiagnosis

Nine of the participants were diagnosed with illnesses other than TB before their doctors finally determined it was TB, making misdiagnosis a common occurrence for participants in this study. These illnesses included asthma, allergies, pneumonia, bronchitis, thyroid cancer, and/or severe colds. The time frame for diagnosing TB was between three months and four years. These patients, who were repeatedly seeking care for their symptoms, were not tested for TB, not asked for a sputum test (i.e., when the phlegm of the person is tested for TB) and did not receive a chest X-ray during their initial visits to the clinic or emergency room for respiratory problems. Participants reported that after doctors diagnosed them with an illness (not TB) they were prescribed medication to treat their presumed condition. In addition to being diagnosed with other illnesses, doctors' referred participants to specialists such as a pulmonologists and oncologists.

To illustrate this theme, we will draw on the case of Beatriz, an 83-year old woman born in Zacatecas, Mexico, with 20 years of legal residency in El Paso, who was interviewed with her daughter Ximena. Beatriz was selected because, while her time to diagnosis of three months was shorter than others with misdiagnosis, the number of diseases she was misdiagnosed with was quite high. Three months before being interviewed, Beatriz began experiencing shortness of breath, coughing, and fatigue. She decided to go to her general practitioner, which was covered by her Medicare and Medicaid, to ask about her symptoms. Her doctor told her that she had severe bronchitis and provided her with antibiotics; but a few days later, Beatriz's symptoms continued. Beatriz then decided to go the hospital because she could not tolerate the symptoms any longer. At the Del Sol Medical Center, Beatriz was first admitted to the emergency room, and after staying overnight, she was again told that she had bronchitis and was treated with several inhalers. Beatriz was released from the hospital, and a few days later, the symptoms continued. Ximena then decided to take her mother to see a doctor in Juárez (Mexico, just across the border from El Paso), because they both felt that the doctors in El Paso were not helping Beatriz. The doctor in Juárez diagnosed Beatriz with asthma and allergies and gave Beatriz two shots. The mother and daughter returned to El Paso, but none of Beatriz symptoms went away. Beatriz returned to her primary doctor in El Paso, and mentioned to her doctor that she had gone to Juárez, where they had given her two shots for asthma and allergies. Beatriz's doctor told her that there was no such a thing as shots for asthma and what she really had was pneumonia. Beatriz could not believe she had pneumonia, but her doctor prescribed her a medication and she returned home.

Beatriz's symptoms did not go away. Ximena said that her mother had been experiencing those symptoms for more than two months by this time, and since the symptoms were worsening, Ximena decided to take her mother to another hospital. At Providence Hospital, Beatriz was treated with inhalers and was told once again that she had pneumonia. After being admitted to the hospital and staying overnight, Beatriz was told that they were going to perform a biopsy because she did not have pneumonia. To do so, they were going to insert a tube through her throat (endoscopy) because they could not identify what she was suffering from.

Three days after being admitted to Providence Memorial Hospital, the doctor told Ximena that her mother had cancer. Ximena said:

> When the doctor came out of the endoscopy, he told me, "I have bad news!" I said, "What's happening?" "Your mother has a cancerous tumor, which was like a pea on her lung." "Are you sure?" And he said, "Yes ... It is cancer." And I said, "What will happen?" "No," he said, "let's do some more studies and let's see what treatment we are going to give her." So I said, "But is it cancer?" "Yes, it is cancer"... I am very ignorant, but I know that to diagnose it, there needs to be various tests, right? But, just telling me, your mother has a cancerous tumor, that was very shocking news to me. The doctor told me not to say anything to my mom, he said "let me do other studies, to see what we are going to do", and I kept insisting "But doctor is it cancer?" And he told me that it was already the lung, which was cancerous, the tumor is cancerous, so when we were told, three, four days later, no, no, it is not cancer, it is tuberculosis. I said bless tuberculosis!
> (*Translated from Spanish*)

Beatriz and Ximena did not quite know how Beatriz was finally correctly diagnosed with TB. Ximena only remembered that one day the doctor told her that her mother had cancer and few days later, Ximena was told that her mother had TB. Ximena did not know how this diagnosis was finally confirmed. She never asked the doctor what he did to determine that it was TB. However, prior to the diagnosis of TB, Beatriz received five different diagnoses: bronchitis, pneumonia, asthma, allergies, and cancer. Ximena said that having her mother diagnosed with TB was a blessing because she knew that TB was curable, and that her mother was not going to die from cancer. Beatriz completed her treatment for pulmonary TB in November of 2010.

Provider Lack of Awareness: TB Test Errors

In addition to repeated misdiagnoses, the lack of awareness of TB by providers was also manifested in their apparent disregard for a patient's TB test results and her subsequent requests to be tested TB, given symptoms. Out of the 15 participants, only one (Alexandra) experienced this; however, we wanted to feature this narrative as a secondary part of the "provider lack of awareness" theme because of the serious implications, both for Alexandra, her social contacts, and her broader social environment.

In February of 2010, Alexandra, a 23-year old woman born in Durango, Mexico found out that she had TB. Alexandra's diagnosis was not easily confirmed because she did not receive a skin test, a sputum test, or X-rays during several visits to the emergency room, despite manifesting symptoms of TB. During the summer of 2009, when Alexandra began to feel sick, she went to the county hospital in El Paso where she mentioned she had night sweats, coughing, and loss of appetite (all TB symptoms). In the emergency room, they told Alexandra that she had pneumonia, and they prescribed her a 10-day course of antibiotics.

Years before, Alexandra's mother had been very concerned because she had an aunt who died of TB when Alexandra was 10 years old. After her aunt's death, her mother took her to Tillman Health Center (a local clinic in downtown El Paso, where people can get TB testing for free) for a TB skin test. In a skin test, the practitioner puts a small amount of TB antigen under the top layer of the skin in the inner forearm. The skin will react to the antigens by developing a firm red bump at the site within two days if the person has been exposed to TB bacteria. At Tillman Health Center, Alexandra's test was positive (indicating LTBI), but they told Alexandra's mother that they could not give her preventative treatment for TB because Alexandra also had Spina Bifida.

Thirteen years later, Alexandra's mother kept insisting that Alexandra go and get checked again for TB even though her doctors had not suggested it, so Alexandra decided on her own to get another skin test at Tillman Health Center. At Tillman, they performed a skin test, and Alexandra was told that she did not have TB, but that she should go to the TB clinic for measurement of her spot and confirmation of TB anyway. Alexandra remembers her spot being so big and red that her mother was concerned about it. Alexandra remembers the spot being about 18 mm in diameter. In a skin test, if the spot is bigger than 10 mm, the person is diagnosed with TB. She said that when she arrived at the TB clinic, they told her that she did not have TB, and that she could go home. Based on Alexandra's account, it appeared as if the TB clinic missed diagnosing her with TB at that time.

Then, Alexandra left the United States to visit her family in Durango, Mexico with the same symptoms of night sweats, and coughing, still believing it was a severe cold. In hindsight, this was very risky, because she could have infected others with her yet undiagnosed active TB disease. When she returned, Alexandra continued some semblance of a normal life until January of 2010, when her symptoms began to worsen. Alexandra returned to the county hospital, with the same symptoms and they told her she had pneumonia. Alexandra specifically told the doctors at the hospital that she had been tested for TB and that her aunt had died from TB, but Alexandra did not receive an X-ray or further examination to see what she was suffering from. Alexandra was released from the hospital and she returned home with antibiotics for 10 days.

Two weeks later, Alexandra once again returned to the county hospital. She explained:

> I came back to the E.R. and I told them the same thing! You know what, I have been coughing, I have night sweats and I lost ten pounds, and I couldn't eat anymore! Everything that I ate, I would just throw up, because I had a pain in my stomach, and that was the reason I went in ... And they told me, you have gallstones and then they asked me, "when was the last time you went to see a doctor?" And I told them, "I was here two weeks ago, for pneumonia!", and they were like okay ... I kept telling them, "I have night sweats; I have been coughing for more than a year." And, when I told my doctor, because she happened to be there, she told me, "What do you mean by night sweats?" And then I told her that I was feeling like that for over a year, and that's when they were like, we need to do more testing.... That was when they told me that they were going to keep me there, just to do all this stuff. Two or three days later, Dr. B. went in to see me, because I saw a lot of doctors, and they didn't know what it was ... And Dr. B. went and touched my neck and said "Oh, okay, yes, you have TB" and then he told me "I just want for you to give me some sputum, but for sure you have it; and that is when they told me I had TB ..."

Alexandra's confirmed diagnosis took about a year and a half. This was in spite of the fact that Alexandra knew that TB was a possibility for her, as her aunt died, and her mother insisted she get checked more than once. It seemed that those associated with the public health system at the TB clinic and the Tillman Health Center ignored the results of her skin test, thus making Alexandra's a case of TB testing errors and ignorance, because her symptoms and results were apparently actively disregarded.

Patient Disadvantage: Fear of U.S. Immigration Authorities

Fear of U.S. immigration authorities, which was accompanied by a lack of health insurance, was another contributing factor to a person's delayed diagnosis, because participants believed that immigration authorities were in hospitals and clinics. Of all participants, two experienced such a fear. This is likely due to undocumented immigrants being less likely to volunteer to participate in the interviews than legal residents and citizens; we believe this fear is relatively common among undocumented immigrants in El Paso (see Heyman et al., 2009).

To illustrate this theme, we will draw on the case of Jorge, who experienced acute fear, which led to his delayed diagnosis. Jorge was a 24-year old born in Ciudad Juárez, Mexico, who had lived 14 years in El Paso at the time of the interview. During the fall of 2009, Jorge went to visit his brother who had been released from jail in Ciudad Chihuahua (Mexico). Jorge recalled that his brother had some gang-related problems in jail. Jorge was aware that being with his brother put him at risk of being attacked too. Jorge said that one day after his brother was released, they were walking, and they were picked up by some men and tied up. The men took the siblings to another place where Jorge and his brother were severely beaten. Telling the story of his brother was not easy for Jorge, in simple terms, he said (*translated from Spanish*): "they killed my brother in front of me and they set me free."

Jorge said that after the death of his brother, he returned to El Paso where he began having health problems. His back hurt most of the time, he was tired and wanted to sleep during the day, he had no appetite, was dizzy, and his nose bled frequently. Jorge did not seek medical attention for these symptoms at any time; in fact he was feeling these symptoms for six months until one day, when he could no longer get out of bed and walk, his wife called the ambulance. At Providence Memorial Hospital, Jorge was rushed to surgery, where the doctor discovered an abscess and TB in his spine. During our interview, Jorge showed the first author his wound. He had a scar from the surgery and remains of the abscess, which made his back look very swollen. Jorge received antibiotics for his abscess at the hospital and then began treatment at the TB clinic.

Jorge asserted that an important reason for him not going to the hospital sooner was fear of immigration officers because he was an undocumented immigrant. Even at his appointments at the TB clinic, Jorge expressed his fear of immigration officers:

> What if I'm illegal? Am I going to be detained there by one of the immigration officers? Seriously, I was afraid of coming to my appointments [at the TB clinic]. I began to investigate this with the nurse who would go to give me my medication; "Do you think they are going to detain me there or something?" And she said, "noooo, no, don't worry, none of that will happen there, Jorge. Go, because the doctor has to see you once a month that will happen for the rest of the year, to take your medicine". But, I tell you, I was afraid, because nobody explained to me that here there was no risk of that, and that was my fear because I have never sought care here or anywhere. That time that the ambulance took me to the hospital from downtown was because, really, I could not get up, and the ambulance had to come for me … I was afraid that they would cure me and then send me to Juarez, or something. (*Translated from Spanish*)

Jorge's fear of immigration officers being in hospitals was still present at the time of the interview. When he finally sought care for his spine, it was the first time Jorge had seen a doctor since he moved to the United States over a decade ago. Jorge considered his doctor at the TB clinic his primary source for care, and he wondered about his health care after he completed his treatment.

During our interview, Jorge indicated that he was worried about his future. After the surgery, Jorge's doctor told him that he could not do any physical activity for two years because that much time was needed to allow his back and body to fully recover from the surgery. As an undocumented immigrant, Jorge used to work picking up rocks at Fort Bliss (local army base); he said that he could not return to that job anyway because it was physically demanding and his body was not the same. He reported feeling weak and that he does not have full strength in his back. Jorge did not know what to do to earn an income to support his wife and children, a five-year old and a one and a half-year old. In the meantime, Jorge helped his sister with her yard work and painted restaurants every once in a while when someone hired him, but he did not have a secure source of income. Jorge was not eligible to receive any type of government assistance such as unemployment because of his immigration status. He hoped for a full recovery, and to feel healthy again to start looking for a job to support his family.

Patient Disadvantage: Few Economic Resources for Health Care

Participants who did not have sufficient economic resources waited until symptoms were severe to seek medical help because of the cost, even when they were not undocumented like Jorge. Their lack of economic resources seemed to facilitate their conclusions that their symptoms were a common cold that could cure itself. Participants reported that symptoms needed to become very severe (e.g., began to cough blood, could not sleep anymore, or the cough interfered with regular activities) for them to seek care. Eight participants reported that the primary reason for not seeking care when they first began to have symptoms was not having health insurance and/or not being able to afford medical services or prescribed medications.

To illustrate this theme, we will describe the story of Marcela because she had the fewest economic resources for care of all people interviewed, and the most extreme consequences associated with not being able to afford care. Marcela was 47-years old and an American citizen. She was a mother to five children: Daniel (21) and Teresa (16) (both American citizens), Mario (28), Maria (13) and Julian (11), who were Mexican citizens.

Back in 2008, Marcela began experiencing weight loss, weakness, hair loss, dehydration, and loss of appetite. At first, Marcela thought it was anemia caused by severe menstrual periods and the extreme summer heat because they did not own an air conditioner. After six months of experiencing these symptoms, Marcela began to have high fevers that would cause her to have lapses of unconsciousness and fainting, so she would stay in bed most of the time. Seeing his mother feeling weak and losing weight, her son Mario told her that she needed to see a doctor, but Marcela refused to go because paying the doctor would take the weekly salary from her son, the only provider in the family. Marcela explained:

> I had no money to pay for the medical testing; it was that, or we ate, that my children ate, because I stopped eating so that my children could eat, or so I could get the medical testing. And when I finally went for the medical testing, it was because I started having a very high temperature. My little girl called my mom, who lives in Juárez, and said: "My mom is very ill, and does not want to get up or eat!" Then my mom came to my home to see me and she said, "I have to take you to the doctor". At the first appointment with the doctor, they did the examination, which took all of the weekly salary of my oldest son and still my mom had to borrow some money. So that's why I did not want to go to get tested, because it was unfair to them to work all week to pay for me. I thought it was anemia, dehydration, I said I had anemia from bleeding so much. (*Translated from Spanish*)

After her son Mario paid for the first appointment, Marcela decided not to return to the doctor because they could not afford all of the testing that her doctor requested. Marcela returned home, and her symptoms continued to worsen. Mario, the provider of this family, knew his mother need to see another doctor in Juárez, where they were living at the time. Mario did not want to take her mother to a hospital because they did not have enough money to pay for the testing and were uninsured. Mario decided to take Marcela to a local pharmacy where they ran some tests, but the pharmacist told them that it was best to take her to a hospital because they did not have the equipment to conduct the necessary exams to determine Marcela's condition. Mario told his mother that it was best if they called Daniel, who lived in El Paso, and for him to bring Marcela to the hospital in El Paso, since Marcela is an American citizen.

Having no other option, Marcela decided go to El Paso, despite great personal risk. At the port of entry, Marcela was arrested because she had a warrant for not completing her time in a half-way house after being released from prison. Marcela had been previously arrested for illegally smuggling people into the United States on the San Diego/Tijuana border. After being arrested that day she tried to cross for health care, Marcela was detained and two weeks later, she was sent to San Diego, where her case originated. Marcela said that at that time she weighed 60 pounds, and while in court, the hand-cuffs were so heavy that she had difficulty walking. Once in federal prison, Marcela was unable to eat because she was weak; she had spells of unconsciousness, had little hair, and not enough energy to move on her own. Marcela indicated that thanks to the help of other inmates, she was able to receive medical attention. One of the other inmates noticed that Marcela was not eating and was very sick. Marcela said that after several months in prison, she fell unconscious and the other inmates called the guard who was able to get medical help for Marcela.

Marcela was then transferred to a hospital outside the prison. At the hospital, Marcela was diagnosed with TB, HIV and syphilis. The doctor told Marcela that she had the HIV virus for more than 15 years, and since she was not eating well or getting the proper care for HIV, her immune system had weakened and TB developed. Marcela did not know she had HIV until that moment and wondered how she could have gotten infected. During our interview, Marcela indicated that she had never done intravenous drugs, and that she only had had only two sexual partners in her life, both of whom were her ex-husbands. Marcela believed that she got infected with the HIV virus from her second partner, and, at the time of the interview, she was still wondering about her two youngest children and whether they are also HIV positive.

After completing her treatment at the hospital, Marcela returned to prison to finish her sentence. Marcela was released from prison and was able to return to El Paso, where she continued her TB treatment at the TB clinic. Unfortunately, neither Marcela nor her son Mario knew, or were told by the doctors or pharmacists in Juárez, that there were places where uninsured people with few economic resources can seek care and receive free treatment and medication for TB and HIV/AIDS in Ciudad Juárez.

Marcela completed her treatment in the fall of 2010. At the end of our interview, Marcela indicated that she needed help from an organization in El Paso that could help her test her children for HIV. The first author was able to refer Marcela to some organizations in El Paso. Marcela also indicated that she wanted to learn English and get a job because she did not have any money to support her children. Marcela looks forward to beginning a new life after completing her TB treatment and finishing the remaining months of her probation.

DISCUSSION

Health narratives, the orienting method for data collection and the presentation of results, was an effective method to describe the impacts of TB on residents of El Paso, Texas undergoing treatment at the TB clinic. In the analysis, we sought to understand TB, not only in terms of how the sick person and members of the family saw TB, but in terms of how they lived with the illness, responded to symptoms, and coped with the illness (these aims were described in Bell, 2000). As a summary of our findings, the narratives presented illustrated how delayed diagnoses impact participants living in El Paso. We found that participants were often misdiagnosed and TB was not even considered by doctors until other diseases were ruled out. Second, participants who sought care, especially in emergency centers, experienced poor quality of care and a lack of knowledge about TB on the part of the doctors. Doctors on both sides of the border (El Paso, and Ciudad Juárez) routinely diagnosed participants with pneumonia (which was also noted in Tsai et al., 2008), and provided an antibiotic. Third, fears related to seeking care because of the presence of U.S. immigration officials at health centers (hospitals and clinics) inhibited participants from seeking care in early stages of the illness leading to severe symptoms of TB and delayed diagnosis. Lastly, having few economic resources was an important factor that delayed diagnosis for TB. Since over half of the participants in this study were uninsured, on the patient side, this contributed to delayed diagnosis.

As reviewed earlier, several studies on TB have suggested that provider lack of awareness (e.g., Gaviria et al., 2010) and patient disadvantage (e.g., Asch et al., 1998)–the two main themes in this analysis- contribute to delayed diagnosis of TB. While the general themes identified in our narratives matched the small quantitative literature on delayed diagnosis, one theme not addressed was the problems with acquiring and interpreting the TB tests than Alexandra experienced. Issues with immigration status have also received scant attention in the delayed diagnosis of TB literature. Future quantitative studies should investigate both of these issues in more detail.

While provider lack of awareness and patient disadvantage have been addressed previously, this health narratives approach provides richness and detail that helps us understand these broad causes. Considering only the four cases presented in detail, one can see the immense personal suffering that occurs when the person with TB continues to live without knowledge of their condition and treatment. This is missed in the quantitative studies. For example, Beatriz faced an unnecessary surgery and a cancer diagnosis; Alexandra suffered for a year without doctors listening to her; Jorge became so sick that he could not get out of bed; and Marcela nearly died, eventually choosing prison over going without health care in Mexico. In addition to causing stress and suffering for family members (consider Beatriz's daughter, Alexandra's mom, Jorge's wife and Marcela's children), individuals in active infection, like those highlighted here, can spread TB to ten or fifteen people before being treated (WHO, 2007).

CONCLUSION

The conclusion will focus on providing policy recommendations related to our two broad themes. Findings from this study suggest that prompt diagnosis of TB could be achieved if medical personnel (doctors, nurses, and specialists) had a higher index of suspicion and recognition of symptoms of TB. This would keep people affected by TB from being misdiagnosed with other illness like pneumonia. Certainly sufficient emphasis in health professionals' training is needed. In the study community, these efforts could be targeted at the local Texas Tech Medical School in El Paso, and the nursing schools at the University of Texas at El Paso and El Paso Community College. Advocacy groups (e.g., Border Health Association in the study community) also have a role to play as they can target medical students, professors, and medical professionals with educational outreach.

We believe that patient narratives, such as those presented in this chapter, could be used to enhance these education efforts.

The results also have implications for public health policies that can better control TB by permitting widespread access to affordable health care regardless of legal status or socioeconomic status. Health policy change must occur in order to defeat these barriers of fear of deportation and the high monetary costs related to medical care that have been shown to delay diagnoses of TB. In addition, available services need to be better promoted, so that people can take advantage of opportunities that already exist. TB clinics are well-positioned to share information about other free and reduced cost health-care options with their patients. In El Paso, this should include information about general health care and TB treatment options in Juárez, Mexico. At the same time, in El Paso (and we assume elsewhere) few people know about the TB clinic and its services. To effectively prevent new infections, TB clinics should take an active role in promoting themselves in the community and offering free TB testing throughout the city in order to identify and treat people with LTBIs. In El Paso, the clinic currently relies on contact tracking (i.e., the method used to locate and test the people closest to a person had been diagnosed with TB) to identify new cases. Identifying latent cases more effectively has the potential to reduce the chances of people getting misdiagnosed or diagnosed late when properly referred to medical services.

ACKNOWLEDGMENTS

We acknowledge Dr. Eva Moya and Dr. Timothy Collins (both at UTEP) for their feedback on earlier versions of this research. We are also grateful to the TB clinic for assisting us in the recruitment of participants, and to participants themselves, who kindly shared their stories with us.

REFERENCES

Araujo Paz, E. P., & Moita Sa, A. M. (2009). The daily routine of patients in tuberculosis treatment in basic health care units: A phenomenological approach. *Latino-am Enfermagem, 17*(2), 180–186.

Asch, S., Leake, B., Anderson, R., & Gelberg, L. (1998). Why do symptomatic patients delay obtaining care for tuberculosis? *American Journal of Respiratory and Critical Care Medicine, 157*, 1244–1248.

Bell, S. E. (2000). Experiencing Illness in/and Narrative. In C. Bird, P. Conrad & A. Fremont (Eds.), *Handbook of medical sociology* (pp. 184–189). Upper Saddle River, NJ: Prentice Hall.

Berk, M. L., & Schur, C. L. (2001). The effect of fear on access to care among undocumented Latino immigrants. *Journal of Immigrant Health, 3*, 151–156.

CDC (Centers for Disease Control and Prevention). (2008). *Tuberculosis elimination and general information. Safer healthier people.* Retrieved from http://www.cdc.gov/tb/. Accessed on January 31, 2012.

Deiss, R., Garfein, R. S., Lozada, R., Burgos, J. L., Brouwer, K. C., Moser, K. S., … Strathdee, S. A. (2009). Influences of cross-border mobility on tuberculosis diagnoses and treatment interruption among injection drug users in Tijuana, México. *American Journal of Public Health, 99*(8), 1491–1495.

De Heer, H., Moya, E. M., Lacson, R., & Sheldin, M. G. (2009). Voices and images. Tuberculosis photovoice in a binational setting. *Cases in Public Health Communication and Marketing, 2*, 55–86.

Derose, K. P., Escarse, J. J., & Lurie, N. (2007). Immigrant and health care: Sources of vulnerability. *Health Affairs, 26*(5), 1258–1268.

Gaviria, M. B., Henao, H. M., Martinez, T., & Bernal, E. (2010). Papel del Personal de Salud en el Diagnostico Tardío de la Tuberculosis Pulmonar en Adultos de Medellín, Colombia. *Revista Panamericana de la Salud Publica, 27*(2), 83–92.

Heyman, M. J., Nunez, G. G., & Talavera, V. (2009). Healthcare access and barriers for unauthorized immigrants in El Paso County, Texas. *Family and Community Health, 32*(1), 4–21.

McEwen, M. M. (2003). *Mexican immigrants understanding and experience of tuberculosis infection.* Ph. D. dissertation, College of Nursing, University of Arizona. Thesis Dissertation: 1–274.

McEwen, M. M. (2005). Mexican immigrants; explanatory model of latent tuberculosis infection. *Journal of Transcultural Nursing, 16*(4), 347–355.

Molloy, M. (2012). Frontera Listerve. New Mexico State University Library. Retrieved from http://groups.google.com/group/frontera-list?hl=en. Accessed on January 29, 2012.

Moya, E. M. (2010). *Tuberculosis and stigma: impacts on health-seeking behaviors and access in Ciudad Juárez, México, and El Paso, Texas.* Thesis dissertation. University of Texas at El Paso.

Moya, E. M., & Lusk, M. (2009). Tuberculosis and stigma: Two case studies in El Paso, Texas and Ciudad Juárez , México. *Professional Development, The International Journal & Continuing Social Work Education, 12*(3), 48–58.

Pan American Health Organization. (2007). *Frontera De Estados Unidos Y México. Salud En Las Americas, Volumen II – Paises.* Retrieved from http://www.paho.org/hia/archivosvol2/paisesesp/Frontera%20de%20Estados%20Unidos%20y%20M%C3%A9xico%20Spanish.pdf. Accessed on January 31, 2012.

Quitugua, T. N., Seaworth, B. J., Weis, S. E., Taylor, J. P., Guillete, J. S., Rosas, I. I., … Cox, R. A. (2002). Transmission of drug-resistant tuberculosis in Texas and México. *Journal of Clinical Microbiology, 40*(8), 2716–2724.

Rivera, J. O., Ortiz, M., & Cardenas, V. (2009). Cross-border purchase of medications and health care in a sample of residents of El Paso, Texas, and Ciudad Juárez, México. *Journal of the National Medical Association, 101*, 167–173.

Tsai, T.-C., Hung, M. S., Chen, I.-C., Chew, G., & Lee, W.-H. (2008). Delayed diagnosis of active pulmonary tuberculosis in emergency department. *American Journal of Emergency Medicine, 26,* 888–892.

US Bureau of The Census. (2012). *Quick facts about El Paso county.* Washington DC. Retrieved from http://quickfacts.census.gov/qfd/states/48/48141.html. Accessed on January 31, 2012.

Wallace, M. R., Kammerer, J. S., Iadermarco, M. F., Althomsons, S. P., Wiston, C. A., & Navin, T. R. (2009). Increasing proportions of advanced pulmonary tuberculosis reported in the United States. Are delays in diagnosis in the rise? *American Journal of Respiratory and Critical Care Medicine, 180,* 1016–1022.

Wells, D. C., Ocana, M., Moser, K., Bergmire-Swat, D., Mohle-Boetani, J. C., & Binkin, N. J. (1999). A study of tuberculosis among foreign-born Hispanic persons in the U.S. states bordering México. *American Journal Respiratory and Critical Care Medicine, 159,* 834–837.

WHO (World Health Organization). (2007). *Global tuberculosis control surveillance, planning, and financing.* WHO Report. (WHO/HTM/TB/2007.306). Retrieved from http://www.who.int/tb/publications/global_report/2007/en/index.html. Accessed on January 31, 2012.

VIEWS OF JAPANESE IMMIGRANT WOMEN ABOUT CARE AS THEY AGE

Atsuko Kawakami and Jennie Jacobs Kronenfeld

ABSTRACT

Scholars have explained how people in Japan feel ashamed when elderly members of the family are cared for by formal services such as day care or government/commercial-based nursing homes due to the cultural norms of the consciousness of social appearance. However, this consciousness of social appearance plays a minimum role when it comes to elderly Japanese immigrant women's preference to utilize formal care services in the United States. They see receiving family based care as a burden on their middle-aged children (or grandchildren) and they prefer purchasing formal long-term care services when they can no longer feel confident about maintaining their independent lives. Elderly Japanese immigrant women hold rather positive views on formal care in the United States, including nursing homes. This chapter suggests that elderly Japanese immigrant women may not consider it shameful to utilize formal care as many previous scholars have suggested.

Keywords: Japan; immigrants; aging; women; care services

Issues in Health and Health Care Related to Race/Ethnicity, Immigration, SES and Gender
Research in the Sociology of Health Care, Volume 30, 67–83
Copyright © 2012 by Emerald Group Publishing Limited
All rights of reproduction in any form reserved
ISSN: 0275-4959/doi:10.1108/S0275-4959(2012)0000030006

Studying the views of elderly immigrants on the various kinds of care and support systems is becoming increasingly important in the United States, a nation of immigrants, with a rapidly aging population. There are several well-designed, detail-oriented, quantitative studies concerning the relationship between the levels of assimilation, ethnic identification, available care systems, and/or self-evaluated well-being among elderly immigrants (e.g., Angel & Angel, 1992; Beyene, Becker, & Mayen, 2002; Jang, Kim, Chiriboga, & King-Kallimanis, 2007; Mui, 1999). Lin-Fu (1988) points out that Asians are one of the smallest but fastest growing populations in the United States due to increasing number of immigrants; however, they "remain one of the most poorly understood minorities and their health-care needs have received relatively little attention" (p. 18). Taylor et al. (2004) found that Asians in their home countries, Asians (immigrants) in the United States, as well as Asian Americans in the United States utilize social support less than European Americans. Taylor et al. (2004) explain that the East Asian cultural norms discourage active engagement in social support networks for the purpose of solving one's problems. It would be considered a selfish motivation if one uses social support for his/her own advantage since Asian culture highly values collectivism. Asian cultural norms also make Asian immigrants and their families turn away from formal services and rely on family care based on filial piety (Min & Moon, 2006). However, Cheung, Kwan, and Ng (2006) argue that filial piety is actually a highly valued concept in both collectivist and noncollectivist cultures. While the collectivistic and filial piety explanations for the underutilization of non-family based support may be accurate and adequate for well-generalized Asian populations, studying the effects of cultural specificity and immigration experiences on elderly individuals' preference of care-giving/receiving is needed. For example, one cannot assume that how elderly Japanese immigrants who became naturalized American citizens several decades ago feel and how the elderly U.S.-born Japanese Americans (children of Japanese immigrants) feel would be the same in terms of their aging and long-term care services. However, due to the lack of sufficient data, scholars often have to combine all "Asians" and "others" as one group in most quantitative studies. Children of immigrants and the first-generation immigrants are often combined and categorized as "immigrants" to have enough cases to find statistical significance, resulting in general explanations such as that East Asian culture discourages utilization of social supports.

Even though scholars are sensitive about the immigration generational differences and ethnic specificity, the textbook description of first-generation elderly Japanese and second-generation Japanese Americans tend to emphasize their preference of filial care for the elderly. Hooyman and Kiyak (2011, p. 638) write:

> For first-generation Japanese, or *Issei*, a value that that transcends that of family is group conscience, characterized by cohesiveness, pride, and identity through devotion to and sense of mutuality among peer-group members. This value has been preserved through the residential and occupational isolation of older Japanese Americans cohorts form mainstream American culture. Even among the second generation, (*Nissei*), the Japanese vision of Buddhism endures in the cherishing of filial devotion and the loving indulgence of the old toward young children. Such interdependence with and respect for elders who have greater life experience, knowledge, and wisdom are widely accepted values. Accordingly, Japanese American old people tend to value intergenerational interactions, hierarchical relationships, interdependency, and empathy – all values that may not characterize formal services.

Asai and Kameoka (2005) argue that Japanese families are often misunderstood about the importance of filial piety as a strong value. Japanese families are perceived to prefer filial care over the formal care systems such as government-based or commercial-based facilities; however, the truth is that the concept of *sekentei* prevents Japanese caregivers from utilizing nonfamily based care systems (Asai & Kameoka, 2005). *Sekentei* can be translated social appearance or social reputation. Inoue (1977) explains that Japanese people's consciousness of their neighbors' surveillance leads to the consciousness of keeping good *sekentei*, or a good social reputation. Traditionally and in almost all cultures, females have been the filial caregivers to the elderly (Abel, 2001), which results in great personal and career sacrifices for females (Hamon, 1992). Japan is no exception as to this tradition. However, the unique case of Japan's filial care system is that daughters-in-law were designated to be filial care-givers by the government. Guided by the former samurai families' style, the Meiji Civil Code of 1898 in Japan outlined the culture of primogeniture in which the first son inherits all properties from his parents (Ishida, 1971; Kondo, 1990, pp. 124–127). In exchange, his wife becomes the caregiver for the husband's parents; this system has prevailed in Japan until recently (Asai & Kameoka, 2005). In other words, the care for the elderly is specifically the responsibility of daughters-in-law (Asai & Kameoka, 2005; Ishida, 1971) based on the idea of family continuity (Kondo, 1990, pp. 124–127). Before the Meiji Civil Code of 1898, inheritance systems and eligibility varied in different geographical areas and social classes (Hayami, 1983; Ishihara, 1981) but after the Meiji Civil Code, the homogenous preference of primogenital inheritance and related cultural practices were adopted across the areas and social classes including the system of filial care by the wife of the first son.

Of course, the Meiji Civil Code of 1898 has been replaced by the new, more egalitarian, laws after World War II; however, the cultural practice has remained. Although Japanese people have shown their attitudinal change about this custom, this system has been the basis for Japan's well-established means of caring for the elderly and acted as a quasi-official social security system for them (Ogawa & Retherford, 1993). Asai and Kameoka (2005) argue that the historical practice of primogeniture and filial care, combined with the *sekentei* consciousness, means that many Japanese families still feel ashamed when elderly members of the family are cared for by nonfamily members or formal services such as day care or government/commercial-based nursing homes (also see Momose & Asahara, 1996).

The elderly Japanese immigrants in the United States are not as restricted by these social expectations and norms from the homeland. Because most of them came to the United States many years ago either by themselves or only with their American husbands, they do not have relatives from their family of origin in the United States. They do not have the well-established means or patterns of the aging process or kin-based support systems that elderly people are expected to have in Japan. It is doubtful if they hold to *sekentei* consciousness with the same intensity in the United States. as they would have in Japan. Research shows that friends can be effective psychological support for the elderly, especially for those without children and those who have lost their spouse (Beckman & House, 1982; Connidis & Davies, 1990). These studies do not necessarily give special attention to the immigrant population, but the friend-based support system can be a valid substitution for filial care among elderly Japanese immigrants who do not have offspring, if they do not bring and hold the social norms of *sekentei* from their homeland and have instead adopted American social norms. Before considering the possibility of substitution for filial care, we have to ask this question first: does *sekentei* confine elderly Japanese immigrants to stay in filial care and prevent utilization of nonfamily based care such as formal government-run/commercial-based care or friend-based care in the United States? What are the ethnic specific factors which influence their preference for the different kinds of care-giving/receiving among elderly first-generation Japanese immigrants? This chapter will, first, discuss reasons why some elderly Japanese immigrants still think filial care is ideal and their plans for care-receiving. Contrary to the stereotypical image of Japanese families, most elderly immigrant women do not plan to be under care linked to children's filial piety. While analyzing elderly Japanese immigrant women's views toward filial care, it becomes clear that they hold rather positive views toward formal care and services. Then, finally we will discuss why other collective cultural values such as avoiding putting burden on others, instead of *sekentei,* have played a more influential role on their decision when it comes to deciding the preferable care receiving styles.

METHODS AND DATA

In order to answer the above questions, it is imperative to figure out what is the preferred ways of care-giving/receiving among elderly Japanese immigrants in the United States. It is also imperative to find out why Japanese people feel the way they feel about a particular care-giving and care-receiving method. In order to do so, qualitative analysis on their views about their preference on care-giving and care-receiving among elderly Japanese immigrants is necessary. By reviewing the related literatures and the data collected, we will analyze what methods of care giving/receiving are preferred and why those preferences exist among elderly Japanese immigrants in the United States.

The data used in this chapter were originally collected between 2007 and 2010 for a larger project on the identity of elderly Japanese immigrant women in the United States. The senior author conducted participant observation in two Japanese women's social groups in a major metropolitan city in a southwest state of the United States. These groups of women held monthly lunch meetings and other events such as semiannual garage sales, a summer retreat at a local hotel, and a Christmas party. Almost all women in these groups are first-generation Japanese immigrant women whose ages were between early 30s and mid 80s; most of them are above 50s who finished raising their children. Most of them are linguistically and socioeconomically well assimilated, but some of them still have difficulty with English.

In addition to the data from participant observation, personal narratives were collected from 31 Japanese women, age 40–84. Median and mean ages for these 31 Japanese women who were willing to share personal narratives were 65 years old. A vast majority of these women came to the United States as young women in the 1950s and 1960s with their American husbands who were serving in the military at that time. Ten of them were members of the social groups mentioned above and 21 of them were not members of either of the social groups. Incorporating the combination of snowball and purposive sampling to select the interviewees, the heterogeneity of personalities is maximized. Also, heterogeneity of participants' social class, marital status, and working experiences are considered.

Summing up the sample, all of them are cognitively healthy, noninstitutionalized, and physically capable to maintain their independent life. Many elderly Japanese women became naturalized American citizens, but they still consider themselves Japanese due to their racial and ethnic heritage and their place of birth. At the same time, most of them are culturally well assimilated and living comfortably in the United States. Some of them have no intention of becoming naturalized American citizens and intend to keep their Japanese citizenship. A vast majority of the women are/were married (mostly to white, American men). Some of them became widows and a few of them became divorced. Most had children. About half of the women (mostly the younger generations) have/had occupations. About 40% of these women, mostly the younger informants, had some college education.

IS IT SEKENTEI OR SOMETHING ELSE?

Although Asai and Kameoka's (2005) study was about *sekentei* (social appearance) and underutilization of formal care among Japanese people in Japan, they extended their scope to include Japanese immigrants and their descendants in the United States for additional consideration. Asai and Kameoka (2005, p. 117) conclude their study as follows:

> The extent to which *sekentei* is relevant to Japanese Americans is unclear. The influence of *sekentei* on the behaviors of third- and fourth-generation Japanese Americans may be diminished yet manifested in more subtle ways and may be extinguished among those who have intermarried. The relevance of *sekentei* among these highly acculturated Japanese Americans, however, remains an important empirical question that needs to be addressed in future research.

To answer their own question about the relevancy of *sekentei* in the United States as the future research agenda, Asai and Kameoka (2005) surmise that the U.S.-born grandchildren and great-grandchildren of Japanese immigrants may not show any significant behavioral differences influenced by *sekentei*. By doing so, Asai and Kameoka (2005) argue that the children (the second generation) of Japanese immigrants and the first-generation Japanese immigrants may restrict themselves to utilizing nonfamily based support systems with the *sekentei* concept even in the United Sates.

We argue that *sekentei* is not a large part of the elderly Japanese immigrants' concern when it comes to their preference of receiving long-term care.

However, it does not mean that the elderly Japanese immigrant women do not share their collectivistic values anymore, but it seems that they have a different way of thinking to show their consideration for "others."

Reasons of Filial Care: Affinity

Some of the elderly Japanese immigrant women still hold the filial care ideology as normative even though this ideal is not necessarily practiced by them as a care-giver or care-receiver. Almost all of the immigrant Japanese women said they do not expect to be cared for by their offspring in their same household. However, some expressed their wish or responsibility to be a care-giver for their own parents in Japan. The motivation for their wish is their affinity for their parents, rather than due to the *sekentei* norm to show that they are dutiful daughters. They did not mention care-giving to their husband's parents. For instance, a well-assimilated, especially linguistically well-assimilated, elderly Japanese woman, Miyuki, said she has no regrets about immigrating to and spending most of her life in the United States except for one thing. She regrets that she could not take care of her aged mother in Japan who was a widow for many decades. Miyuki was already in the United States when her mother became ill. Following the social norms of filial care in Japan, Miyuki's sister-in-law (her elderly brother's wife) took care of her sick mother at their home, but her mother and her sister-in-law did not get along well. Miyuki was the youngest among her siblings, and Miyuki had the closest relationship with her mother during her childhood as compared with her siblings. Now Miyuki is in her 70s, but she is not worried about her own aging in a foreign country because, as she described "I know the retirement system here. I don't even know how Japan's social security system works. I have to re-learn Japanese life again. But I know I can survive here. I have confidence and experiences ... I am not rich, but the house is paid off, and I am doing OK financially." Miyuki wanted to take care of her parents, but she is not expecting her child to take care of her. She said she can purchase the services if her health deteriorates.

Another informant mentioned not only living close to her sibling's family in Japan but also staying close to her children in the United States. Those who mentioned the possibilities of living close to their siblings and children did not indicate their consciousness for the *sekentei* and keeping a good social appearance as their reason. They are not planning to depend on those relatives. However, they are not necessarily refusing to consider their children and siblings as resources for support as they age. Again, the consciousness for the good *sekentei* is not the reason, but rather wanting the companionship of relatives. That is their main reason for mentioning the possibility of living with or close to children, siblings, and relatives.

Another Reason of Filial Care: Obligation

Naomi was divorced twice in America. After her bitter experiences of two failed marriages, she went back to Japan to take care of her aging mother and her father, who was very sick at that time. She said "as a human being, avoiding filial care for sick parents deviates from the way of being human." Naomi's primary reason for taking care of her parents indicates her duty; "not to deviate from the way of being human." While Naomi was taking care of her dying parents in Japan as a dutiful daughter who provides filial care in the culture of origin, she said, she heard her own voice in English. The voice said, "I don't belong here." After she took care of her parents to fulfill what she thought was her obligation of filial piety, Naomi came back to the United States. Naomi stayed in an apartment of her grown-up daughter and her son-in-law right after coming back to the United States; however, this living arrangement was uncomfortable for all of them. Naomi had to rent her own apartment. She is still working part time at a retail store and living alone in her late 60s. There is no one she is closely associated with in Japan anymore. Returning to Japan one more time does not look like a very attractive choice for her, but she has, at least, her daughters in the United States. Although, Naomi took care of her parents to fulfill what she thought was her obligation of filial piety, she is not expecting her daughters to do the same for her. She does not have a definite plan for her future in terms of monetary preparation for utilizing a nursing home or assisted living, but she said she is going to stay in the United States for good. She said "what else can I do?" Again, the *sekentei* ideology seems to play a minimal role in Naomi's choice, at least, in the United States. If *sekentei* still had influence on Naomi and her daughter, Naomi would not be a part time worker in her late 60s and living in an apartment by herself.

Another elderly Japanese woman, Ryoko, who immigrated to the United States in her mid 40s made a comparison between aging in the United States and Japan:

> Here [in the U.S.], you spend your own money to go to nursing home instead of leaving money for children and children taking care of you. Compared to Japan, parent-child relationships are independent. Having children in America does not mean you have a security for your age at all. ... You cannot say you are safe (*anshin*) because you have a

child. You have to take care of yourself. It is very clear. (*Totemo assari siteiru.*) So, the necessary, concrete steps I have to take are either downsizing the house until I have to live in the nursing home. But [because of the clear expectation of self-sufficiency for old age in the U.S.] you will not let other people say that what you are doing [such as not leaving property for children or sending your parents to a nursing home] is wrong. In Japan, it will not be that clear and easy. You have a strong wind against you (*kazeatari ga tsuyoi*) if you do something like that. I don't think Japan has yet reached that point [in terms of independency between parents and children].

Ryoko is concerned about her *sekentei* (social appearance) and its criticism for her if she would return to Japan and would use all of her savings for a more expensive nursing home there, instead of leaving some money to her children and family for their future. She thinks she will have to face "a strong wind (criticism) against [her]" if she purchases nonfamily based care without leaving an inheritance in Japan. However, Ryoko does not think purchasing nonfamily based care would create criticism against her in the United Sates. She is not concerned about how it would appear in the United States if she would stay in an American nursing home at the last stage of her life.

AVOIDING PUTTING BURDEN ON OFFSPRING

The influence of *sekentei* (social appearance) seems to be minimal among these elderly Japanese immigrant women in the United States when it comes to their choice in filial care or nonfamily based care. One elderly woman said "Both of my daughters are living [on the east coast]. I see them maybe once or twice a year, at most. [Because the current situation already lacks the frequent visits,] then, it does not make any difference even if I live in Japan. But if I live in Japan, then, they have to travel even more [distance to see me] than they do now and I don't want to cause such a burden for them (*meiwaku kaketakunai*). ... Then, the *best* way is being in a nursing home close to my daughter's place [on the east coast]."

Because this woman feels she is not well assimilated in the United States, linguistically and culturally, she is worried about living in an American nursing home. She said "Someday my health becomes deteriorated and I cannot be functional .... Children are living far away and not many people visiting me in the nursing home ... I wonder if I can make new friends there or not."

This elderly woman's concern for making new friends at a new place seems to be appropriate since she still has not established social networks with any particular groups of people since she came to the United States. Her anxiety is exacerbated by her disconnection from the society as well as the geographical distance from her daughters. Yet, she is concerned that living with one of her daughters is putting too much of a burden on her daughter. She thinks staying in the nursing home near her daughter's area might be the best option.

Contrary to this woman, Aki is a socioeconomically and linguistically well-assimilated elderly Japanese immigrant woman in her 80s. She has grandchildren in the same community where she lives and she maintains close relationships with them. Aki is a widow and a naturalized American citizen who lost her only son in a car accident many years ago. She refuses to live with and depend on her grown-up grandchildren. It is not even an option for her to think about counting on her grandchildren if (when) her health starts deteriorating. She said "No! I do not want to depend on them at all. I have always been independent. I do not want to put a burden on them." She has already checked on several independent living homes with her friends. She wanted to sell her condominium in the up-scale neighborhood last year, but the housing market has been so undesirable for the sellers that she decided to stay in the condo one more year. She laughed and said "I may stay here longer. When I cannot go upstairs to my bedroom, then I really will have to move. But right now I can jump up and go [to the upstairs] (*pyon, pyon ikeru*)." Aki thinks an independent assisted-living home is an ideal form for the elderly because "I would rather pay fees and be cared for by the professionals. ... You have your own living space with kitchen, bath, everything, but if you don't want to cook, you don't have to cook. There is a cafeteria too."

If Aki would care about her *sekentei,* she would not choose assisted living because someone who cares about her *sekentei* might imagine that utilizing assisted living will give the impression of herself as a neglected grandmother by her grandchildren. Such a thought does not even occur to Aki. She does not talk about her fear of utilizing the formal commercial-based support system nor does she talk negatively about the institution itself. However, she did mention her wish to avoid putting a burden on her grandchildren several times.

As Asai and Kameoka (2005, p. 117) pointed out, it is important to consider empirically how relevant the *sekentei* concepts are in the United States in terms of utilization of supports for old age among children of Japanese immigrants. Asai and Kameoka (2005) speculate that U.S.-born descendants of Japanese immigrants may not show any significant behavioral differences, but *sekentei* may make the first-generation Japanese immigrants reluctant to utilize nonfamily based supports even in the U.S. environment. However, this research indicates that even among the first-generation Japanese immigrants in the United States, *sekentei* does not seem to have much significant influence. The main reason these women do not care about *sekentei* is that they are in the United States, where they do not feel such Japanese social pressures.

As Aki explained her reason for not counting on her grandchildren to live with her is that she feels comfortable asking help and support from her friends. She said:

> I do not want to be [restricted by] paying attention [to grandchildren's feelings to keep the harmony with them] ("*Ki wo tsukai taku nai.*"). ... I don't want to put a burden on my grandchildren ("*Meiwaku wo kaketakunai.*"). They have their lives. I would rather ask my friends for a little help. I am really happy when my friends are close to me and giving me a helping hand.

Aki said she does not want to count on her grandchildren's help, because it may be troublesome, or put a burden on her grandchildren, but it is "*ureshii*" (happy) when she is receiving her friends' help. She does not feel she is causing trouble or "putting a burden on" her friends. This view is not a representation of distance from her grandchildren or selfishness in taking advantage of her friends. It is because of her consideration for the timing of the life course her grandchildren are going through right now as young parents. Aki and other informants said that they feel their middle-aged children or grandchildren are too busy to provide help, but their friends who are in their similar age cohort may have more time and flexibility, which makes them feel more comfortable in asking them for help. Many elderly Japanese immigrant women who feel comfortable in aging in the United States expressed their easy feelings of utilizing friends' help. Some of them described that they think people in the United States know how to take someone's help when they need it and know how to offer help when they can as a part of everyday life; thus, there is no special effort or sense of burden between the two parties.

This pattern of thinking could be based on the practical matter of whether their middle-aged children are available to care for them rather than on the elderly immigrant women's train of thinking based on their assimilation. However, the *sekentei* consciousness in Japan does not recognize an importance in being sensitive to the timing of the life course of one's children and grandchildren in its expectations of filial piety care. A person with a strong *sekentei* consciousness in Japan would assume that they would receive help from their middle-aged daughter-in-laws or female children regardless of their busy work schedule. In that sense, the pattern of thinking that Aki and other informants hold is distinct from the *sekentei* consciousness in Japan.

POSITIVE VIEW TOWARD FORMAL CARE

As described above, two opposite types of elderly Japanese women used the same expressions *"meiwaku kaketakunai"* ("I don't want to cause a burden [for (grand) children]"). In fact, regardless of one's level of socioeconomic, linguistic, and cultural assimilation, almost all immigrant women mentioned their plan of utilizing assisted living facilities and nursing homes, or at least thinking about utilizing these services. Yoko and her American husband do not have children. She used to work at a restaurant, but she can no longer be a server with her rheumatism. Yoko is very concerned about the time when she may not be functional in the future in everyday life. She said "but, being worried [about the future] does not create extra money. If it did, I would worry more, but it doesn't. So, I am worried, but I try not to think about it." Since she thinks that financial resources determine a comfortable retirement, she feels she cannot even *think* about concrete plans for a comfortable life in old age. She kept repeating how expensive the formal (commercial based) support system in the United States would be and how she cannot afford to utilize it. Then, she returns to her conclusion of "not to think about it" to mitigate her anxiety for aging. Her comments indicate not only her view in which the readiness for old age depends on financial resources but also her subconscious idea that purchasing high-quality services from a formal support system such as commercial based organizations would be ideal for the elderly.

Machiko, in her mid 60s, also mentioned utilizing a formal (nonprofit or commercial-based) support system and described the importance of friendship and social networks.

> I am not worried about [getting old]. When you are still healthy, you have a good time with other people, lunch, and gatherings. If you cannot sustain your household, you can go to assistant living. Then, when you really cannot move yourself, you can go to a nursing home and wait until the time comes. There are many institutions and systems to go through here. If you don't have money, you are not going to live in a very nice retirement place, but still, there are some places you can go. It's better to have money so that you can stay in a nicer facility, but if not, you can still find some places. The government will help you out if you have very little money. So, I am not worried about it. ... Have small gatherings and lunch with your friends and have fun. ... I think all the elderly people who reside here are living like that, making groups, join a church group ... I didn't save much money, even when I was in my 40s or 50s, but I still feel everything will be OK.

This much trust and optimism in the host country's retirement and social security system is unusual for the immigrant Japanese women, especially given the fact that she did not save much when she was young. However, Michiko's comments indicate that one's financial security may not be the biggest safety net for the elderly immigrant women in the host country, but friendship based supports may hold the key to understanding the elderly immigrant women's safety net. Many of them mentioned that having frequent lunches or gatherings with friends and having "a good time" will help their widowhood or compensate for not having offspring. One of them said that "Japanese people still hold the misconception that a senior home or assistant living is a horrible, lonely place, but it is possible to have a good time in a senior home."

Images of Nursing Home in Japan and the United States

Most immigrant women see the assisted living facility or nursing homes in a positive manner; however, there are some elderly immigrants who see it differently. One elderly woman in her mid 60s mentioned that her linguistic limitations and dietary differences between the United States and Japan make her wonder if she can bear to live in an American nursing home. If she thinks about these issues, a Japanese nursing home sounds more bearable for her, although she foresees different kinds of difficulties in a nursing home in Japan. Even though she would not have a problem with the language and food in a Japanese nursing home, she has a critical view toward the culture of Japanese nursing homes. She is not sure about Japan's common customs to keep a quasi-family atmosphere in formal care institutions for the elderly such as nursing homes and day-care centers in Japan. She said "in Japan, nursing homes and other institutions try to bring more domestic, home-like environments" but this elderly woman thinks being called "Grandma" or "Grandpa" by the nurses and staff members actually encourages elderly people to play the sick role in the nursing home, and so the elderly person becomes someone to be cared for by others. To make her point about respect for individuality in the United States and separation between the institution and the family, she said "here [in the U.S.], even if the elderly person is asinine, the staff members call the person with his name. ... Japan is not like that. I don't know if it is a good thing or bad, but it is supposed to be like that ...."

The anxiety among some immigrant women may be caused by their fear of the "unknown." Another immigrant woman gets almost panicky when her American husband tries to explain how the American social security system works. She gets even more panicky and repeats "I don't understand!" when her husband tries to explain how the pension and social security are transferable between Japan and the United States if she wishes to return to Japan after becoming a widow. It seems to be a daunting task for many immigrant elderly women to apply for enrollment in governmental or commercial retirement plans internationally, especially when one has depended on the spouse in terms of financial management and other household maintenance issues for such a long time.

Sometimes the fear of the "unknown" is created by over-generalization in the media, such as stories about small numbers of criminals scamming the elderly. This results in mistrust of American institutions in general, including nursing homes.

> When you think about all these situations [such as Japan's high cost of living, lack of available nurses, and drastic decreasing of the young population], Japan is also [a] difficult [place to live] in the future. ... Then the feasible plan would be living in an American nursing home. ... But, ... , you hear about too many perverts, like pedophiles becoming teachers here [in the U.S.] ... The quality [of teachers and caregivers] here is too unequal between the high-quality places (institutions) and low-quality places (institutions) ...

Although some informants expressed their concerns for institutionalization, most elderly Japanese immigrant women did not express their opinions toward nursing home and assisted living as negatively as previously thought. Likewise, filial care is not as highly valued as the stereotypical image of Asian families suggests. At least, there is no *sekentei* consciousness to confine themselves to family care in the host country.

CONCLUSION

We have discussed how the consciousness of social appearance, *sekentei,* plays a minimum role when it comes to these elderly Japanese women's preference or decision to utilize formal care services. However, it does not mean that immigrant women do not share the collectivistic cultural values anymore. They see receiving family based care as a burden on their middle-aged children (or grand children) and they prefer purchasing formal long-term care services when it comes to the time they can no longer feel confident about maintaining their independent lives. They feel they have to be conscious about how their children and grand children would feel all the time and pay attention to their needs first before their own needs if they would receive filial care from their children. In such situations, the elderly member of the family refrains from requesting small but frequent help or services. This situation will put the elderly members in an inactive mode. In turn, filial care will result in minimum services for the elderly in the name of maintenance of family harmony. Since there is very little influence of *sekentei* existing in the United States, the elderly Japanese women would prefer purchasing services and being able to act freely and more independently.

In addition, avoiding putting one's burden on others (*"Meiwaku wo kakenai"*) is one of the most emphasized collectivistic values among Japanese people. "Others" do not include family members, therefore, all the burden of filial care have been carried by the family, namely daughters-in-law or female middle-aged children. However, in the individualistic culture, one's own children are also considered "others" too. One of the interviewees articulated: "Here [in the U.S.] ... parent-child relationships are independent. ... You have to take care of yourself. It is very clear. ... In Japan, it will not be that clear and easy ... I don't think Japan has yet reached that point [in terms of independency between parents and children]." With this in mind, it is easier for the elderly immigrant women to support each other with similar aged friends while they are still functional in everyday life. When it comes to the time they can no longer support their independent life, purchasing services from professional nursing home staff is a more attractive choice instead of feeling bad about asking assistance from their middle aged children who are in the midst of their busy period in their life course.

Elderly Japanese immigrant women do hold rather positive views on formal care in the United States, including nursing homes. Since most of the informants in this study were elderly immigrant women who have been living in the United States for most of their lives, this chapter did not focus on whether there are differences based on current age or length of stay in the United States in responses about aging care. The length of stay in the United States may affect how they feel on care as they age. In fact, some childless Japanese immigrant women in their early 30s who have been living in the United States for less than 10 years did express their anxiety for utilizing nursing homes and fear for possible social isolation at the old age in the host country when they should become a widow. However, they did not necessarily express their feelings of "shame" or bad "social appearance" (*sekentei*) in responses to utilization of formal care.

After all, this chapter suggests that most elderly Japanese immigrant women do not consider it shameful to utilize formal care as many previous scholars have suggested. This is a contribution of this study. There have not been many other studies with Asian populations aging in the United States in general, nor with aging Japanese immigrants in specific. Of course, the women in this study were all living independently at this point in time. What we can learn from this study is that these elderly Japanese immigrants, most without much of an extended family from Japan, but only U.S. relatives of their husband's family or their own children and grandchildren, may not regard filial care as the best care nor view it to be as highly preferred as previously thought.

Another topic not addressed in this study is whether elderly first-generation immigrant Japanese individuals who have been institutionalized in a formal care facility hold similar opinions about filial care and formal care, since the participants of this study were all cognitively and physically healthy enough to maintain their independent life. It is also unknown if services of formal long-term care institutions actually meet with satisfaction from currently institutionalized immigrant Japanese elderly. Future studies could explore those issues with those populations.

REFERENCES

Abel, E. K. (2001). Historical perspectives on caregiving: Documenting women's experiences. In A. J. Walker, M. Manoogian-O'Dell, L. McGraw & D. L. White (Eds.), *Families in later life: Connections and transitions* (pp. 83–88). Thousand Oaks, CA: Pine Forge.

Angel, J. L., & Angel, R. J. (1992). Age at migration, social connections, and well-being among elderly Hispanics. *Journal of Aging and Health, 4*, 480–499.

Asai, M. O., & Kameoka, V. A. (2005). The influence of sekentei on family care giving and underutilization of social services among Japanese caregivers. *Social Work, 50*, 111–118.

Beckman, L., & House, B. (1982). The consequences of childless on the social-psychological well-being of older women. *Journal of Gerontology, 37*, 243–250.

Beyene, Y., Becker, G., & Mayen, N. (2002). Perception of aging and sense of well-being among Latino elderly. *Journal of Cross Cultural Gerontology, 17*, 155–172.

Cheung, C.-K., Kwan, A. Y.-H., & Ng, S. H. (2006). Impacts of filial piety on preference for kinship versus public care. *Journal of Community Psychology, 34*, 617–634.

Connidis, I. A., & Davies, L. (1990). Confidants and companions in later life: The place of family and friends. *Journal of Gerontology: Social Sciences, 45*, 141–149.

Hamon, R. R. (1992). Filial role enactment by adult children. *Family Relations, 41*, 91–96.

Hayami, A. (1983). The myths of primogeniture and importable inheritance in Tokugawa Japan. *Journal of Family History, 8*, 3–25.

Hooyman, N. R., & Kiyak, H. A. (2011). *Social gerontology: A multidisciplinary perspective* (9th ed.). Boston, MA: Allyn & Bacon Boston.

Inoue, T. (1977). *Sekentei no Kozo (The structure of sekentei)*. Tokyo: Nihonhoso shuppankyokai.

Ishida, T. (1971). *Japanese society*. New York, NY: Random House.

Ishihara, K. (1981). Trends in the generational continuity and succession to household directorship. *Journal of Comparative Family Studies, 12,* 351–363.

Jang, Y., Kim, G., Chiriboga, D., & King-Kallimanis, B. (2007). A bidimensional model of acculturation for Korean American older adults. *Journal of Aging Studies, 21,* 267–275.

Kondo, D. K. (1990). *Crafting selves: Power, gender, and discourses of identity in a Japanese workplace.* Chicago, IL: University of Chicago Press.

Lin-Fu, J. S. (1988). Population characteristics and health care needs of Asian pacific Americans. *Public Health Reports, 103,* 18–27.

Min, J. W., & Moon, A. (2006). Older Asian Americans. In B. Berkman (Ed.), *Handbook of social work in health and aging* (pp. 257–272). New York, NY: Oxford University Press.

Momose, Y., & Asahara, K. (1996). Relationship of 'sekentei' to utilization of health, social and nursing services by the elderly. *Nihou Koshu Eisei Zasshi, 43,* 209–219.

Mui, A. C. (1999). Living alone and depression among older Chinese immigrants. *Journal of Gerontological Social Work, 30,* 147–166.

Ogawa, N., & Retherford, R. D. (1993). Care of the elderly in Japan: Changing norms and expectations. *Journal of Marriage and the Family, 55,* 585–597.

Taylor, S. E., Sherman, D. K., Kim, H. S., Jarcho, J., Takagi, K., & Dunagan, M. S. (2004). Culture and social support: Who seeks it and why? *Journal of Personality and Social Psychology, 87,* 354–362.

TWO SIDES OF THE POTOMAC: A QUALITATIVE EXPLORATION OF IMMIGRANT FAMILIES' HEALTH CARE EXPERIENCES IN VIRGINIA AND WASHINGTON, DC

Colleen K. Vesely, Marriam Ewaida and
Katina B. Kearney

ABSTRACT

In this chapter we examine how micro- and macro-level issues including access to child-only or family public health insurance shape low-income immigrant families' health care experiences in two policy contexts in the Washington, DC metropolitan area.

This qualitative study includes 40 in-depth interviews with first-generation, low-income immigrant Latin American and African mothers in DC and Northern Virginia.

The majority of families living in Virginia had child-only health insurance, whereas most of the families living in Washington, DC, had family health insurance. Regardless of these insurance differences, all mothers had access to free health care for prenatal care. Pregnancy, for most, was

Issues in Health and Health Care Related to Race/Ethnicity, Immigration, SES and Gender
Research in the Sociology of Health Care, Volume 30, 85–112
Copyright © 2012 by Emerald Group Publishing Limited
All rights of reproduction in any form reserved
ISSN: 0275-4959/doi:10.1108/S0275-4959(2012)0000030007

their entry into the U.S. health care system. Families' ongoing health care experiences differed in relation to insurance access, and culture, including parents' previous experiences with health care in their countries of origin.

Future research should consider the experiences of other immigrant groups, mental health experiences of immigrants, and fathers' experiences with health care.

Future initiatives to address health care should focus on providing family health care to low-income immigrant families across the country, improving access to mental health services for immigrant families, and creating more culturally and linguistically appropriate health care services.

This study points to the importance of family health care for immigrant families, as well as care that is culturally and linguistically competent.

This study illustrates the need for public family health insurance for low-income immigrant families, and the importance of culturally competent health care for immigrants.

Keywords: Immigrant families; health care policy; low-income families

One in eight individuals in the United States is foreign born. Children of immigrants comprise about one-quarter of all children in the United States and are the fastest growing segment of the child population in the United States (Hernandez, 2009). Consequently, immigrant families are a larger part of U.S. society than in previous decades. Immigrant families, particularly those who have recently arrived in the United States, tend to experience greater levels of poverty, higher rates of unemployment and underemployment, as well as lower wages (Harwood, Leyendecker, Carlson, Asencio, & Millar, 2002) than their native-born counterparts. In addition to these serious economic challenges, low-income immigrant families also experience disparities in health status (Dey & Lucas, 2006) and access to health care (Huang, Yu, & Ledsky, 2006).

Immigrant families' health care situations are complex for micro-level reasons including country of origin (COO) health care experiences; cultural and linguistic barriers; and shifting health care needs based on acculturation and length of time in the United States. Additionally, a number of macro-level changes in terms of health care policy shifts in recent years make these families' situations even more complex. Specifically, mixed documentation status of immigrant families in which children may be U.S.-born citizens eligible for Medicaid and Children's Health Insurance Program (CHIP) with parents who are undocumented creates situations in which coverage of eligible children may be compromised because only the child has access to public health care (Guendelman, Wier, Angulo, & Oman, 2006). Further, five-year waiting periods faced by some documented immigrants to receive Medicaid shape these families' unique situations. Health care policies continue to shift across states as we move toward full implementation of the *Affordable Care Act* passed in March 2010. In turn, health care experts assert that immigrant families, and particularly those in which children are eligible for Medicaid or CHIP, and parents for reasons of documentation or waiting periods, are ineligible for public coverage, require, "special consideration for their complex situations" (McMorrow, Kenney, & Coyer, 2011, p. 8). Consequently, it is important to make known the experiences of low-income immigrant families with mixed public health care eligibility statuses due to documentation as well as timing of immigration, such that we can better understand how different policy contexts shape these families' utilization of and experiences with health care in the United States. In this chapter, we explore the health care experiences of both documented and undocumented immigrants from Latin America and Africa living in two policy contexts – child-only coverage and family coverage – in the Washington, DC metropolitan area.

HEALTH CARE AMONG IMMIGRANT FAMILIES IN THE UNITED STATES

Despite experiencing lower rates of morbidity and mortality compared to native-born families, immigrants living in the United States for longer periods tend to have higher rates of chronic diseases like obesity, hypertension, and cardiovascular disease than their recently immigrated counterparts (Dey & Lucas, 2006). In addition, as a result of the many traumas and stressors faced by immigrants and refugees, they have been found to be at high risk for developing mental health problems, especially depression and anxiety disorders (Pumariega, Rothe, & Pumariega, 2005). Risk factors including poverty, low parental education, unemployment, and poor physical health that immigrant families disproportionately face, affect the severity of depression and anxiety faced by individuals.

In addition to their health status declining over time, as well as mental health challenges, low-income immigrant families indicate lower access to health care than low-income native-born families (Sternberg & Barry, 2011) and are also less likely to have a usual source of care or a regular care provider (Dey & Lucas, 2006; Huang et al., 2006). In particular, low-income immigrants are twice as likely to be uninsured as low-income U.S. citizens (Huang et al., 2006). Further, research using the National Survey of American Families found that immigrant children were four times less likely to have health insurance than children with native-born parents. These same children were 40–80% less likely to have visited a doctor or a dentist in the previous year (Huang et al., 2006). Limited access to health care services for children and/or parents can ultimately affect these families' overall well-being.

Finally, research indicates cultural barriers to care including language, as well as limited understanding of health care in the United States, leave immigrants, "less connected with the health care system" (Huang et al., 2006, p. 634). Further, noncitizen parents, compared to their citizen counterparts, were least likely to know how to navigate the health care system, and naturalized citizen parents were less knowledgeable of where to go for health care support compared to U.S.-born citizens (Yu, Huang, Scwalberg, & Kogan, 2005).

Despite the wealth of demographic research on immigrant children and adults in terms of disparities in health status and health care access, there is limited research considering the experiences of immigrant *families*. Specifically, there are few, if any, studies that provide insight into the lived experiences of parents as they adjust to being in the United States and negotiate the health care system. The health care experiences of immigrant parents and their children are unique from those of native-born families not only because of language and cultural barriers faced by immigrants, but also because of the mixed documentation and citizenship status of many immigrant families. Recent research shows parents' immigrant status shapes their U.S.-born children's participation in public health care coverage, with citizen children of immigrants being less likely than children of native-born parents to be enrolled in Medicaid or CHIP (Kenney, Lynch, Cook, & Phong, 2010).

SHIFTING FEDERAL HEALTH CARE POLICY AND IMMIGRANT FAMILIES

The social production of disease/political economy of health framework, espoused by the Commission of the Social Determinants of Health with the

World Health Organization, indicates a connection between income inequalities and population that can be traced to political and economic structures (Solar & Irwin, 2007). For immigrant families who experience higher rates of poverty than their native-born counterparts (Hernandez, 2009) as well as poorer health status over time (Dey & Lucas, 2006), political structures or policies, including eligibility criteria for public health care, are likely contributing factors to these families' health. Consequently, it is important to understand how these policies shape immigrant families' experiences in terms of health care.

The signing of the *Children's Health Insurance Reauthorization Act* in February 2009 led to insurance coverage for 4 million additional children, including those who were documented immigrant children and pregnant women with no waiting period. Despite increasing much needed coverage for children and pregnant women in low-income families across the country, 10% of children in the United States in 2010 remained uninsured (Children's Defense Fund, 2011). The expansion of CHIP was focused on children and pregnant women only, and thus, 17% of nonelderly adults in the United States remained uninsured, with a fair percentage of these being immigrant parents.

Regardless of family income and being in the United States lawfully, only certain categories of immigrants are eligible for Medicaid coverage prior to having lived in the United States for five years. Specifically, the federal government indicates that states are required to provide Medicaid to documented immigrants who migrated to the United States for humanitarian reasons (refugees and asylees, Cuban, Haitian, Iraqi, and Afghan special entrants, Amerasians, victims of severe human trafficking), legal permanent residents meeting certain work criteria, members of the military and veterans, and individuals receiving Supplemental Security Income (SSI) (Fortuny & Chaudry, 2011). States can choose to fund other categories of immigrants not deemed qualified by the federal government.

The most recent health care legislation, the *Patient Protection and Affordable Care Act*, passed in March 2010, will not be fully implemented until 2014. As a result, many nonelderly U.S. adults remain uninsured. Additionally, the *Affordable Care Act* will not change health care access for low-income undocumented immigrant parents even though their U.S. citizen children are covered by CHIP. Finally, there are 3 million Medicaid/CHIP-eligible children who have undocumented parents and 0.5 million Medicaid/CHIP-eligible children whose parents are legal U.S. residents but have been here for fewer than five years. Some health care experts worry that these children's unique situations may impact their receipt of public health care coverage despite being eligible (McMorrow et al., 2011). Consequently, it is necessary to understand as much as possible about these families' health care experiences such that we ensure these eligible children remain enrolled in Medicaid and CHIP.

Some assert that a way to increase children's use of social programs is to improve their parents' access to these same social programs. According to Dubay and Kenney (2003), providing family health care coverage – or providing coverage to children *and* parents – rather than child-only coverage led to Medicaid use among eligible children that was 20 percentage points higher than in states that offered child-only coverage. Other studies show that child-only coverage may contribute to more gaps in health care among children as well as children attending fewer well-child visits (Guendelman & Pearl, 2004). This line of research is extremely important to increase our understanding of the importance of family health care coverage rather than child-only; however, the literature in this area is mostly quantitative and thus offers limited insight into the lived experiences of families in these distinct policy situations. Moreover, it does not illustrate how access to child-only versus family insurance shapes families' health care experiences. Consequently, in this chapter we aim to shed light on the experiences of immigrant mothers living in these distinct health care policy contexts in the DC metropolitan area.

Local Policy Contexts

Health care in Virginia (VA)

Family Access to Medical Insurance Security (FAMIS) program primarily includes the CHIP and Medicaid. CHIP is specifically for low-income working families in VA who earn too much to qualify for Medicaid but cannot afford private insurance for their children. To be eligible for CHIP, children must live in VA, be younger than age 19, and be U.S. citizens. Their families must be at or below 200% of the federal poverty level (FPL). It is not necessary that the parents be citizens for their children to qualify. Medicaid provides health care coverage to children (at or below 133% FPL), parents, the elderly and individuals with disabilities. In addition to CHIP and Medicaid, FAMIS MOMS makes special provisions for pregnant women such that if a woman is pregnant she receives Medicaid coverage for the duration of her pregnancy (Virginia Department of Medical Assistance Services, 2010). Immigrants' eligibility for Medicaid and FAMIS MOMS depends on their documentation and date of entry into the United States. Consequently for many immigrant families, the public health care coverage offered in VA is child-only coverage. At the local level, low-income families in many VA communities have access to health clinics run by the city's health department. Primarily, these clinics provide services related to pregnancy, HIV case management, chronic or acute illnesses, mental health counseling, pharmaceutical, dental, and pediatric primary care services.

In 2009 approximately 13% of Virginians were without health insurance. In the wake of the economic downturn that began in the fall of 2008, the number of uninsured adults grew by 44,000 between 2008 and 2009, the year in which the data for this study were collected. Also during this same year, the number of uninsured *children* dropped by 7,000 because of increased access to the CHIP (Macri, Coyer, Lynch, & Kenney, 2011). However, the number of uninsured children ages one to five increased by 6,000 children (1 percentage point). Still, adults in VA are more likely to lack coverage than children. Finally, noncitizen adults residing in VA are more than three times likely to be uninsured as their U.S. citizen counterparts (Macri et al., 2011).

Health Care Coverage in Washington, DC (DC)
Public health care coverage in DC is provided by Medicaid and DC HealthCare Alliance (Alliance). Medicaid, which in DC includes CHIP, can be accessed by DC residents who fall into one of the following demographic groups: children under age 19 with family incomes less than 300% FPL; youth, 19–20 years old with incomes less than 200% FPL; pregnant women with incomes less than 300% FPL; elderly who are blind or disabled with incomes less than 100% FPL; adults, ages 21–64 with incomes less than 200% FPL. The federal government covers 70% of the cost of Medicaid and 79% of the cost of CHIP (DC Medicaid Annual Report, 2008). Individuals who reside in DC but do not qualify for Medicaid or Medicare qualify for Alliance if they have no other health insurance, have incomes below 200% FPL, and have belongings and savings that are less than $4,000 for an individual and $6,000 for a family (DC Department of Health Care Finance, 2011). This program is available to both documented and undocumented immigrants regardless of how long they have been in the United States. The services provided by DC Health Care Alliance include preventative care, health screenings, prescription drugs, dental services, family planning services, urgent and emergency care, immunizations, prenatal care, well-child care, and hospital care. It is paid for solely by the DC government (DC Medicaid Annual Report, 2008). In turn, for many low-income immigrant families, the public health care coverage offered in DC is family coverage.

In DC in 2008, Medicaid, including CHIP, covered, on average, 2% more people per month than were covered in 2007. Spending per beneficiary in DC was also 23% higher than the national average in 2006. In fact, DC

Medicaid children received higher percentages of recommended screenings than national averages. Alliance also saw an increase in people covered from 2007 to 2008. In fact, together, Medicaid and Alliance provided health insurance to one in three Washingtonians in 2008. In contrast to other states, DC has tried to minimize the differences among Medicaid, CHIP and Alliance so that despite changes in age and income, individuals experience continuity in coverage (DC Medicaid Annual Report, 2008).

This chapter aims to describe the health care experiences of low-income immigrant mothers with young children living in the United States particularly in terms of their initial entry into the system, and their ongoing experiences with the health care system in terms of health insurance and providers. Specifically, we explore micro-level issues including language, culture, and COO experiences as these shape families' health care in the United States. In addition, by studying immigrants living in two different policy contexts, we show how macro-level issues including whether families have access to child-only or family public health insurance shape families' health care experiences.

METHODS

The findings in this chapter come from 40 in-depth interviews with low-income, immigrant mothers from Latin America ($n = 21$) and Africa ($n = 19$) with young children between the ages of three and five. Mothers were part of a larger study focused on immigrant mothers' adjustment to parenting in the United States, and their experiences with the health care system was one aspect of this larger research project. The richness of the qualitative data and in turn, the findings from this research, provide insight into the lived experiences and processes of immigrant mothers as they navigated health care systems in different policy contexts in the DC metro area. Just under half of the mothers lived in DC and the rest lived in a city in Northern Virginia at the time of the interviews. Despite living in neighboring communities surrounding the nation's capital, mothers in DC and VA, based on divergent health care policies, had different health care experiences.

Recruitment of Immigrant Mothers

Mothers were recruited to participate in this study from three publically funded, means-tested early childhood care and education (ECCE) programs in the DC metro area in which a high percentage (over 70%) of immigrant families from a variety of countries were enrolled. The first author spent approximately an academic year in each field site, meeting teachers, children, and parents, as well as observing in classrooms.

Recruitment efforts commenced after receiving Institutional Review Board (IRB) approval of the study. Inclusion criteria for this study were being a mother of a child who was enrolled in one of the ECCE programs mentioned above; having children who would begin kindergarten between fall 2010 and fall 2011; and being a first-generation immigrant (i.e., the mother was born outside of the United States and arrived in the United States after age 16). These eligibility criteria allowed for purposeful sampling or asking certain "information-rich" immigrant mothers to participate (Patton, 2002). Interviewing mothers ceased when saturation, or no longer hearing new information, themes, or stories regarding mothers' experiences, was reached.

Data Collection

During the informed consent process, participants were informed verbally and in writing that their interviews would be digitally audio-recorded. In addition, participants were made aware that they could ask questions about the study before, during, and after the interview, as well as discontinue the interview and/or withdraw from the study at any time. Each participant received a copy of the consent form to keep for their records.

There are various estimates of the number of interviews necessary to achieve saturation, or the point at which there is no new conceptual and theoretical information being gleaned from each interview (Daly, 2007), which range from 20 (Daly, 2007) to 30 (Isaac & Michael, 1981). Because families were recruited from three field sites in two geographic areas, it was necessary to conduct more than 30 interviews such that saturation could be reached in each subgroup. Specifically, data were collected from 40 mothers, 17 of whom lived in DC and 23 who lived in VA. Most Africans lived in VA and the majority of Latina participants resided in DC.

Most interviews were conducted in mothers' homes, while seven interviews took place at one of the field sites out of convenience for the mother. All of the interviews were digitally audio-recorded, and focused on the following topics, which were pertinent to the analyses and findings presented in this chapter: demographic background (age, number of children, marital status, house-hold data, COO), immigration experiences, mothers' ideas and interactions with the health care system in the United States and their countries of origin, as well as their health beliefs, and finally, any advice they would share with other immigrants. Interviews lasted one to three hours, with the average interview lasting approximately two hours.

All of the African mothers were interviewed in English, and the Latina mothers were interviewed in Spanish with the assistance of undergraduate research assistants (UGRAs) who were bilingual and bicultural. Following the interviews, the UGRAs transcribed the interviews in Spanish, and then translated these to English for analyses. The UGRAs randomly checked each other's transcriptions and translations for accuracy.

Data Analyses

Utilizing a modified grounded theory approach, formal data analyses were divided into three phases: open coding, axial coding, and selective coding (LaRossa, 2005). Field notes and transcribed interviews were loaded into Atlas.ti, a software program designed to assist qualitative researchers with data management. During open coding, each interview was read and initially coded using both sensitizing concepts (Van den Hoonard, 1997) as well as ideas that emerged from the data (LaRossa, 2005). The sensitizing concepts with which coding began were related to mothers' health care experiences and interactions including mothers' experiences of the health care policy context; COO health care experiences; first experience with health care in the United States; and family members' health statuses. A constant comparison method was used throughout open coding, such that paragraphs of text were read and then compared with previous blocks of text to determine if the new block of text was an indicator of an existing category or if a new category needed to be created (Glaser & Strauss, 1967). This aspect of the analyses yielded additional codes related to mothers' experiences with doctors in the United States; barriers and facilitators to health care use; and role of culture and language in experiences with doctors and health care in the United States.

During the second phase of analyses, axial coding, each of the salient categories or codes that emerged during open coding were examined by looking across cases to understand the various dimensions of each category (LaRossa, 2005). For example, to fully understand the dynamics of mothers' first experiences with the health care system in the United States, all of the coded text for this code was compiled using Atlas.ti. Next, all the pieces of text related to "first experience with health care in the U.S." were read to understand and code for the various dimensions of this code. Ultimately, what emerged during this phase of coding related to the code "first experience with health care in the U.S." were not only the reasons for initially looking for a doctor in the United States, but also how mothers selected doctors through the use of both social and organizational connections.

Finally, during selective coding, the last phase of analyses for this study, the main "story underlying the analysis" (LaRossa, 2005, p. 850) emerged reflecting various facets of immigrant mothers' interactions with the health care system. Specifically, a description of how immigrant mothers' health care experiences are shaped not only by micro-level factors including language, culture and their experiences in their COOs with health care, but also by macro-level issues in terms of disparities based on access to health care among parents emerged.

SAMPLE DESCRIPTION

The sample for this study consisted of 40 first-generation, low-income immigrant mothers who had children at one of three public ECCE programs located in Washington, DC, and Northern Virginia. All of the mothers in the study were low-income and lived below the federal poverty threshold. Nineteen mothers hailed from various African countries (Ethiopia, $n = 8$; Ghana, $n = 5$; Sudan, $n = 2$; Egypt, $n = 1$; Eritrea, $n = 1$; Morocco, $n = 1$; Somalia, $n = 1$) and 21 were from Latin American countries (El Salvador, $n = 9$; Mexico, $n = 7$; Guatemala, $n = 2$; Argentina, $n = 1$; Dominican Republic, $n = 1$; Ecuador, $n = 1$). They migrated to the United States nine years (minimum $= 2$; maximum $= 21$) before they were interviewed for this study, on average, and were 32 years old (minimum $= 21$; maximum $= 46$) at the time of the interview. They had two children (minimum $= 1$; maximum $= 4$), on average. Mothers' levels of education varied, with the majority having at least a high school degree ($n = 29$) and 11 mothers with less than high school. For 21 mothers, this was their first child. The majority of mothers in the sample ($n = 31$) were married or cohabiting, with the percentage of single mothers (around 25%) being similar among both the African and Latina mothers. Thirty mothers were employed, eight were not employed, and two were unemployed and looking for work.

All but one of the focal children in the study had health insurance and they attended regularly scheduled medical exams. Sixteen of the mothers lacked health insurance, with the majority of these mothers living in VA.

Among the mothers with health insurance, seven (six of whom were in VA) utilized private, employment-sponsored health insurance. See Table 1 for additional descriptive demographic data.

Table 1. Participant Characteristics (Frequencies).

	Total Mothers ($n = 40$)	DC Mothers ($n = 17$)	Virginia Mothers ($n = 23$)
Maternal age			
Mean age (in years)	32.25	31.23	33.00
20–29	15	9	6
30–39	18	5	13
40–49	7	3	4
Maternal education			
Less than high school	11	6	5
High school	14	4	10
Some college	13	6	7
College	2	1	1
Income			
Income less than 100% of federal poverty threshold	40	17	23
Maternal employment			
Employed	30	15	15
Not employed	10	2	8
Maternal time in United States			
Average years	9.08	9	9.13
Region of origin			
Africa	19	1	18
Latin America	21	16	5
Child characteristics			
Average number of children	2.22	2.23	2.21
Couple relationship			
Married/cohabiting	31	12	19
Single	9	5	4
Health insurance coverage			
Public child-only health insurance	15	1	14
Public family health insurance	17	15	2
Private family health insurance	7	1	6
No family or child health insurance	1	0	1

FINDINGS

Mothers' health care experiences in the United States began with initial entries into the health care system. This was generally their introduction to health insurance options. Their experiences also consisted of ongoing health care needs, coupled with their access to and use of child-only or family health insurance as well as interactions with health care providers. Almost all of the children in this study were insured by either public or private insurance, and regardless of where they lived, in DC or VA, they seemed to have similar and fairly positive interactions with both insurance companies and pediatricians. However, mothers' experiences related to their own health care varied based on where they lived, and in turn, the public health insurance eligibility, as well as their COO experiences, language, and culture.

Entry into the U.S. Health Care System

For the majority of mothers in this study, their first interactions with the U.S. health care system were during pregnancy. Many did not go to the doctor until they were pregnant because they believed that if they felt well there was no reason to seek health care. For some, as Marisol, a mother of one from Virginia, indicated, this was coupled with having limited time.

> My first visit ... I think it was when I was pregnant. Before that I hadn't gone ... . It's just when you feel fine ... and when I came I had two jobs, I worked 12 hours a day ... when I started to get thirsty, very thirsty and tired. And they would tell me, "you're pregnant." That's when I went to the doctor – but when you feel fine, you don't go.

For the majority of mothers in this study, clinics and doctors in their COOs were not as accessible as health care they utilized in the United States. Consequently, having access to doctors and services while being pregnant in the United States was support that exceeded most mothers' expectations. They described family and friends in their COOs who walked for two to three hours at a time to another city for monthly prenatal exams, as well as gave birth in their homes because hospitals and clinics were too far away. Paola, a Mexican mother of two living in DC, described this difference:

> In Mexico, you'd be on your own. But here, no – here when you are in your first months they want to see you every 15 days at the clinic to check the baby, and make sure everything is okay ... over there you would have [the baby] on your own in a house.

Additionally, specific negative health care experiences in their COOs led some mothers to be sure to utilize health care and particularly prenatal care in the United States. Maria, a Salvadorian mother of one living in VA who had a miscarriage in El Salvador, was vigilant about seeing a doctor in the United States when she suspected she was pregnant again.

> When I was 19 I got married, and six months after that I found myself pregnant. My stomach was growing and everything ... the problem was that I never went to the doctor, even though I was thinking I was pregnant, I never went. When I was six or seven months supposedly pregnant, I had a strong pain in my stomach so I went to the emergency room. They told me I had a tumor that was growing instead ... it was a pregnancy but the tumor had eaten it.

However, a few mothers described their health care experiences in their COOs to be very similar to their experiences with the U.S. health care system, particularly during pregnancy. They recalled having a similar number of visits before giving birth, but a couple of mothers did mention that the use of ultrasound technology was something new to them, as it was not used in their COOs.

Many of the mothers who ultimately used public insurance throughout their pregnancy did not have insurance until their initial early pregnancy visit. The health care professionals at local clinics, where the majority of these mothers sought care, usually assisted mothers in completing paperwork to receive Medicaid coverage for their prenatal care. This insurance was available to mothers who qualified financially in both DC and VA. Most mothers had insurance by the time they were due for their three-month prenatal visit. However, Esmeralda, a Mexican mother of one living in DC at the time of her pregnancy, indicated that her insurance coverage did not come through until she was five months pregnant. Consequently, she had to pay for her initial prenatal exam, which cost $150.

Mothers who did not qualify financially for Medicaid in either DC or VA during their pregnancies were covered by private insurance they or their spouses received through employment. However, Halima, an Egyptian mother of four who lived in VA without private insurance or Medicaid at the time of her first child's birth, did not know anything about insurance or health care in the United States, and ultimately paid out of pocket for a private doctor and a hospital in DC.

> Yeah, when I gave birth to the first baby I didn't know anything and went to a private doctor, to a wonderful woman in Washington, DC. But we pay a lot of money, because we didn't know anything about [insurance]. Even after the baby came we pay for shots for [the baby]. I pay cash for the sonograms and when the bills came my husband wrote a check ... for the second one we tried to do this again but it was too much. [Interviewer:

Did you keep track of how much money you spent [on health care] during that time?] We spent a lot. For the hospital, I still have the bill ... more than $4,000 or $5,000.

Compared to other mothers in this study, Halima's experiences were certainly unique as all of the other mothers received health care coverage for their prenatal and delivery care.

Only a couple of mothers' initial interactions with the health care system were for routine, annual visits either for themselves or children who were born in their COOs. Perla, a Mexican mother of two living in DC, indicated a history of breast cancer in her family, and thus her first visit to a doctor in the United States was for a mammogram four years after immigrating. In describing her health care experiences in the United States, she mentioned a negative experience with a private clinic in Mexico. Specifically, when she was 26 and still living in Mexico, she went to the doctor because she felt a lump in her breast. After conducting a brief "test" the doctor told Perla she needed surgery. This surprised Perla because the doctor did not indicate any other possibilities in terms of managing the possible tumor. Ultimately, Perla refused the surgery and did not mention this interaction with the doctor to her mother or anyone else in her family. When she was able to see a doctor in the United States a few years after arriving, she asked her U.S. doctor about what her doctor in Mexico had said. The U.S. doctor, with whom Perla ultimately developed a trusting relationship that spanned more than a decade, told her that she did not need surgery, and that "sometimes doctors want the money because [she] went to a private clinic." Utilizing DC Alliance, Perla continued to visit the same doctor at the same clinic. Even when she moved over the border into Maryland, Perla chose to pay out of pocket to continue to come to the same clinic as she had built such a trusting relationship with the clinic staff and the doctor.

There were mothers who arrived in the United States with children, both documented and undocumented, and it was for these children's annual exams that mothers initially connected with the U.S. health care system. Alejandra, a Salvadorian mother of two who lived in VA and was undocumented, initially interacted with the U.S. health care system when her oldest daughter was 18 months old and needed to be vaccinated. Alejandra had been trained as a nurse in El Salvador and knew the importance of being vaccinated as a young child. This was evidenced not only by the fact that Alejandra found a clinic where her daughter could be vaccinated for free but also by her bringing Melissa's vaccination cards from El Salvador – despite traveling on foot, through the desert and grueling conditions. When asked about the cost of this visit, Alejandra indicated,

... they gave her a checkup as well. Well, they gave us the check up for free because they told us that children with or without papers, all children have the right to vaccinations and the right to a check-up. You only have to apply, what you make ...

Finally, for one mother, her first experience with the U.S. health care system was due to an emergency illness. Yenee, an Ethiopian mother of one living in VA, had been in the United States for one year when she fell ill with gastritis at work as a nanny. Despite her employer bringing her to the hospital, it was challenging because none of the staff or doctors with whom she interacted spoke Amharic, her native tongue.

You know I am really sick and my English was not like now, it was like poor. So [my employer] took me to the hospital ... and still you know he only speaks English and they think he speaks my language. Then they asked him, "why are you here?" Then he said, "I will understand her, you know." Sometime I want to say something he won't know but he'll say, "is this the word you are trying to say?" and that was my first experience.

Ultimately, with the help of her employer, Yenee successfully told the doctors and the staff what her symptoms were such that they were able to prescribe her appropriate medication. As Yenee later indicated, at the time she did not have health insurance because she was working – it was not provided by her employer and she earned too much to qualify for Medicaid.

Regardless of when or why mothers first sought health care, whether it was due to pregnancy, a routine exam, or an emergency, they utilized social, organizational, and geographic connections to find both providers and insurance. Social connections included friends and family members, as well as acquaintances and neighbors who linked these mothers with clinics as well as public and private doctors. Esmeralda described, "The first time I went to the clinic was when I became pregnant about four years ago. It was good. They were good to me. It was a clinic and the lady I used to live with showed me." Organizational connections included doctors, public health clinics, and insurance programs, with doctors and clinics linking mothers with public insurance, and health clinics connecting mothers with both doctors and public health insurance. These organizational connections were most common among mothers in DC who had access to free health care through DC Alliance. Finally, geographic connections were links to health care that were based on where mothers lived. For example, a few mothers mentioned initially visiting a clinic they knew about because it was in their neighborhood. This was particularly common among mothers living in DC. Isabel, a Mexican mother of three living in DC, discussed her experiences finding a clinic, which reflected a geographic connection based on where she lived, and then she used the clinic as an organizational connection to enroll in DC Alliance.

> When I was pregnant with my daughter, I went to ask at the clinic. Since I live nearby and I'd catch the bus to go to work, I noticed there was a clinic there. So I went and asked what I needed to apply for insurance and they helped me there, and told me what I needed and helped me fill out the forms.

Mothers entered the health care system for a variety of reasons with pregnancy being the most common. In thinking about their experiences with health care in the United States, many mothers reflected on their health care experiences in their COO, indicating greater access to better health care in the United States. However, some mothers mentioned the similarity across health care systems in their COO and the United States. Finally, mothers utilized three different types of connections to link with the health care system in terms of learning more about insurance and providers: social, organizational, and geographic.

Ongoing Use of the Health Care System

Families' ongoing use of the health care system as well as their interactions with health care providers were shaped by the health status of parents and children and their access to child-only public or family public or private insurance. At the time of the study, three of the mothers in this study were either ill and/or 16 mothers had at least one child who was suffering from a chronic and in some cases, a life-threatening illness, and had varied health care experiences. Some mothers discussed continuing to use health care for annual exams and minor health issues, while others did not see a doctor unless they were sick. Finally, there were a couple of mothers who discussed mental health issues for which only one mother sought care.

For Isabel, a Mexican mother of three living in DC, whose daughter was diagnosed with Leukemia when she was four years old, easy and inexpensive access to doctors and hospitals were aspects of the American health care system that were extremely important to her. Both she and her daughters utilized public health care in DC.

> She is going on three years of being on treatment so she goes every month just like the doctors would tell me. They said, after one year it'll be every month, then two years – every two months but she would have to keep up with the treatment. What scares me is leaving to México and her getting sick while we're over there. I'm not scared of it coming back while we're here because any little thing that happens I can take her to the hospital in a hurry.

Isabel feared returning to Mexico would hinder her daughter's progress and would result in her daughter not receiving the immediate attention of doctors – something she was thankful for in the United States. However, not only did Isabel have to care for her eldest daughter, but her youngest daughter was later born prematurely and with several heart problems. For Isabel, life revolved around spending time in and out of doctor's offices.

Some families' experiences with the health care system, despite having children with debilitating diseases, were not as positive. Sharon, a mother from Ghana living in VA, explained how two of her three children have sickle cell, a disease of the blood that causes a lot of pain, particularly when it is cold. One of the children with sickle cell lives in Ghana. Sharon discussed her experiences when her daughter was first diagnosed.

> It was like during the winter time she said she was having chest pains. Yea so we took her to the emergency room. They had to really monitor what to do, whether there was a problem with her heart or something since she said she was having chest pains. And she started having, in her joints, she was having pains in her joints too. I think she wasn't able to walk for like a week or so. Her legs too, she was having problems with her legs. They were ... I mean she's on medication, on antibiotics.

Neither of Sharon's children in the United States had public health insurance, despite qualifying financially. Sharon explained that her children had been on Medicaid but when she went to renew it she was assigned a new caseworker, and ran into issues regarding the documentation needed. She thought it had to do with her own visa papers not being in order. Sharon was concerned about lack of coverage not only for her daughter, but also for her son, because her son's illness could result in passing illness on to his sister who had a compromised immune system.

> Yea for the kids and because she has sickle cell, she needs, she needs to be covered all the time because I don't know when she is going to break down. So when I took her to the doctor, he said [not receiving insurance] doesn't make sense cause of her. And even if [her brother], because he is related to her he is also supposed to be covered with [insurance] because if he has any disease like a flu or something and I don't take him to the hospital to be treated, then she will get it from him ... I had a different case worker and as soon as I switched to that case worker, he started being difficult. Asking for our passport papers ... I have a friend who we have the same case worker now, and she is also considering not applying for Medicaid again because he is also making it even more difficult.

Without Medicaid coverage for her children, Sharon would utilize the emergency room if necessary and would pay out of pocket for the medications her daughter needed for her sickle cell, as well as for both of her children's annual exams.

Some mothers described health challenges of their own that required ongoing medical attention. Marisol suffered from diabetes. Her case was challenging because the disease had affected her teeth as well as her reproductive system. Marisol mentioned seeing a doctor and nutritionist at a local clinic on a regular basis despite having to pay out of pocket for these services because she did not have insurance for herself. Yenee discovered through a complicated pregnancy that she had an ovarian cyst that needed to be removed, compounded with thyroid problems and anemia. Doctors urged Yenee to remove her uterus; however, she declined because she was still considering having more children, and she did not have health insurance or the means to be sure that her son, Lebna, would be cared for during her recovery.

> My son does have [insurance] and I used to have Medicaid but I'm working right now and they say I'm not qualified but that's you know make me ... it's like to buy insurance it is very expensive and so like if I have a medical issue now I don't know. I have thyroid problems and it's just complicated ... I need to remove my uterus also they told me that. [So when you went to a clinic they told you that?] Yeah, first they told me that I had a cyst, you know ovary cyst – they removed that you know ... I started this job in September-October and ... if you do this kind of surgery ... I have to stay home and make sure who is going to take care of Lebna. So, I said you know let me be with the pain. [It's painful?] Every month when I get my period, oh my god it's painful, it is really, really painful. [So do you go to the ER or a clinic for this?] Just take the medicine, take it off work and stay home. Sometimes yeah I have, when I have a heavy bleeding and I'm anemic also, so that really scare me.

Other mothers, particularly those without health insurance, only sought health care when they faced a particular health issue. Esmeralda, who had child-only coverage, usually did not go to the doctor because she did not have health insurance. However, she described a recent visit to a local clinic to mend an ingrown toe nail:

> No I haven't gone to the doctor's [since I have been without insurance]. I don't go. Friday I did have to go because an ingrown nail and I had to take it out. It was a clinic, I don't remember what it is called. No, you have to pay – the appointment was $55 and everything else will be around $200.

Finally, mothers with child-only coverage were discouraged from going to the doctor regularly because of the challenges they faced making an appointment to see a doctor if they did not have insurance and were utilizing a clinic. Emilia, an Ecuadorian mother of two living in VA, described her frustrations, which reflected the challenges mothers in VA faced.

> But sometimes when you don't have health insurance, you don't have the money to pay a private doctor – I have to do my pap test and I got three years that I haven't done it

because I don't have the money to pay for the test. I try to make an appointment at the health clinic and they say, "Oh call in two months." They've been like that ... I don't know what to do ... there I would pay $15. I'm worried about that because if I have to go to a private doctor to pay I don't know how much it will be – maybe $500. I don't have money like that – so it's hard ... it's very different if you have insurance ...

Among mothers in this study who reported that their physical health was generally good, there was variation based on whether mothers had access to family health insurance or not. Mothers without family insurance, like Kassa, an Ethiopian mother of four living in VA, admitted she was fearful of getting sick because they lacked health insurance. Kassa described coping with this worry: "I'm praying every day that I don't get sick – [because] no insurance." It was this fear that hovered over several of these women who could not confidently describe their current health status. Despite feeling okay mothers who lacked health insurance were worried that they were ill with a disease and did not yet know it. A comment from Aster, an Ethiopian mother of three living in VA, illustrated this fear:

But with me, a health clinic, I don't have one doctor. Sometimes I worry that maybe I have breast cancer and some type of cancer or something, but I don't know because I don't have a general check-up. Just raising my kids. I am not watching about myself.

Certainly, mothers with child-only coverage could visit their local health care clinics for their own health care needs, but these mothers were often deterred from scheduling annual exams because of the cost of coverage despite utilizing a public clinic. Finally, some mothers discussed utilizing the emergency room as their back-up plan in case they faced any major health issues while being uninsured. A few mothers had already used the emergency room and accrued large bills for which they ultimately sought the financial support of the hospital to pay off the bills. Makeda, an Ethiopian mother of one living in VA at the time of the interview, described a recent experience:

Yea, I was sick like six months ago and I just stayed in the emergency room here, and they took care of me. When I got better they asked me to pay them and I told the manager that I couldn't afford to pay the hospital bill. They gave me a number and I talked to them and they told me they were going to send a charity paper to fill out ... I sent it back and they approved me. [Interviewer: How much was the bill?] It was like $6,000.

Makeda went on to explain that the hospital would help low-income individuals pay their bills regardless of how many times they requested support. She mentioned friends who had asked the hospital three and four times and each time the hospital paid their bills.

Not only did some of the mothers in this study describe physical health concerns, they also highlighted emotional and psychological health issues that played a role in their daily lives. These mothers had elevated psychological symptoms that were exacerbated due to pregnancy and general stressors, including the health of their children and lack of emotional support, all of which affected their overall mental health status. However, none of the mothers with these mental health concerns had health insurance that would cover mental health care.

Isabel's children's health problems, especially her daughter's Leukemia diagnosis, impacted Isabel's mental health such that she eventually sought mental health counseling. Isabel described how her daughters' health issues took a toll on her mental health:

All the treatment was really strong so yeah at that point I felt really bad and went to a psychologist and she wanted me to take anti-depressants. I spoke with Melissa [a doctor] of Parents and Children Together who told me not to because they would make me really sleepy and that I needed to be awake for my daughters.

Even though Isabel chose not to take the anti-depressants, her families' health played a significant role in affecting her mental and emotional health. Constantly going back and forth to doctor's appointments as well as consistent worry whether her daughter would survive, let alone live a healthy, intervention-free life, exhausted Isabel physically, mentally, and emotionally.

Some mothers discussed experiencing post-partum depression and going without treatment because they did not realize that they were suffering from anything that could be treated. Emilia described her experiences:

That you feeling you don't want that baby, that's postpartum. And I cried a lot, a lot, a lot because when you are alone with the baby and you don't know what to do. Because I didn't know ... . Right now I know you can go to class, and they can teach you things, but back then I didn't know.

The mothers who sought mental health care did so through community-based agencies or paid out of pocket because these services were not covered within most of their health insurance plans.

Mothers' experiences with health care providers were varied and tended to diverge based on race–ethnicity due to mothers' language needs and abilities as well as their access to health insurance. Many of the Latinas discussed the importance of finding either a Latina care provider or at least someone who spoke Spanish. Compared to the mothers from Africa, finding bilingual providers was something that Latinas mentioned far more frequently. In discussing the importance of finding a bilingual provider, mothers pointed to both convenience and comfort as reasons. First, as Guadalupe, a Salvadorian mother of one living in DC, pointed out, if her doctor spoke Spanish she would not need to find a family member or friend to come with her to her appointment to translate. Second, mothers described the comfort they felt with a provider who spoke their language. Mercedes, a Salvadorian mother of three living in DC, shared her initial experiences with a health clinic in the United States.

> My experience was really good because everybody was welcoming and there were people who spoke Spanish. The doctor that checked me spoke Spanish and was friendly. I liked it a lot because I was comfortable.

Emilia was not as fortunate, such that as much as she wanted a bilingual provider, because of where she lived there were none available that would take her insurance.

All of the African mothers indicated that having a doctor who spoke their language or was of their cultural, racial, or ethnic background was not necessarily important to them. Even for mothers who initially did not speak English very well, they brought their husband or other family members with them to appointments to translate for them.

Mothers who had access to health insurance for themselves, whether it was public or private, were able to complete their annual exams and tended to see the same providers year after year. Continuity of care is one of the reasons mothers particularly appreciated having access to DC Alliance, as it provided them with opportunities to maintain health care coverage, and access to their providers even during shifts in employment in which they experienced temporary losses of private health insurance. In other words, mothers in DC were able to have continuous coverage even when they lost employment and were employed at companies that had a waiting period before health insurance could be accessed. For some, this was the only time they utilized public health care in DC. Mothers with access to insurance maintained longer relationships with their doctors and nurses, and consequently felt more comfortable with their providers. Some even mentioned learning a lot from their regular providers, compared to mothers who saw a different doctor or nurse each time they faced a health issue. Camila, a Mexican mother of two living in DC who utilized Alliance, indicated feeling well informed by her doctor:

> ... [the doctors] explain everything to you ... you have more options and you know something has more consequences – that this can give you that ... we go to the clinic for everything and they explain it to us there.

This is the kind of relationship that was particularly important as mothers learned to navigate the health care system.

A number of mothers living in VA reflected on their access to child-only health insurance. These mothers had family and friends in DC or worked in DC, and consequently knew about Alliance, and the access to family health care they would have if they moved to the other side of the Potomac River. However, despite understanding that some of the benefits in DC were better than in VA, families' social ties in VA, the cost of moving, as well as a strong education system kept families in VA. Halima described her reasons for living in VA:

> Yeah, my friend told me that in DC they have insurance even if you don't have documents – she has no documents and has health insurance. But we cannot go to DC because of our kids, VA is better for school. We say it is better to pay out of pocket for doctor and have our kids safe [in school] here.

Further, even though the system was far from perfect for some of the VA families, it was a system that mothers had learned and now, for the most part, understood. Moreover, only seeing the doctor when they were ill without considering preventative annual exams was something that was fairly normative in some of these mothers' COOs, so even having access to child-only insurance was more than what they anticipated having in their COO.

DISCUSSION

In this study, we described the health care experiences of low-income immigrant families, particularly mothers from Latin America and Africa and their U.S.-born young children, living in two distinct health care policy contexts in the DC metropolitan area. At the time of the interviews, 23 of the families lived in Virginia and thus had access to child-only public health care through CHIP or health insurance that covered only the children in the family, and 17 families lived in DC with access to family health care – insurance coverage for parents and children – through CHIP, Medicaid, and/or DC Alliance. Based on the social production of disease/political economy of health framework, it is important to understand these families' differential access to health insurance and in turn, health care due to political constraints.

Considering health care experiences of immigrant families with child-only and family health care may provide insight into the processes that underlie the connection between income inequalities, political and economic structures, and immigrants' health (Solar & Irwin, 2007). Moreover, recognizing when this divergence in health insurance and in turn, health care experiences occurs, whether it is during pregnancy, pediatric care, or when parents need care, is important to uncover so that policy and programmatic changes can be made in the most effective ways possible. Given this, we outlined families' initial entry into the U.S. health care system, which for the majority of families was when mothers were pregnant with their first U.S.-born children. Nearly all of the mothers had access to health insurance and health care for prenatal care. Further, we considered families' ongoing health care needs and use of the health care system to manage their families' physical and mental health. We illustrated how families' health care experiences were shaped by micro-level factors (COO experiences of parents, language, and culture), and macro- or policy-level factors (access to child-only or family public or private insurance).

For the majority of the mothers in this study, regardless of whether they lived in DC or VA, or were Latina or African, pregnancy was generally the reason they initially sought health care in the United States. All but one mother in the study had access to public or private health care for the majority of prenatal care as well as labor and delivery. It was during these earliest prenatal visits that mothers learned how to apply for health insurance from the providers at the local health clinics. For some mothers, their prenatal experiences were similar to what they believed their experiences in their COOs would be, while for others they shared stories of limited or no prenatal support in their COOs. A couple of mothers entered the health care system for either routine or emergency health care procedures.

For the majority of mothers, their prenatal health care experiences, as well as their children's health care experiences, regardless of living in VA or DC, were fairly similar. Overall, mothers felt as though they were well taken care of when they were pregnant and were generally pleased with their children's health care experiences. However, families' experiences diverged in relation to parents', and specifically mothers', nonprenatal health care experiences based on insurance access, as well as language and culture. Mothers with child-only insurance tended to worry about their health and avoided visiting doctors unless they were ill or pregnant. In turn, it was not uncommon for these mothers to see different doctors or health care providers each time they needed health care. Alternatively mothers living in DC with family health insurance indicated that they saw their providers for routine exams and thus, over time, built trusting relationships with their providers. These relationships provided mothers not only with physical health care, but also important health care information that families utilized in their daily lives. For mothers in families with child-only health insurance, they lived in constant fear of illness because if they were to get sick they would not be able to afford care. In addition, mothers who did not have health insurance also put off getting the care they needed for ailments diagnosed previously.

In addition to health insurance, families' cultural backgrounds, particularly in terms of language played a role in families' health care experiences. Latina mothers especially made note of the importance of having access to health care providers who spoke Spanish and for some mothers, they were particularly interested in having doctors who were of Latin American descent. African mothers did not have a preference for African or American providers. When asked about any language challenges they faced when they first arrived to the United States, they indicated regularly bringing a family member to appointments for translation assistance.

Finally, there were a couple of mothers who mentioned mental health struggles. For these mothers, whether they had access to child-only or family coverage, they did not receive financial support for mental health care through their health insurance. Only one utilized community-based mental health programs for free mental health care. For many of the mothers in this study, mental health challenges were fairly stigmatized in their COOs and thus it was not until someone else in the United States urged them to seek care for mental health issues. The second mother who mentioned mental health issues only realized, in retrospect, that she needed mental health counseling.

Limitations

Despite the strengths of this study including gathering an in-depth understanding of low-income immigrant mothers' health care experiences in two policy contexts, there are some limitations that must be noted. First, as with all qualitative research the findings from this study cannot be used to generalize to other populations. However, the level of detail of information gathered from these families can help shape future quantitative research in this area, such that we continue to understand the importance of family public health care availability, particularly for immigrant families. Second, this research focuses only on Latina and African immigrants, and thus does not offer any insight into how these experiences might vary across immigrant groups. Future work in this area should examine Asian American and/or Middle Eastern families' experiences with child-only and family public insurance. Finally, this study focused on the experiences of mothers and children. To gain an even richer understanding of families' experiences, including fathers will be important in future research in this area.

Implications for Policy and Practice

This research has a few implications for both policy and practice. First, the findings indicate the toll child-only or no insurance can have on both the physical and mental health of parents. In particular, mothers who could not afford insurance for themselves consistently worried about their health and for some they put off having important health procedures done. Also, mothers without family health insurance did not have a regular doctor they utilized, reducing their abilities to build trusting and informative relationships with their doctors. Moreover, it was not uncommon for these mothers to utilize the emergency room when they were really ill and then use the financial aid of the hospital to pay the bill. If these mothers had access to preventative care, some of these pricy emergency room visits could likely be avoided, and families could have the opportunity to build trusting relationships with their providers, leading to information sharing and other potential health benefits. These findings illustrate the importance of states working toward providing family health care to families living below the FPL.

A second implication of this work is improved access to mental health services, particularly for immigrant families. Immigrants face elevated mental health challenges due to traumatic COO and immigration experiences, and the limited resources they have access to in the United States tend to compound these issues (Pumariega et al., 2005). A couple of mothers discussed needs for these services, but none was able to get these services covered by insurance. Thus, one mother relied on a community-based program, and one mother noted going untreated. Consequently, it is important to continue to make these community-based programs available and known while health care policymakers need to work to ensure mental health issues are covered by public insurance for all families, including immigrants.

A third implication of this research is the importance of culturally and linguistically appropriate health care services for immigrant families. It is necessary to move beyond solely providing translators, particularly for Latino families, as the Latina mothers were most adamant about finding providers who not only spoke Spanish but also were of Latin American descent. In addition, the findings suggest the importance of providing existing health care providers with cultural competency training such that they are able to understand how COO experiences as well as culture and language shape these families' health care experiences. Finally, these findings show a need for working to increase the number of Latino health care providers.

Finally, the findings from this study reiterate the importance of hospitals and clinics being hubs of information and support, especially for low-income immigrant families. A number of mothers relied on these organizations to apply for public health care, as well as to learn more about health care in general. If more families had access to health insurance, they may utilize health care providers more regularly, not only for improving their physical and mental health, but also for health care information.

The combination of micro- and macro-level issues, including child-only and family health insurance, plays a vital role in examining low-income immigrant families' experiences as they relate to health care. Understanding the lived experiences and processes of immigrant mothers as they navigated health care systems in varying policy contexts is a step forward in reducing health care disparities in the United States.

REFERENCES

Children's Defense Fund. (2011). *Who are the uninsured children, 2010: Profile of America's uninsured children*. Retrieved from http://www.childrensdefense.org/child-research-data-publications/data/data-unisured-children-by-state-2010.pdf. Accessed on January 3, 2012.

Daly, K. J. (2007). *Qualitative methods for family studies and human development*. Los Angeles, CA: Sage.

DC Department of Health Care Finance. (2008). *Working together for health: Medicaid annual report, FY 2008*. Retrieved from http://www.dc-medicaid.com/dcwebportal/documentInformation/getDocument/1225. Accessed on January 18, 2012.

DC Department of Health Care Finance. (2011). *What do you need to know: DC Medicaid and Alliance*. Retrieved from http://dhcf.dc.gov/dhcf/frames.asp?doc=/dhcf/lib/dhcf/pdf/dc_medicaid_and_alliance_eligiblity_factsheet.pdf. Accessed on January 20, 2012.

Dey, A. N., & Lucas, J. W. (2006). Physical and mental health characteristics of U.S. and foreign-born adults: United States, 1998–2003. *Advance Data, 369*, 1–19.

Dubay, L., & Kenney, G. (2003). Expanding public health insurance to parents: Effects on children's coverage under Medicaid. *Health Services Research, 38*(5), 1283–1301.

Fortuny, K., & Chaudry, A. (2011). *A comprehensive review of immigrant access to health and human services*. Washington, DC: Urban Institute.

Glaser, B., & Strauss, A. L. (1967). *The discovery of grounded theory: Strategies for qualitative research*. Chicago, IL: Aldine Publishing Company.

Guendelman, S., & Pearl, M. (2004). Children's ability to access and use health care. *Health Affairs, 23*(2), 235–244.

Guendelman, S., Wier, M., Angulo, V., & Oman, D. (2006). The effects of child-only insurance coverage and family coverage on health care access and use: Recent findings among low-income children in California. *Health Research and Educational Trust*, 41, 125–147.

Harwood, R. L., Leyendecker, B., Carlson, V. J., Ascncio, M., & Millar, A. M. (2002). Parenting among Latino families in the U.S. In M. H. Bornstein (Ed.), *Handbook of parenting, Vol. 4, Social conditions and applied parenting* (2nd ed., pp. 21–46). Mahwah, NJ: Lawrence Erlbaum Associates.

Hernandez, D. J. (2009, March). Generational patterns in the U.S.: American Community Survey and other sources. Paper presented at a national conference on children and adolescents from immigrant families, "The immigrant paradox in education and behavior: Is becoming American a developmental risk?" Providence, RI.

Huang, Z. J., Yu, S. M., & Ledsky, R. (2006). Health status and health service access and use among children in U.S. immigrant families. *American Journal of Public Health, 96*(4), 634–640.

Isaac, S., & Michael, W. B. (1981). *Handbook in research and evaluation: A collection of principles, methods, and strategies useful in planning, design, and evaluation of studies in education and the behavioral sciences.* San Diego, CA: EDITS Publishers.

Kenney, G. M., Lynch, V., Cook, A., & Phong, S. (2010). Who and where are children yet to enroll in Medicaid and the Children's Health Insurance Program? *Health Affairs, 29*(10), 1920–1929.

LaRossa, R. (2005). Grounded theory methods in qualitative family research. *Journal of Marriage and Family, 67*, 837–857.

Macri, J., Coyer, C., Lynch, V., & Kenney, G. (2011). *Profile of Virginia's uninsured.* Washington, DC: Urban Institute.

McMorrow, S., Kenney, G., & Coyer, C. (2011). *Addressing coverage challenges for children under the affordable care act.* Washington, DC: Urban Institute.

Patton, M. Q. (2002). *Qualitative research & evaluation methods* (3rd ed.). Thousand Oaks, CA: Sage.

Pumariega, A. J., Rothe, E., & Pumariega, J. B. (2005). Mental health of immigrants and refugees. *Community Health Journal, 41*(5), 581–597.

Solar, O., & Irwin, A. (2007). *A conceptual framework for action on the social determinants of health.* Geneva: World Health Organization.

Sternberg, R. M., & Barry, C. (2011). Transnational mothers crossing the border and bringing their health care needs. *Journal of Nursing Scholarship, 43*(1), 64–71.

Van den Hoonard, W. (1997). Talking distance from the data and Constructing sensitizing concepts. In *Working with sensitizing concepts: Analytical field research* (Vol. 41). Qualitative Research Methods Series. Thousand Oaks, CA: Sage.

Virginia Department of Medical Assistance Services. (2010). *Medicaid and FAMIS-plus handbook.* Richmond, VA: DMAS.

Yu, S. M., Huang, Z. J., Scwalberg, R. H., & Kogan, M. D. (2005). Parental awareness of health and community resources among immigrant families. *Maternal and Child Health Journal, 9*(1), 27–34.

ETHNICITY AND THE USE OF "ACCEPTED" AND "REJECTED" COMPLEMENTARY/ALTERNATIVE MEDICAL THERAPIES IN CANADA: EVIDENCE FROM THE CANADIAN COMMUNITY HEALTH SURVEY

Christopher J. Fries

ABSTRACT

Research is needed that uses large enough samples to facilitate disaggregation of users by specific types of complementary/alternative medical (CAM) practices and by ethnicity in order to examine possible patterns in the use of CAM therapies not accorded efficacy by family physicians. The objective of this study is too use data from a large population health survey to determine the relationship ethnicity, measured with multiple indicators, has with the use of CAM therapies classified as "accepted" or "rejected" by family physicians in terms of efficacy. Using data from the Canadian Community Health Survey (CCHS) Cycle 1.1, logistic regression models estimate the factors influencing the use of the two binary categories of CAM therapy. Measures of ethnicity available in

Issues in Health and Health Care Related to Race/Ethnicity, Immigration, SES and Gender
Research in the Sociology of Health Care, Volume 30, 113–131
Copyright © 2012 by Emerald Group Publishing Limited
All rights of reproduction in any form reserved
ISSN: 0275-4959/doi:10.1108/S0275-4959(2012)0000030008

the CCHS are used to focus on ethnic origin, comparing North American and Foreign born, and on ethnic identification, comparing Whites with Asians, South Asians, Blacks, Latin Americans, Aboriginals, and others. Whites and North American born had higher odds of using "accepted" therapies, whereas immigrant visible minorities and those with Asian ethnic identities were more likely to use "rejected" therapies. This research confirms that ethnicity constitutes a cultural resource upon which users of CAM draw as they make their health-care decisions, sometimes despite the recommendations of family physicians.

Keywords: Complementary/alternative medical practices; ethnicity; Canada

INTRODUCTION

Population-based studies have identified correlates of the overall use of CAM therapies: women marginally outnumber men as users; usage peaks in the West of North America; users are slightly more affluent, better educated, and have more chronic diseases than the general population; and the use of CAM is supplemental to biomedical health care (Astin, 1998; Eisenberg et al., 1993, 1998; Millar, 1997, 2001; Nazeem, Neudorf, & Martins, 2000). At the same time, ethnicity has been identified as a determinant of health behavior (Aspinall, 2001; Leduc & Proulx, 2004; Pachter, 1994). Because many CAM therapies (such as Traditional Chinese Medicine, Ayurveda, Indigenous Systems of Healing, and Homeopathy) originate in cultural traditions distinct from the Western biomedical tradition, ethnicity may influence the use of therapies the efficacy of which Western medicine often questions (Angell & Kassirer, 1998; Fontanarosa & Lundberg, 1998). At the same time, research finds that patients' beliefs regarding their physicians' perceptions of the efficacy of CAM influences disclosure of CAM use (Stevenson, Britten, Barry, Bradley, & Barber, 2003). It has also been shown that over half of CAM users do not discuss their use of these therapies with their physicians (Eisenberg et al., 2001) and that ethnic minority populations have particularly low rates of disclosure, which varies by ethnicity and type of CAM (Chao, Wade, & Kronenberg, 2008). Physicians need to be aware of the use of CAM by their patients because of the risks posed by adverse events associated with the interactions of these treatments with conventional care (Chao et al., 2008; Hsiao et al., 2006). In the Canadian context, physicians report experiencing "growing multiculturalism" as "becoming a major medical challenge" in medical encounter communications (Mackay, 2003). A study of Asian Americans who disclosed their use of CAM to their physicians found that such disclosure, while uncommon, was positively correlated with higher ratings of health-care quality (Ahn, Ngo-Metzger, & Legedza, 2006). Research is needed that considers how ethnicity is related to the use of CAM therapies lacking in perceived medical efficacy (Chao et al., 2008).

While there is information on the relationship of ethnicity to overall CAM use (Bair et al., 2002; Kakai, Maskarinec, Shumay, Tatsumura, & Tasaki, 2003; Keith, Kronenfeld, Rivers, & Liang, 2005; Roth & Kobayashi, 2008), less is known about how ethnicity influences the patterns of use of different types of CAM (Hsiao et al., 2006). A 1998 US study found that ethnic differences did not predict use of alternative medicine (Astin, 1998). Since then, other population-based research finds that a substantial proportion of the use of particular CAM therapies cannot be accounted for by the ethnicity of users (Ahn et al., 2006; Bair et al., 2002; Barnes, Powell-Griner, McFann, & Nahin, 2004; Graham et al., 2005; Grzywacz et al., 2007; Kakai et al., 2003; Keith et al., 2005; Mackenzie, Taylor, Bloom, Hufford, & Johnson, 2003; Roth & Kobayashi, 2008). The U.S. Institute of Medicine has concluded, "In large surveys with representative samples, there is a need for better, more culturally sensitive questions that will provide more accurate data about CAM use among minority populations" (2005). By employing ethnic-specific measures Hsiao and colleagues identified patterns of CAM use across ethnic groups in a cross-sectional survey representative of the California population that differ from the predictors of overall CAM use in the general population (2006). However, an unresolved question is the extent to which the ethnicity of users relates to the use of CAM therapies not accorded efficacy by Western medicine. Research is needed that uses large enough samples to facilitate disaggregation of users by specific types of CAM and into ethnic groups in order to examine possible patterns in the use of CAM therapies not accorded efficacy by family physicians.

Explaining that "the reasons for defining modalities as 'CAM therapies' are not only scientific but also political, social, and conceptual" (2005) the U.S. Institute of Medicine concludes, "Given the lack of a consistent definition of CAM, some have tried to bring clarity to the situation by proposing classification systems that can be used to organize the field" (2005). Sociologists (Fries & Menzies, 2000) propose classifying CAM therapies into the binary categories of "accepted" and "rejected" by Western biomedicine in order to address what they outline as a central policy and practice question: Why do some patients use therapies whose effectiveness is questioned by conventional physicians? The present study employs a binary classification CAM therapies developed in a study of

Canadian family physicians who were asked to rate the efficacy of 14 modalities of CAM therapy listed in the CCHS (Fries, 2008).

Ethnicity is a multidimensional concept that is generally understood to include elements such as race, origin or ancestry, shared group identity, language, religion, or some intermixture of these elements (Aspinall, 2001). My purpose is to use data from a large population health survey to determine the relationship ethnicity, measured with multiple indicators, has with the use of CAM therapies identified in the Canadian study as "rejected" by Western physicians (Fries, 2008). Because health beliefs and behaviors are influenced by ethnocultural factors (Aspinall, 2001; Leduc & Proulx, 2004; Pachter, 1994) it was hypothesized that respondents reporting ethnic origins and identifications would be more likely to use rejected CAM therapies than accepted therapies as compared to those born in North America.

METHODS

Data Source

This analysis is based on cross sectional data (118,336 cases age 18 or older) from cycle 1.1 of the CCHS. This national probability sample covers the household population aged 12 and older in all provinces and territories except persons living on Indian Reservations, on Canadian Forces bases, in institutions (prisons, hospitals, universities) and in some remote areas. The dataset contains 16 questions pertaining to CAM use and two questions pertaining to ethnic origin and ethnic group identification. Specifically, CAM use was measured by responses to the following questions: *In the past 12 months, have you seen or talked to an alternative health-care provider such as an acupuncturist, homeopath or massage therapist about your physical, emotional or mental health? If yes, who did you see or talk to-Massage therapist? Acupuncturist? Homeopath or naturopath? Feldenkrais or Alexander teacher? Relaxation therapist? Biofeedback teacher? Rolfer? Herbalist? Reflexologist? Spiritual healer? Religious healer? Other? Number of consultations-Alternative health-care provider? Chiropractor?* Ethnic origin is measured by the question: *In which country (were/was) (you/he/she) born? Canada, China, France, Germany, Greece, Guyana, Hong Kong, Hungary, India, Italy, Jamaica, Netherlands/Holland, Philippines, Poland, Portugal, United Kingdom, United States, Vietnam, Sri Lanka, Other (specify).* Ethnic group identification is measured by the question: *People living in Canada come from many different cultural and racial backgrounds. Are (you/he/she):*

White, Chinese, South Asian, Black, Filipino, Latin American, Southeast Asian, Arab, West Asian, Japanese, Korean, Aboriginal, or Other (specify). Detailed descriptions of the CCHS design, sample, and interview procedures are available (Beland, 2002).

Data Analysis

Multinomial logistic regression permits assessment of the association between the measures of ethnicity and the use of accepted and rejected therapies while adjusting for other variables that influence the use of CAM. Further, it allows assessment of interaction effects between two variables that have independent impacts on the dependent variable to be combined to determine whether they also have a combined effect. An interaction effect is when the effect of one independent variable on the dependent variable varies as a function of a second independent variable. In this case, the multiplicative effect of Place of Birth times Visible Minority Status. Analysis was conducted using Stata Statistical Software (Stata, 2003).

The CCHS sampling design can lead to problems in the estimation of variances using conventional tests of statistical significance. In order to estimate population characteristics, I used Stata survey estimation techniques that account for sample design effects when calculating standard errors (Piérard, Buckley, & Chowhan, 2004). Sample weights, which were adjusted to sum to the sample size, are used in all data analyses to account for the unequal probabilities of selection as a results of the multistage sampling design employed in the CCHS. These procedures provide a more reliable estimate of variance by adjusting for the unequal probabilities of selection.

"Accepted" and "Rejected" CAM

Multinomial logit models (Tables 1–3) are used to estimate the factors that influence the use of CAM therapies classified by family physicians in previous research (Fries, 2008) as either accepted or rejected. The dependent variable is equal to 0 (no use) if the respondent reported not using any CAM therapy in the year prior to the survey, 1 (accepted use) if the respondent reported using either chiropractic, acupuncture, massage therapy, relaxation therapy, biofeedback, and spiritual or religious healing or any one or some combination of all and 2 (rejected use) if the respondent reported using any

Table 1. Odds Ratios (95% Confidence Intervals) for the Use of Accepted and Rejected Complementary/Alternative Medical Practices Compared to Nonuse, by Measures of Ethnic Origin, Aged 18 or Older, Canada, 2000/2001.

		Accepted	Rejected
Base model			
Sex	Men[a]	1.000[b]	1.000[b]
	Women	1.141[c] (0.029)	1.790[c] (0.099)
Age	18–24	1.553[c] (0.084)	1.869[c] (0.212)
	25–44	2.170[c] (0.088)	2.330[c] (0.208)
	45–64	1.781[c] (0.071)	2.314[c] (0.198)
	65 +[a]	1.000[b]	1.000[b]
Province	Newfoundland[a]	1.000[b]	1.000[b]
	Prince Edward Island	1.315 (0.180)	1.693 (0.464)
	Nova Scotia	1.242 (0.154)	1.896 (0.464)
	New Brunswick	1.465[c] (0.174)	1.642 (0.402)
	Quebec	3.681[c] (0.381)	5.516[c] (1.18)
	Ontario	3.740[c] (0.382)	4.285[c] (0.914)
	Manitoba	6.393[c] (0.576)	4.046[c] (0.921)
	Saskatchewan	5.401[c] (0.576)	4.412[c] (0.987)
	Alberta	5.804[c] (0.608)	5.231[c] (1.14)
	British Columbia	5.365[c] (0.554)	6.444[c] (1.38)
	The North	3.073[c] (0.385)	3.060[c] (0.762)
Years since	Less than two	0.584[c] (0.110)	0.452 (0.129)
immigration	Three to five	0.756 (0.121)	0.811 (0.208)
	Six to ten	0.741 (0.098)	1.273 (0.286)
	Eleven to fifteen	0.724 (0.089)	1.025 (0.212)
	Sixteen to twenty	0.925 (0.125)	1.593 (0.335)
	More than twenty[a,d]	1.000[b]	1.000[b]
Urbanity	Rural[a]	1.000[b]	1.000[b]
	Urban	0.840[c] (0.023)	0.825[c] (0.041)
Education	< High school graduation[a]	1.000[b]	1.000[b]
	High school graduation	1.266[c] (0.050)	1.621[c] (0.148)
	Some postsecondary	1.601[c] (0.080)	2.103[c] (0.202)
	Postsecondary degree	1.537[c] (0.053)	2.413[c] (0.173)
Income	Low[a]	1.000[b]	1.000[b]
	Lower-middle	1.014 (0.041)	1.191 (0.094)
	Upper-middle	1.284[c] (0.046)	1.274[c] (0.092)
	High	1.507[c] (0.059)	1.399[c] (0.107)
Chronic	None[a]	1.000[b]	1.000[b]
conditions	One	1.435[c] (0.049)	1.344[c] (0.095)
	Two	1.583[c] (0.060)	1.491[c] (0.112)
	Three +	1.779[c] (0.070)	2.120[c] (0.172)
Chronic pain	No[a]	1.000[b]	1.000[b]
	Yes	1.480[c] (0.047)	1.421[c] (0.084)

Table 1. (*Continued*)

		Accepted	Rejected
Unmet	No[a]	1.000[b]	1.000[b]
health-care	Yes	0.817[c] (0.027)	0.559[c] (0.032)
needs			
Medical	None[a]	1.000[b]	1.000[b]
consultations	One	1.271[c] (0.056)	1.043 (0.096)
	Two	1.458[c] (0.065)	1.100 (0.099)
	Three to five	1.583[c] (0.067)	1.183 (0.100)
	More than six	1.663[c] (0.072)	1.531[c] (0.129)
Predictors			
Ethnic origin	North America[a]	1.000[b]	1.000[b]
	South/Central America and Caribbean	0.719 (0.091)	0.475 (0.144)
	Europe	0.779[c] (0.040)	0.890 (0.089)
	Africa	0.518[c] (0.087)	0.434 (0.159)
	Asia	0.608[c] (0.057)	1.273 (0.181)
	Oceania	1.012 (0.321)	0.744 (0.289)

Data source: Canadian Community Health Survey Cycle 1.1 (2000–2001).
[a]Reference category for which odds ratio is always 1.00.
[b]Not applicable.
[c]Significantly different from reference category, $p < 0.05$.
[d]Includes native-born Canadians.

one or all of homeopathy/naturopathy, Feldenkrais/Alexander Technique, Rolfing, herbalism, reflexology, or "others" in the year prior to the survey. Those respondents who used both accepted and rejected therapies were classified as users of rejected medicine. A check on the multinomial logit model's requirement of independence from irrelevant alternatives (IIA) using Small and Hsiao's test found no violation of this assumption with the "accepted" and "rejected" users constituting two separate categories that can be assumed to be distinct for the purposes of statistical analysis (Long & Freese, 2001).

Measures of Ethnicity

Our analytic strategy takes advantage of the multiple measures of ethnicity available in the CCHS to first focus on ethnic origin (Tables 1 and 2) and then on ethnic group identification (Table 3). The base model includes control variables that previous population-based research suggests are correlates of

Table 2.   Odds Ratios (95% Confidence Intervals) for the Use of
Accepted and Rejected Complementary/Alternative Medical Practices
Compared to Nonuse, by Place of Birth and Visible Minority Status,
Aged 18 or Older, Canada, 2000/2001.

		Accepted	Rejected
Base model			
Sex	Men[b]	1.000[d]	1.000[d]
	Women	1.143[a] (0.029)	1.788[a] (0.010)
Age	18–24	1.591[a] (0.086)	1.888[a] (0.214)
	25–44	2.193[a] (0.081)	2.315[a] (0.207)
	45–64	1.791[a] (0.072)	2.210[a] (0.197)
	65 +[b]	1.000[d]	1.000[d]
Province	Newfoundland[b]	1.000[d]	1.000[d]
	Prince Edward Island	1.317 (0.180)	1.692 (0.453)
	Nova Scotia	1.252 (0.155)	1.912 (0.468)
	New Brunswick	1.464[a] (0.174)	1.639 (0.401)
	Quebec	3.674[a] (0.371)	5.433[a] (1.16)
	Ontario	3.779[a] (0.386)	4.295[a] (0.917)
	Manitoba	6.529[a] (0.706)	4.155[a] (0.946)
	Saskatchewan	5.504[a] (0.587)	4.475[a] (1.00)
	Alberta	5.881[a] (0.616)	5.325[a] (1.16)
	British Columbia	5.457[a] (0.564)	6.672[a] (1.43)
	The North	3.555[a] (0.457)	3.420[a] (0.865)
Years since	Less than two	0.565[a] (0.107)	0.473 (0.134)
immigration	Three to Five	0.737 (0.120)	0.843 (0.215)
	Six to Ten	0.737 (0.099)	1.300 (0.294)
	Eleven to Fifteen	0.715 (0.089)	0.984 (0.200)
	Sixteen to Twenty	0.919 (0.123)	1.553 (0.331)
	More than Twenty[b,c]	1.000[d]	1.000[d]
Urbanity	Rural[b]	1.000[d]	1.000[d]
	Urban	0.842[a] (0.023)	0.828[a] (0.042)
Education	<High School Graduation[b]	1.000[d]	1.000[d]
	High School Graduation	1.258[a] (0.050)	1.612[a] (0.148)
	Some postsecondary	1.601[a] (0.080)	2.083[a] (0.203)
	Postsecondary Degree	1.529[a] (0.053)	2.400[a] (0.171)
Income	Low[b]	1.000[d]	1.000[d]
	Lower-middle	1.011 (0.041)	1.182 (0.094)
	Upper-middle	1.274[a] (0.455)	1.265[a] (0.092)
	High	1.493[a] (0.058)	1.394[a] (0.107)
Chronic	None[b]	1.000[d]	1.000[d]
conditions	One	1.431[a] (0.488)	1.349[a] (0.095)
	Two	1.579[a] (0.060)	1.492[a] (0.112)
	Three +	1.771[a] (0.070)	2.195[a] (0.173)

Table 2. (*Continued*)

		Accepted	Rejected
Chronic pain	No[b]	1.000[d]	1.000[d]
	Yes	1.475[a] (0.047)	1.415[a] (0.084)
Unmet health	No[b]	1.000[d]	1.000[d]
care needs	Yes	0.817[a] (0.028)	0.560[a] (0.032)
Medical	None[b]	1.000[d]	1.000[d]
consultations	One	1.270[a] (0.056)	1.040 (0.096)
	Two	1.452[a] (0.065)	1.099 (0.099)
	Three to Five	1.578[a] (0.066)	1.182 (0.100)
	More than Six	1.658[a] (0.072)	1.530 (0.129)
Predictors			
Birth	N.A. Born[b]	1.000[d]	1.000[d]
	Foreign Born	0.777[a] (0.038)	0.829 (0.081)
Visible minority	White[b]	1.000[d]	1.000[d]
	Visible Minority	0.661[a] (0.057)	0.671 (0.099)
Birth × visible	Interaction	1.197 (0.144)	1.877[a] (0.379)
minority			

Data source: Canadian Community Health Survey Cycle 1.1 (2000–2001).
[a]Significantly different from reference category, $p < 0.05$.
[b]Reference category for which odds ratio is always 1.00.
[c]Includes Native Born Canadians.
[d]Not applicable.

the use of CAM. Ethnic origin is added as a predictor to the analysis by comparing North American born with those born in five other regions of the globe where "North America" is the referent category (Table 1). Then, I treat ethnic origin as a dichotomous variable ("Place of Birth") where those born in North America serve as the referent category and add the measure of "Visible Minority" provided by Statistics Canada (Table 2). Those respondents answering "White" make up the referent category compared with those indicating a visible minority cultural and racial background. This model also includes an interaction effect between place of birth and visible minority status added into analysis. It is important to note that several analysts have pointed towards conceptual difficulties associated with the unproblematic use of "visible minority" in a theoretical context (Bourhis, 2003). Visible Minority Status is a blunt measure of the respondents' self reported cultural background and/or group identification. The final model (Table 3) uses a finer measure of ethnic identification where those reporting a White cultural background and/or identification serve as the referent category compared

Table 3. Odds ratios (95% Confidence Intervals) for the Use of Accepted and Rejected Complementary/Alternative Medical Practices Compared to Nonuse, by Ethnic Identity, Aged 18 or Older, Canada, 2000/2001.

		Accepted	Rejected
Base model			
Sex	Men[b]	1.000[d]	1.000[d]
	Women	1.148[a] (0.029)	1.783[a] (0.010)
Age	18–24	1.679[a] (0.091)	1.905[a] (0.213)
	25–44	2.293[a] (0.092)	2.403[a] (0.213)
	45–64	1.831[a] (0.073)	2.366[a] (0.210)
	65 +[b]	1.000[d]	1.000[d]
Province	Newfoundland[b]	1.000[d]	1.000[d]
	Prince Edward Island	1.319 (0.180)	1.656 (0.450)
	Nova Scotia	1.258 (0.156)	1.947 (0.482)
	New Brunswick	1.467[a] (0.175)	1.669 (0.413)
	Quebec	3.650[a] (0.378)	5.616[a] (1.21)
	Ontario	3.679[a] (0.376)	4.298[a] (0.928)
	Manitoba	6.450[a] (0.699)	4.072[a] (0.938)
	Saskatchewan	5.506[a] (0.589)	4.555[a] (1.03)
	Alberta	5.804[a] (0.609)	5.346[a] (1.18)
	British Columbia	5.298[a] (0.548)	6.398[a] (1.39)
	The North	3.459[a] (0.448)	3.400[a] (0.877)
Years since	Less than two	0.473[a] (0.088)	0.447[a] (0.122)
immigration	Three to Five	0.647 (0.102)	0.797 (0.193)
	Six to Ten	0.649[a] (0.083)	1.274 (0.264)
	Eleven to Fifteen	0.617[a] (0.073)	0.999 (0.188)
	Sixteen to Twenty	0.815 (0.105)	1.396 (0.283)
	More than Twenty[b,c]	1.000[d]	1.000[d]
Urbanity	Rural[b]	1.000[d]	1.000[d]
	Urban	0.831[a] (0.022)	0.822[a] (0.042)
Education	<High School Graduation[b]	1.000[d]	1.000[d]
	High School Graduation	1.250[a] (0.050)	1.582[a] (0.145)
	Some postsecondary	1.600[a] (0.080)	2.056[a] (0.201)
	Postsecondary Degree	1.522[a] (0.053)	2.367[a] (0.171)
Income	Low[b]	1.000[d]	1.000[d]
	Lower-middle	1.006 (0.040)	1.183 (0.093)
	Upper-middle	1.265[a] (0.045)	1.242[a] (0.090)
	High	1.487[a] (0.058)	1.363[a] (0.105)
Chronic	None[b]	1.000[d]	1.000[d]
conditions	One	1.432[a] (0.049)	1.353[a] (0.096)
	Two	1.573[a] (0.060)	1.494[a] (0.113)
	Three +	1.769[a] (0.070)	2.182[a] (0.172)
Chronic pain	No[b]	1.000[d]	1.000[d]
	Yes	1.476[a] (0.047)	1.400[a] (0.083)

Table 3. (*Continued*)

		Accepted	Rejected
Unmet health	No[b]	1.000[d]	1.000[d]
care needs	Yes	0.815[a] (0.028)	0.555[a] (0.034)
Medical	None[b]	1.000[d]	1.000[d]
consultations	One	1.274[a] (0.056)	1.062 (0.099)
	Two	1.455[a] (0.065)	1.092 (0.099)
	Three to Five	1.590[a] (0.067)	1.218 (0.104)
	More than Six	1.670[a] (0.073)	1.581[a] (0.134)
Predictors			
Ethnic identity	White[b]	1.000[d]	1.000[d]
	Asian	0.719[a] (0.065)	1.573[a] (0.206)
	South Asian	0.647[a] (0.065)	0.858 (0.188)
	Black	0.502[a] (0.075)	0.444 (0.169)
	Latin Am.	0.908 (0.234)	0.611 (0.289)
	Aboriginal	0.592[a] (0.059)	0.741 (0.137)
	Other	0.824 (0.100)	0.508 (0.142)

Data source: Canadian Community Health Survey Cycle 1.1 (2000–2001).
[a]Significantly different from reference category, $p < 0.05$.
[b]Reference category for which odds ratio is always 1.00.
[c]Includes Native Born Canadians.
[d]Not applicable.

with those respondents identifying themselves as Asian, South Asian, Black, Latin American, Aboriginal, or Other. By using multiple measures of ethnicity I hoped to be able to address some ambiguities in the current research concerning the effect ethnicity has of the use of particular types of CAM therapies (Ahn et al., 2006; Astin, 1998; Bair et al., 2002; Barnes et al., 2004; Chao et al., 2008; Fries & Menzies, 2000; Graham et al., 2005; Grzywacz et al., 2007; Hsiao et al., 2006; Institute of Medicine, 2005; Kakai et al., 2003; Keith et al., 2005; Kronenberg, Cushman, Wade, Kalmuss, & Chao, 2006; Mackay, 2003; Mackenzie et al., 2003; Roth & Kobayashi, 2008).

RESULTS

Population Characteristics by Accepted and Rejected CAM

In the twelve months prior to the CCCS an estimated 16% of Canadians aged 18 and over, or about 3.7 million people, visited accepted CAM providers, meaning they had at least one consultation with chiropractors

(11.6% of Canadians, or about 2.7 million people), massage therapists (7% of Canadians, or about 1.6 million people), acupuncturists (2.1% of Canadians, or about one half million people), relaxation therapists (about 34 thousand Canadians), biofeedback practitioners (about 6 thousand Canadians), and spiritual/religious healers (about 41 thousand Canadians). About 4% of Canadians, or just under one million people, visited rejected CAM providers, meaning they saw such practitioners as homeopaths or naturopaths, Feldenkrais or Alexander teachers, rolfers, herbalists, reflexologists, or "others." The most consulted rejected CAM therapists were homeopaths or naturopaths (visited by an estimated 2.3% of Canadians, or approximately half a million people). The remaining rejected therapies were each consulted by less than one tenth of 1% of Canadians.

Factors Associated with the Use of Accepted and Rejected CAM

Tables 1–3 report the results of the multinomial logit estimation for each of the models computing the various the odds for the use of accepted and rejected CAM therapies, by selected characteristics, relative to those who did not consult CAM practitioners.

In terms of the base model, the odds of females using accepted therapies are approximately 14% higher than males while the odds of women using rejected therapies are approximately 79% higher than they are for men. Those respondents with the highest reported income level had approximately 50% higher odds of using accepted practices and 40% higher odds of using rejected therapies. The highest odds of using either form of CAM were reported for those respondents with postsecondary degrees. These same, highly educated respondents had nearly two and a half times greater odds of using rejected therapies than did those respondents with less than high school graduation. The odds are almost 80% higher of consulting an accepted practitioner and over two times greater of consulting a rejected practitioner for those with three or more chronic conditions, compared with those with no chronic illness. Those who report chronic pain have 48% higher odds of consulting accepted practitioners and 42% higher odds of consulting rejected practitioners. Those who reported self perceived unmet health-care needs with 18% lower odds of using accepted CAM therapies and 44% lower odds of using rejected therapies compared to those with no perceived unmet health-care needs. For those who reported more than six medical consultations, the odds of using accepted therapies were 65%

greater compared to those with no medical consultations and the odds of using rejected therapies were 53% higher.

With regard to ethnic origin, Table 1 shows that those who immigrated to Canada less than two years before being surveyed had approximately 42% lower odds of using accepted therapies. For accepted therapies, those born in Europe had 22% lower odds of use while those born in Asia had 39% lower and African born had 48% lower odds of consulting an accepted practitioner, compared with North American born respondents.

Table 2 reports the results when treating ethnic origin as a dichotomous variable comparing those born in North America and "Foreign born" and adding Visible Minority Status into the model. There was no statistically significant difference in the odds of using rejected therapies while foreign born had 22% lower odds of using accepted therapies compared to North American born. Visible minorities were 34% less likely to use accepted CAM compared with "Whites." The addition of an interaction term between place of birth and visible minority status showed that visible minority members born outside of North America were 88% more likely to use rejected therapies than native born members of visible minority groups.

Table 3 reports the odds ratios while treating ethnic identity as the primary independent variable. Asians had 57% higher odds of using rejected CAM compared with those who reported a White identity. Consistent with the findings for ethnic origin, as compared with Whites, Asians had 28% lower odds, South Asians 35% lower odds, Aboriginals 40% lower odds, and Blacks 50% lower odds of using accepted therapies.

DISCUSSION

By employing the binary classification of CAM therapies developed in a previous study (Fries, 2008) the current population-based research provides insight into the relationship between ethnicity and the use of CAM therapies lacking physician perceived medical efficacy. Consistent with earlier findings (Bair et al., 2002; Fries & Menzies, 2000; Wade, Chao, Cushman, Kronenberg, & Kalmuss, 2008) respondents who were female, young adults or middle aged, live in the Western part of the continent, had higher levels of education, higher income, and greater incidence of chronic disease and chronic pain, and more medical consultations reported higher rates of using CAM therapies whose efficacy has been questioned by physicians. Women have much higher odds of using rejected therapies than men but only slightly higher odds of using accepted therapies. Other studies looking at the relationship among CAM use, gender, and ethnicity have reported similar results (Bair et al., 2002; Kronenberg et al., 2006; Wade et al., 2008). There continue to be marked regional differences in the use of CAM and especially so for rejected therapies, with Quebec and British Columbia having the highest odds of using rejected therapies, followed closely by the three Prairie provinces and Ontario. As in previous studies (Fries & Menzies, 2000; Mackenzie et al., 2003; Wade et al., 2008), higher levels of education are associated with higher odds of using of CAM, especially rejected therapies; those with at least some level of postsecondary education having more than two times greater odds of using rejected therapies compared to those with less than high school graduation. As in other studies (Barnes et al., 2004; Eisenberg et al., 1993; Grzywacz et al., 2007; Millar, 2001; Nazeem et al., 2000), the incidence of chronic disease conditions and chronic pain remain important predictors of the use of CAM. Those respondents who reported more chronic illness or pain had higher odds of using both types of CAM and those with three or more chronic conditions had twice the odds of using rejected therapies compared with those without chronic illness. Another study using Canadian data found that those who reported themselves to have perceived unmet health-care needs had 51% higher odds of using CAM therapies relative those with no perceived unmet health-care needs (Millar, 2001). In contrast, the present study found a reversal of this pattern. In keeping with previous research (Barnes et al., 2004; Eisenberg et al., 1993; Kronenberg et al., 2006), consultations with both types of CAM providers occur as an adjunct to biomedical care.

As Kronenberg and colleagues (2006) found, "CAM use among racial/ethnic groups is complex and nuanced"; varying by measure of ethnicity, ethnic group membership, and type of CAM therapy. The contribution of the present study lies in unpacking the inconsistencies and ambiguities around CAM use and ethnicity, by using more nuanced measures of ethnicity and a conceptual classification of CAM as either "accepted" or "rejected" by biomedicine. This study shows that Whites and North American born are more likely to use accepted therapies whereas immigrant visible minorities and those with Asian ethnic identities are more likely to use rejected therapies. Our findings find support from existing epidemiological research, which reports descriptive statistics for 31, 014 cases weighted to represent the US population, showing that Whites use chiropractic and massage therapy at higher rates than Blacks or Asians and that Asians have slightly higher rates of using Ayurveda, acupuncture, homeopathy, and naturopathy than do Whites (Barnes et al., 2004). Other research has demonstrated similar demographic patterning of the use of CAM with particular ethnicities using particular therapies (Graham et al., 2005; Grzywacz et al., 2007; Hsiao et al., 2006; Mackenzie et al., 2003). These results are consistent with research which found that as immigrants to the US acculturate their patterns of CAM use converge with those of the general population (Lee, Goldstein, Richard Brown, & Ballard-Barbash, 2010). Further, these findings are in keeping with research which found that White CAM users preferred Western bioscientific sources of health information whereas Asians used lay referral and popular media health information sources (Kakai et al., 2003). Our findings must be considered in light of limitations of the present research.

Limitations

As Aboriginals living in First Nations reservation communities are not included in Statistics Canada survey frames, the findings related to Aboriginals reported here pertain only to those living off reservation. This might have a particular effect on "Spiritual and Religious Healing," given that residents of First Nations reservation communities use such healing practices.

In relying upon the classification based upon family physicians' ratings of the efficacy of particular CAM therapies published in previous research (Fries, 2008) it is important to remember that the opinion of physicians while obviously an important feature of the physician-patient communication regarding CAM, is not the sole arbiter of the bioscientific efficacy of particular CAM therapies. The conceptual premise of the classification employed by the present research is that the distinction between accepted and rejected CAM is socially constructed: It does not depend on the actual effectiveness of treatments offered (Fries & Menzies, 2000). For example, in Canada, homoeopathy is rejected CAM as most biomedical practitioners view it as ineffective (Fries, 2008). However, in countries such as the Netherlands homeopathy is an accepted therapy as many family physicians practice it and it receives state funding (Menges, 1994). As socially constructed, any distinction between accepted and rejected CAM is necessarily specific to the particular cultural and historical contexts under study. Future research wishing to investigate the factors influencing the use of CAM therapies not accorded bioscientific efficacy must be cognizant that with changes in the cultural and scientific context more CAM therapies are likely to be regarded as legitimate health-care options.

In interpreting these results, it should be remembered that Statistics Canada does not include Traditional Chinese Medicine in the CCHS and acupuncture was classified as an accepted therapy (Fries, 2008). This means that Asians had higher odds of using: homeopathy/naturopathy, Feldenkrais/Alexander Technique, Rolfing, herbalism, reflexology, or "others." Most of this CAM utilization can be accounted for by the high use of herbalism among Asians (Lai & Chappell, 2007).

Future Research

The *Handbook of Alternative and Complementary Medicine* classifies nearly 70 CAM therapies under 18 different headings (Fulder, 1996). Obviously, such a list is far too comprehensive to be included in a population-based survey. The CCHS is one of two population health surveys conducted by Statistics Canada that collects information on the use of CAM therapies. (The other is the longitudinal household survey, the National Population Health Survey). A major drawback of the CCHS data is the grouping of disparate therapies in single response categories while there appears no conceptual reason for doing so. Also problematic, is that the list, omits several important and culturally relevant therapies such as Ayurvedic and Traditional Chinese Medicines. Several definitional and interpretive difficulties result from these errors and omissions. Future population health research that seeks to disaggregate CAM into individual therapies to discern the correlates of the use of particular therapies will need to rely on data from sources other than Statistics Canada until such time as the list of CAM therapies originally included in the NPHS and transferred to the CCHS receives substantial conceptual clarification and updating.

CONCLUSION

These findings confirm that ethnicity constitutes a cultural resource upon which users of CAM draw as they make their health-care decisions, sometimes despite the recommendations of their family physicians. Future research is needed to understand the intersections of health beliefs and behavior with ethnicity, income, gender, and education, and needs to examine the correlates of the use of particular CAM therapies by particular subpopulations and how this relates to disclosing this information to physicians. This information can improve patient health care by allowing physicians to better understand the role that the ethnicity of their patients' plays in motivating the use of different CAM therapies.

REFERENCES

Ahn, A. C., Ngo-Metzger, Q., Legedza, A. T. R., et al. (2006). Complementary and alternative medical therapy use among Chinese and Vietnamese Americans: Prevalence, associated factors, and effects of patient-clinician communication. *American Journal of Public Health, 96*(4), 647–653.

Angell, M., & Kassirer, J. P. (1998). Alternative medicine: The risks of untested and unregulated remedies. *New England Journal of Medicine, 339*(12), 839–841.

Aspinall, P. J. (2001). Operationalising the collection of ethnicity data in studies of the sociology of health and illness. *Sociology of Health & Illness, 23*(6), 829–862.

Astin, J. A. (1998). Why patients use alternative medicine: Results of a national study. *The Journal of the American Medical Association, 279*(19), 1548–1553.

Bair, Y. A., Gold, E. B., Greendale, G. A., Sternfeld, B., Adler, S. R., Azari, R., & Harkey, M. (2002). Ethnic differences in use of complementary and alternative medicine at midlife: Longitudinal results from SWAN participants. *American Journal of Public Health, 92*(11), 1832–1840.

Barnes, P., Powell-Griner, E., McFann, K., & Nahin, R. (2004). Complementary and alternative medicine use among adults: United States. In Hyattsville, MD: National Center for Health Statistics 343, pp. 1–19.

Beland, Y. (2002). Canadian community health survey-methodological overview. *Health Reports: Statistics Canada, 13*(3), 9–14.

Bourhis, R. (2003). Measuring ethnocultural diversity using the Canadian Census. *Canadian Ethnic Studies, 35*(1), 9–32.

Chao, M. T., Wade, C., & Kronenberg, F. (2008). Disclosure of complementary and alternative medicine to conventional medical providers: Variation by race/ethnicity and type of CAM. *Journal of the National Medical Association, 100*(11), 1341–1349.

Eisenberg, D. M., Davis, R. B., Ettner, S. L., Appel, S., Wilkey, S., Van Rompay, M., & Kessler, R. C. (1998). Trends in alternative medicine use in the United States, 1990–1997: Results of a follow-up national survey. *The Journal of the American Medical Association, 280*(18), 1569–1575.

Eisenberg, D. M., Kessler, R. C., Foster, C., Norlock, F. E., Calkins, D. R., & Delbanco, T. L. (1993). Unconventional medicine in the United States: Prevalence, costs, and patterns of use. *New England Journal of Medicine, 328*(4), 246–252.

Eisenberg, D. M., Kessler, R. C., Van Rompay, M. I., Kaptchuk, T. J., Wilkey, S. A., Appel, S., & Davis, R. B. (2001). Perceptions about complementary therapies relative to conventional therapies among adults who use both: Results from a national survey. *Annals of Internal Medicine, 135*(5), 344–351.

Fontanarosa, P. B., & Lundberg, G. D. (1998). Alternative medicine meets science. *The Journal of the American Medical Association, 280*(18), 1618–1619.

Fries, C. J. (2008). Classification of complementary and alternative medical practices: Family physicians' ratings of effectiveness. *Canadian Family Physician, 54*(11), 1570-1.e1–1570-1.e7.

Fries, C. J., & Menzies, K. S. (2000). Gullible fools or desperate pragmatists? A profile of people who use rejected alternative health care providers. *Canadian Journal of Public Health, 91*(3), 217–219.

Fulder, S. (1996). *The handbook of alternative and complementary medicine.* London: Oxford University Press.

Graham, R. E., Ahn, A. C., Davis, R. D., O'Connor, B. B., Eisenberg, D. M., & Phillips, R. S. (2005). Use of complementary and alternative medical therapies among racial and ethnic minority adults: Results from the 2002 National Health Interview Survey. *Journal of the National Medical Association, 97*(4), 535–545.

Grzywacz, J. G., Suerken, C. K., Neiberg, R. H., Lang, W., Bell, R. A., Quandt, S. A., & Arcury, T. A. (2007). Age, ethnicity, and use of complementary and alternative medicine in health self-management. *Journal of Health and Social Behaviour, 48*(1), 84.

Hsiao, A.-F., Wong, M. D., Goldstein, M. S., Yu, H.-J., Andersen, R. M., Richard Brown, E., ... Wenger, N. S. (2006). Variation in complementary and alternative medicine (CAM) use across racial/ethnic groups and the development of ethnic-specific measures of CAM use. *Journal of Alternative & Complementary Medicine, 12*(3), 281–290.

Institute of Medicine. (2005). *Complementary and alternative medicine in the United States.* Washington, DC: National Academies of Science.

Kakai, H., Maskarinec, G., Shumay, D. M., Tatsumura, Y., & Tasaki, K. (2003). Ethnic differences in choices of health information by cancer patients using complementary and alternative medicine: an exploratory study with correspondence analysis. *Social Science & Medicine, 56*(4), 851–862.

Keith, V. M., Kronenfeld, J. J., Rivers, P. A., & Liang, S.-Y. (2005). Assessing the effects of race and ethnicity on use of complementary and alternative therapies in the USA. *Ethnicity & Health, 10*(1), 19–32.

Kronenberg, F., Cushman, L. F., Wade, C. M., Kalmuss, D., & Chao, M. T. (2006). Race/ethnicity and women's use of complementary and alternative medicine in the United States: Results of a national survey. *American Journal of Public Health, 96*(7), 1236–1242.

Lai, D., & Chappell, N. (2007). Use of traditional Chinese medicine by older Chinese immigrants in Canada. *Family Practice, 24*(1), 56–64.

Lee, J. H., Goldstein, M. S., Richard Brown, E., & Ballard-Barbash, R. (2010). How does acculturation affect the use of complementary and alternative medicine providers among Mexican- and Asian- Americans? *Journal of Immigrant and Minority Health, 12*(3), 302–309.

Leduc, N., & Proulx, M. (2004). Patterns of health services utilization by recent immigrants. *Journal of Immigrant and Minority Health, 6*(1), 15–27.

Long, J. S., & Freese, J. (2001). *Regression models for categorical dependent variables using Stata.* College Station, Texas: Stata Press.

Mackay, B. (2003). Changing face of Canada is changing the face of medicine. *Canadian Medical Association Journal, 168*(5), 599.

Mackenzie, E. R., Taylor, L., Bloom, B. S., Hufford, D. J., & Johnson, J. C. (2003). Ethnic minority use of complementary and alternative medicine (CAM): A national probability survey of CAM utilizers. *Alternative Therapies in Health and Medicine, 9*(4), 50–56.

Menges, L. J. (1994). Beyond the anglophone world: Regular and alternative medicine: The state of affairs in the Netherlands. *Social Science & Medicine, 39*(6), 871–873.

Millar, W. J. (1997). Use of alternative health care practitioners by Canadians. *Canadian Journal of Public Health, 88*(3), 154–158.

Millar, W. J. (2001). Patterns of use-alternative health care practitioners. *Health Reports, 13*(1), 9–22.

Nazeem, M., Neudorf, C., & Martins, K. (2000). Concurrent consultations with physicians and providers of alternative care: Results from a population-based study. *Canadian Journal of Public Health, 91*(6), 449–453.

Pachter, L. M. (1994). Culture and clinical care: Folk illness beliefs and their implications for health care delivery. *The Journal of the American Medical Association, 271*(9), 690–694.

Piérard, E., Buckley, N., & Chowhan, J. (2004). Bootstrapping made easy: A Stata ADO file. *The Research Data Centres Information and Technical Bulletin, 1*(1), 20–36.

Roth, M. A., & Kobayashi, K. M. (2008). The use of complementary and alternative medicine among Chinese Canadians: Results from a national survey. *Journal of Immigrant and Minority Health, 10*(6), 517–528.

Stata. (2003). *Stata statistical software.* College Station, Texas: Stata Corporation.

Stevenson, F. A., Britten, N., Barry, C. A., Bradley, C. P., & Barber, N. (2003). Self-treatment and its discussion in medical consultations: How is medical pluralism managed in practice? *Social Science & Medicine, 57*(3), 513–527.

Wade, C., Chao, M. T., Cushman, L. F., Kronenberg, F., & Kalmuss, D. (2008). Medical pluralism among American women: Results of a national survey. *Journal of Women's Health, 17*(5), 829–840.

RACIAL RESIDENTIAL SEGREGATION AND ACCESS TO HEALTH-CARE COVERAGE: A MULTILEVEL ANALYSIS

Kathryn Freeman Anderson and Andrew S. Fullerton

ABSTRACT

A developing body of research has demonstrated the impact of racial residential segregation on a variety of negative health outcomes. However, little is known about the effect of residential segregation on access to health care.

This study utilizes multilevel binary logit models based on individual-level health data from the 2008 Behavioral Risk Factor Surveillance System linked to metropolitan-area level data to examine the association between Black-White segregation in 136 metropolitan statistical areas in the United States and health-care coverage.

Overall, an increase in Black-White segregation is related to a decrease in the likelihood of having health insurance for Black residents and an increase in the Black-White gap in health-care coverage. These effects are substantial even when controlling for the effects of educational, social, and economic factors.

Issues in Health and Health Care Related to Race/Ethnicity, Immigration, SES and Gender
Research in the Sociology of Health Care, Volume 30, 133–158
ISSN: 0275-4959/doi:10.1108/S0275-4959(2012)0000030009

This study is the first to examine the impact of segregation on an individual's ability to access health-care coverage, which is an essential starting point for accessing health care in the United States.

Keywords: Segregation; health care; race/ethnicity

INTRODUCTION

Significant differences in health outcomes persist between racial and ethnic groups in the United States. African Americans in particular have the lowest health status of all racial and ethnic groups, and they experience some of the most detrimental health outcomes and environments of any group since the foundation of the United States, especially when compared to Whites (Byrd & Clayton, 2001, 2002; Patterson, 2009; Shavers & Shavers, 2006; Williams & Jackson, 2005). A growing body of literature focuses on documenting the differences in health and health-care access among racial groups in the United States. Researchers in this field consider several approaches to understanding why health disparities exist. More recently, this research emphasizes the mechanisms of racism as it relates to health and health care. Several previous studies consider residential segregation as a form of structural racism to view its impact on a variety of health indicators. However, few have undertaken to study the role that health-care access plays in these health disparities. Access to health care is the leading indicator of a population's health status (U.S. Department of Health and Human Services, 2000). Although access to health care is a multifaceted issue, in this study we specifically examine access to health insurance. Health-care coverage is the main gateway to accessing full and sufficient medical care in the United States. It is increasingly more difficult for Americans in general to access care due to the rising costs of health care and in turn health insurance. For example, 18% of the nonelderly U.S. population has no health-care coverage of any sort (Hoffman & Paradise, 2008). Racial and ethnic minorities in particular make up over half of the uninsured (Hoffman & Paradise, 2008). We posit that racism, in particular residential segregation, exacerbates these problems for the Black community. Furthermore, problems of health-care access may be a strong explanatory factor for the Black-White health gap in the United States.

We address two major research questions in this study. First, is residential segregation related to reduced health-care access for Black residents? Second, does residential segregation contribute to the Black-White gap in health-care coverage? More specifically, we will first examine the impact of residential segregation on access to health care for Black respondents in order to determine whether Black residents of segregated cities are less likely to have health-care coverage compared to Black residents of less segregated cities. To address this first research question, we examine data from Black residents drawing on Massey and colleagues' geographic concentration of poverty theory of segregation. Our hypothesis is that racial residential segregation is related to decreased health-care access. We also test several hypotheses related to different potential mechanisms for the hypothesized link between segregation and health-care access. Specifically, we expect that segregation, as it concentrates poverty and the social problems associated with poverty, will affect access to health-care coverage through reduced educational opportunities, social breakdown, and limited economic opportunity.

The second research question goes beyond the within-group analysis of segregation for the Black community, examining the differences between Blacks and Whites in health insurance coverage. We hypothesize that White residents of segregated cities will not be subject to any potentially negative effects of racial residential segregation because segregation buffers the racially dominant White group from the effects of concentrated poverty in segregated areas. Therefore, we expect that residential segregation will contribute to the Black-White gap in health-care coverage.

Although numerous studies have examined race and access to health care, the role of residential segregation has not been examined using data spanning several regions within the United States. Furthermore, few of the studies that examine race, place, and health-care use a traditional measure of segregation. Instead, previous studies tend to use a measure of the racial make-up of a city or place, which does not directly account for how racial groups are distributed throughout a geographical area. This study contributes to this burgeoning body of literature by examining one of the fundamental barriers to care in the United States, access to health insurance, and the role of racial residential segregation using multilevel models based on individual- and contextual-level data spanning 136 metropolitan statistical areas (MSAs) in the United States.

THEORETICAL FRAMEWORK AND LITERATURE REVIEW

The Geographic Concentration of Poverty Theory of Segregation

While there are many explanations for the persistence of racial differences in health, this research focuses on the role of racial residential segregation as a form of systematic racism in creating a variety of social inequities, including disparities in health and health-care access. The theoretical basis of this study is rooted in Massey and colleagues' geographic concentration of poverty theory of segregation (Massey, 1990; Massey & Denton, 1993; Massey & Fischer, 2000). While residential segregation is no longer legally enforced, it remains an important and persistent part of the racial landscape of the United States. As a mechanism of racism, residential segregation has important consequences for those living in segregated areas. Massey and colleagues' overarching theoretical argument is that as poverty is more highly concentrated in the Black population of the United States, when Blacks are geographically concentrated in one area of a city, poverty and the effects of poverty are also concentrated within that group (Iceland & Wilkes, 2006; Krivo, Peterson, Rizzo, & Reynolds, 1998; Massey & Denton, 1993; Massey & Fischer, 2000). Conversely, they demonstrate that as poor Whites are much more evenly distributed throughout society, the effects of White poverty are also more evenly distributed (Massey & Denton, 1993; Massey, Gross, & Shibuya, 1994).

Furthermore, Massey and Denton (1993) assert that the concentration of poverty within Black segregated areas then produces a variety of social problems and the creation of an "underclass." The effect of segregation is not merely limited to the concentration of poverty, but poverty is always accompanied by a number of social problems resulting from economic disenfranchisement (Massey & Denton, 1993). Furthermore, like poverty, the resulting social ills are geographically and spatially concentrated and continually reproduced within a specific community (Massey & Denton, 1993). A robust literature empirically demonstrates Massey and Denton's (1993) contention on the social problems that result from concentrated poverty in segregated neighborhoods. These studies show that segregated areas are subject to lower quality education (Collins & Williams, 1999; Hummer, 1996), limited employment and economic opportunities (Krivo et al., 1998; Wilson, 1987, 1996), and higher rates of social disorder, such as criminal activity, substance abuse, family breakdown, and female-headed households (Greenberg & Schneider, 1994; Shihadeh & Flynn, 1996; Testa, Astone, Krogh, & Neckerman, 1993; Wilson, 1987). Furthermore, studies demonstrate that segregation may lead to physical disorder, such as poorer housing quality, decreased access to services, housing code violations, vacant lots, broken windows, litter, graffiti, and abandoned buildings (Chang, Hillier, & Mehta, 2009; Shihadeh & Flynn, 1996; Williams, 1999), increased exposure environmental hazards and toxins (Bullard, 2005), limited access to nutritional foods, and greater access to junk foods, fast foods, tobacco, and alcohol (Bahr, 2007; Chang et al., 2009; Grier & Kumanyika, 2008; Kwate, 2008; Larson, Story, & Nelson, 2009; LaVeist & Wallace, 2000). More recently, scholars have turned their attention to the impact that segregation and the resulting social conditions can have on health and health-care outcomes. A growing body of literature empirically examining these issues is reviewed here and informs the present study on access to health-care coverage.

Segregation, Health, and Health Care

Issues related to segregation play a central role in much of the work on racial health disparities. The literature above on the various impacts of segregation considers obvious health implications, such as environmental hazards and physical disorder that reduce access to safe, green space for recreation and exercise, lack of adequate spatial access to nutritional foods, and an increased access to foods of poor nutritional quality (Bahr, 2007; Bullard, 2005; Chang et al., 2009; Grier & Kumanyika, 2008; Kwate, 2008; Larson et al., 2009; LaVeist & Wallace, 2000; Shihadeh & Flynn, 1996; Williams, 1999). In addition, many researchers have directly examined the impact of residential segregation on health. Such scholarship tends to focus on mortality and life expectancy, infant mortality rates, birth weight, overall health, and nutrition and obesity (Chang, 2006; Collins, 1999; Ellen, Cutler, & Dickens, 2000; Grady, 2006; Hart, Kunitz, Sell, & Mukamel, 1998; Hearst, Oakes, & Johnson, 2008; Hummer, 1996; LeClere, Rogers, & Peters, 1997; Polednak, 1991; Polednak, 1997; Subramanian, Acevedo-Garcia, & Osypuk, 2004; Williams & Collins, 2001).

Although many studies have examined the effect of residential segregation on the health of the Black community, few studies have examined the differences in health-care access and health-care use as a result of segregation. As health-care access is so intimately tied to health outcomes, segregation's effect on health-care access may be a strong explanatory factor for the association between segregation and negative health outcomes. The extant literature on segregation and health care demonstrates that the relationship between racial residential segregation and health-care access is multifaceted. Segregation may limit access to the health-care system initially because of the economic and educational factors as described above. Sufficient health care is expensive and because of the concentration of poverty in these areas, access may be limited due to economic forces (Williams & Collins, 2001). Additionally, most Americans receive health insurance through their places of employment, and because of the higher rates of unemployment and job instability in segregated areas, they may be less likely to have access to health insurance in that capacity. Also, due to lower rates of educational attainment, people may be less informed of the need to access medical care, especially preventative care (Kposowa, 2007). Furthermore, medical facilities are less likely to be located in or near segregated areas, which creates a physical barrier to access. This is especially true of more advanced or specialty facilities (Hayanga, Waljee, Kaiser, Chang, & Morris, 2009; Hayanga et al., 2009; Rodriguez et al., 2007). This barrier to health-care access may also be exacerbated if the individual does not have adequate transportation. The health facilities located in segregated neighborhoods also tend to be worse in quality with fewer resources (Smith, Feng, Fennel, Zinn, & Mor, 2007). Additionally, racial segregation persists within and across health-care facilities, especially long-term health facilities (Clarke, Davis, & Nailon, 2007; Sarrazin, Campbell, Richardson, & Rosenthal, 2009; Smith et al., 2007).

Only two studies have directly examined the impact of residential segregation on an individual's ability to access health care, which is the emphasis of this research. However, neither study has examined health-care coverage specifically. The first study found that Black and Hispanic respondents living in counties with a higher percentage of the same racial or ethnic group were less likely to perceive barriers to access to care (Haas et al., 2004). They found a result opposite to what is hypothesized here. However, they were examining variation in health-care access by the percentage of racial and ethnic groups in each county, rather than examining how those groups are distributed throughout a county, such as with a segregation score (Haas et al., 2004). Another study, conducted by Gaskin, Price, Brandon, and LaVeist (2009), found an association between neighborhood racial integration and an increased likelihood of Black residents of those areas to have a health-care visit. This fits with the prior research on segregation and health, and contributes to our understanding of how segregation can impact health care (Gaskin et al., 2009). However, their analysis of an integrated neighborhood only involved one area in Baltimore, MD

(Gaskin et al., 2009). Multiple single-city studies or nation-wide studies would be necessary to systematically examine the relationship between segregation and access to health care.

Analytical Framework and Hypotheses

This study examines one main outcome for assessing segregation's impact on health-care access, access to health-care coverage or insurance. Specifically, we examine health-care coverage because it is the fundamental starting point for accessing health care in the United States. Many health researchers have proposed that equal access to health insurance, or universal coverage, would eliminate many of the social sources of health-care access disparities (Andrulis, 1998). People without insurance are less likely to have access to the entire health-care system. They are less likely to have a usual source of care when needed, less likely to access and use preventative care, more likely to have unmet health needs, and less likely to properly manage chronic health conditions (Hoffman & Paradise, 2008). Furthermore, those without health-care coverage experience diminished health-care outcomes when they are able to access sources of care (Hoffman & Paradise, 2008). They experience higher rates of illness and pain, trips to the emergency room, premature mortality, late-stage cancer diagnosis, and are more likely to experience preventable hospitalizations (Hoffman & Paradise, 2008). Thus, having health insurance is an important indicator of accessing health care in the United States, and furthermore experiencing better health-care treatment and results.

Access to health-care coverage is a complex and multifaceted issue. The health-care system in the United States utilizes both public and private sources of insurance, and individuals may receive their health care through a variety of sources, such as their employer, a family member, or through government programs. However, as the United States primarily relies on an employer-based system, most (61% of the working age population) receive their health-care coverage through their employer (Hoffman & Paradise, 2008). This system, though, has begun to erode in the United States through the changing nature of labor relations, and the extreme rise in the cost of health care (Hoffman & Paradise, 2008). Many low-wage workers are not able to receive coverage through their employers, and health-care coverage is unaffordable for many on the open market (Andrulis, 1998; Hoffman & Paradise, 2008). For example, 36% of the poor, and 30% of the near-poor are uninsured (Hoffman & Paradise, 2008). Racial and ethnic minorities make up a disproportionate amount, over 50%, of the uninsured in the United States (Hoffman & Paradise, 2008). Therefore, we hypothesize that segregation, in this manner, may affect access to health-care coverage. Segregation, as it concentrates poverty and its effects, into one area and among one population, may limit access to health-care coverage for Black residents in such neighborhoods. In addition, we test three effects of concentration of poverty, which may play a role in access to care, particularly through employer-based access. The three facets of concentration of poverty and their effect on access to health insurance are discussed further below.

In this study, we examine the impact of Black-White residential segregation on the ability of Black individuals to obtain health-care coverage. We test several hypotheses regarding the influence of residential segregation on health-care coverage for Black residents and potential explanations for this relationship. The first hypothesis is:

H_1. Black residents of segregated cities, compared to Black residents of less segregated cities, will have diminished access to health insurance.

Furthermore, related to our first research question, in addition to examining the impact of residential segregation itself, we isolate the negative effects that residential segregation produces, affecting Black residents' ability to access health insurance. Following from concentration of poverty theory, we formulated the following three hypotheses on the sources of differing access to health care as a result of segregation. Although other sources of social problems from the concentration of poverty are described above, we chose three factors we thought most pertinent to the outcome of health-care coverage specifically. Our three hypotheses are as follows:

H_2. Segregation affects access to health-care coverage because it can limit educational opportunities, which can impact upward mobility and access to higher quality occupations.

H_3. Segregation affects access to health-care coverage because it can lead to social and family breakdown, which can limit access to health insurance through social and family ties.

H_4. Segregation affects access to health-care coverage because it can limit economic opportunity, which can reduce access to jobs that provide comprehensive benefits, including health insurance.

First, as detailed above, segregation can impact an individual's ability to access quality education at all levels. Education could increase one's access to health care through improved job opportunities, health-care education, and the general upward mobility that education often provides. Our first hypothesis is that the negative effects of lower educational attainment in segregated areas, such as lower rates of college education and higher high school dropout rates, could reduce access to health care for individuals in segregated areas.

Second, as shown above, prior research indicates that segregation can compound the problems of social disorder leading to family instability and breakdown. As many people receive health insurance through a spouse or family member, we examine the impact of family breakdown, through the percentage of married-couple households and female-headed households, as a possible explanatory factor for the impact of residential segregation. Our second hypothesis is that lower marriage rates and higher rates of female-headed households in segregated areas can lead to a decrease in access to health insurance.

Finally, because the prior research on segregation demonstrates that there are lower rates of economic opportunity, we examine the impact of these economic factors on segregation and access to health care. As both the access to employment and quality of jobs available are important factors, we will examine income and poverty, unemployment, type of employment available, and union membership, as those jobs more often provide full benefits like health insurance. As many people receive health insurance through their places of employment, our second hypothesis is that Black residents of segregated areas will have reduced access to health care because of higher rates of poverty, unemployment, and lower quality jobs available. This study examines the impact of racial residential segregation on the ability of Black Americans to access health insurance, and additionally examines each of these three hypotheses in an attempt to understand the more specific effect that residential segregation can have on a variety of negative health outcomes.

Moreover, with regards to our second research question, we examine whether segregation affects the ability of Black residents to access health-care coverage compared to their White counterparts within the same metropolitan area. We also formulated one final hypothesis regarding the influence of residential segregation on racial disparities in health-care coverage:

H₅. Black residents of segregated cities, compared to their White counterparts, will have reduced access to health-care coverage.

DATA

We test these hypotheses using individual-level data from the 2008 Behavioral Risk Factor Surveillance System (BRFSS) and contextual data from several publicly available sources. The BRFSS is an annual survey conducted by the Centers for Disease Control and Prevention (CDC) to monitor trends in health risk behaviors and illness in the United States. The survey is collected by telephone interviews with noninstitutionalized adults using random sampling in all U.S. states and territories. We use the selected metropolitan/micropolitan area risk trends (SMART) version of the data, which organizes the data geographically by MSAs and only includes those areas with 500 or more respondents. The MSAs are comprised of groups of counties that contain at least one urbanized area of 50,000 or more inhabitants. The original BRFSS data set included identifiers for micropolitan statistical areas, which are areas with a population less than 50,000, but still greater than 10,000. These were not included in this study as level 2 data was not available for these geographic divisions. Additionally, the data set included geographical units called Metropolitan Divisions, which are smaller divisions of particularly large MSAs. We combined some of these areas into the original, larger MSA in order to match the segregation data. After dropping cases due to missing data, the final sample sizes are 14,633 Black respondents and 106,679 White respondents nested within 136 MSAs.

Individual Level

The dependent variable, *health-care coverage*, is a binary indicator for whether or not the respondent has any kind of health-care coverage or insurance (1 = yes, 0 = no). The questionnaire item is specifically worded as, "Do you have any kind of health-care coverage, including health insurance, prepaid plans such as HMOs, or government plans such as Medicare?" As the health-care coverage variable includes government health programs such as Medicare, we limited the sample to the working age population (ages 25–64) to remove the effect of Medicare, which is a nearly universal health-care program for those older than 65. We control for several socio-demographic independent variables at level 1, including *age* (in years), *female* (gender: 1 = female, 0 = male), *education* (in years), *income* (binary variables for <$15K [reference], $15K to <$25K, $25K to <$35K, $35K to <$50K, $50K or more, and don't know or refused), *married* (marital status: 1 = married, 0 = else), *employment status* (binary variables for wage/salary worker [reference], self-employed, unemployed, and not in labor force), and *city center* (metropolitan area status: 1 = inside city center, 0 = else). We also control for *general health status*, which reflects the respondent's self-assessment of their general health. The variable ranges from excellent (1) to poor (5). We control for health-care status as poor health status or chronic health problems may be a barrier to affordable care and health insurance coverage.

Metropolitan Area Level

The key independent variable in this study, segregation, is conceptualized as having five dimensions: evenness, exposure, concentration, centralization, and clustering (Massey & Denton, 1988, 1989). The most commonly used of these is evenness, and the most commonly used measure of evenness is the index of dissimilarity, which numerous other studies on segregation and health have used (Ellen et al., 2000; Farley, 2005, 2008; Hart et al., 1998; Polednak, 1991). However, more recent studies suggest that the exposure indices are better measures to capture the social isolation from segregation and the health effects it could produce (Collins & Williams, 1999; Subramanian et al., 2004). In this study, we use one such exposure index, *Black isolation*, which measures the extent to which a Black resident of a MSA is likely to be in contact with another Black resident based on residence. A higher likelihood of within-group contact indicates higher levels of racial segregation and group isolation. Therefore, the index measures the extent to which Blacks as a group are isolated from the rest of the population. For the purpose of this study, we used the calculations of the Black isolation index for each MSA as published by the Lewis Mumford Center (2002). The Black isolation index was calculated using the following formula:

$$\text{Black Isolation}_j = 100 \times \sum \left(\frac{B_{ij}}{B_j}\right)\left(\frac{B_{ij}}{T_{ij}}\right) \tag{1}$$

where B_j is the Black population in metropolitan area j, B_{ij} is the Black population of tract i in metropolitan area j, and T_{ij} is the total population of tract i in metropolitan area j (Lewis Mumford Center, 2002). Black isolation ranges from 0 to 100, with a higher score indicating higher amounts of Black isolation, or more racial residential segregation. We also estimated the models using the index of dissimilarity and found very similar results.

We also include several MSA-level independent variables in order to test the hypotheses we introduced earlier. We compiled the MSA-level data from the 2000 U.S. Census, the Lewis Mumford Center, the U.S. Department of

Commerce, American Factfinder, Diversity Data, City and County Extra, and Union Stats. We use the Black isolation index to test Hypotheses 1 and 5. For Hypothesis 2 (educational opportunities), we include *bachelor's degree* (% of residents with a four-year college degree) and *high school dropout* (% of residents who dropped out and did not complete high school) in order to capture the positive effects of higher education and negative effects of educational breakdown, respectively. In order to test Hypothesis 3 (social and family breakdown), we include *married couples* (% of households that are married couples) and *female-headed households* (% of households that are single-parent with a female head of household). For Hypothesis 4 (economic opportunity), we include *percent poverty* (% of households at or below the official poverty level), *unemployment* (% of workers not employed but looking for work), *percent manager/professional* (% of workers employed in managerial or professional occupations), *percent manufacturing* (% of workers employed in the manufacturing sector), and *union density* (% of workers that are union members). Finally, we also control for *population size* (logged), *median income per capita* (logged), and *population density* (population per square mile) in the statistical models.

METHOD

We examine the relationship between residential segregation and health-care access using multilevel binary logit models, which simultaneously account for the multilevel nature of the data (i.e., individuals nested with metropolitan areas) and the fact that the outcome is binary rather than continuous (Raudenbush & Bryk, 2002). The multilevel binary logit models include a random intercept and fixed slopes. Hypotheses 1 through 4 focus on the relationship between segregation and health-care access for Black residents. Therefore, we restrict the sample to Black respondents in the first set of models in order to test these hypotheses. Hypothesis 5 refers to the racial gap in health-care coverage. As a result, we also estimate the final model for White respondents in order to test this hypothesis.

RESULTS

We present descriptive statistics for the individual- and metropolitan area-level variables in Table 1. On average, Blacks are less likely to have health-care coverage from any source (83%) compared to Whites (92%) before

Table 1. Descriptive Statistics for Variables Used in Multilevel Binary Logistic Regression Models of Health Insurance.

Variable Name	Blacks Mean	Blacks SD	Whites Mean	Whites SD	Range	Description
Dependent variable						
Health-care coverage	0.83	0.38	0.92	0.28	0–1	1 = insured, 0 = not insured
Independent variables						
Level 1						
Age	46.30	10.76	48.08	10.35	25–64	Age in years
Female	0.69	0.46	0.61	0.49	0–1	1 = female, 0 = male
Education	14.08	2.93	15.28	2.82	0–18	0 = no school, 5 = elementary, 10 = some high school, 12 = high school, 14 = some college, 18 = college graduate
Income						
<$15,000 (reference)	0.15	0.36	0.05	0.21	0–1	1 = less than $15,000, 0 = else
$15,000 to $25,000	0.18	0.39	0.08	0.26	0–1	1 = $15,000 to $25,000, 0 = else
$25,000 to $35,000	0.12	0.33	0.07	0.25	0–1	1 = $25,000 to $35,000, 0 = else
$35,000 to $50,000	0.15	0.35	0.13	0.33	0–1	1 = $35,000 to $50,000, 0 = else
$50,000 or more	0.31	0.46	0.60	0.49	0–1	1 = $50,000 or more, 0 = else
Don't know/Refused	0.08	0.28	0.08	0.27	0–1	1 = don't know/refused, 0 = else
Married	0.35	0.48	0.65	0.48	0–1	1 = married, 0 = else
Employment status						
Employed (reference)	0.59	0.49	0.63	0.48	0–1	1 = employed for wages, 0 = else
Self-employed	0.06	0.23	0.11	0.31	0–1	1 = self-employed, 0 = else
Unemployed	0.09	0.29	0.05	0.21	0–1	1 = unemployed/out of work, 0 = else
Other	0.26	0.44	0.22	0.41	0–1	1 = homemaker/student/retired/unable to work, 0 = else
City center	0.65	0.48	0.40	0.49	0–1	1 = live in city center, 0 = else
General health status	2.70	1.09	2.29	1.03	1–5	1 = excellent, 2 = very good, 3 = good, 4 = fair, 5 = poor

Table 1. (*Continued*)

Variable Name	Mean	SD	Range	Description
Level 2				
Black isolation	31.88	22.86	0.64–79.02	0 = no isolation, 100 = complete isolation (LMC)
Bachelor's degree	16.86	3.92	7.18–31.17	Percent with a bachelor's degree in MSA (AF)
High school dropout	9.62	2.83	4.16–18.25	Percent of high school dropouts in MSA (AF)
Married couples	51.28	3.82	39.8–69.8	Percent of married couple households in MSA (AF)
Female-headed households	12.19	2.32	7.7–18.9	Percent of female-headed households in MSA (AF)
Percent poverty	11.46	3.42	5.6–25.4	Percent of population in poverty of MSA (AF)
Unemployment	3.87	2.61	1.6–29.9	Unemployment rate of MSA (CCE)
Percent managerial/Professional	34.18	4.93	22.2–50.2	Percent manager/professional occupations in MSA (DD)
Percent manufacturing	12.67	5.69	2–39.4	Percent manufacturing occupations in MSA (AF)
Union density	11.62	6.29	0–31.1	Percent union membership in MSA (US)
Population size	14.39	1.05	11.11–16.07	Log of population size in number of people (LMC)
Median income per capita	10.39	0.18	9.79–11.01	Log of median household income in dollars (USDC)
Population density	532.62	789.74	12.5–8158.7	Population per square mile of land area of MSA (AF)

Note: Black Model: Level 1 $N = 14,633$ and Level 2 $N = 136$. White Model: Level 1 $N = 106,679$ and Level 2 $N = 136$. Level 1 data come from the 2008 Behavioral Risk Factor Surveillance System. Level 2 data come from the 2000 United States Census, the Lewis Mumford Center (LMC), the United States Department of Commerce (USDC), American Factfinder (AF), Diversity Data (DD), City and County Extra (CCE), and Union Stats (US). The source of each level 2 variable is indicated in parentheses in the variable description.

accounting for the impact of place and segregation. This difference is statistically significant ($p < .001$). When race was included in a binary logistic regression model of health insurance (not shown in the tables), being Black, compared to White, decreased the odds of having health insurance by 53%. Black respondents are also more likely to be in poor health (2.70 compared to 2.29 for Whites). Blacks are far more likely to be unemployed compared to Whites (9% vs. 5%). Blacks in this sample are also much less likely to be married compared to Whites (35% vs. 65%). Additionally, they are more likely to live in an urban setting, are overrepresented in the lower income groups, and are underrepresented in the higher income groups. We can see from the descriptive statistics that Blacks are in a disadvantaged social position compared to Whites.

The level 2 results for Black respondents from all six multilevel binary logistic regression models can be found in Table 2. We control for several socio-demographic variables at level 1 but do not show those results in the tables (the results are available upon request). In Model 1, we include Black isolation with no additional level 2 variables, and we add control variables in Model 2. The effect of Black isolation is negative and statistically significant in both models, and the effect actually gets stronger when the control variables are added. Based on the results in Model 2, we see that a one standard deviation increase in Black isolation is predicted to decrease the average odds of health-care coverage by a factor of 0.81 (or 19%).

In Models 3 through 6, we attempt to explain this relationship between segregation and health-care coverage using measures related to educational opportunities, social and family breakdown, and economic opportunities. In Model 3, we add the educational opportunity variables to the model. Metropolitan areas with higher rates of high school dropouts have significantly lower average odds of health-care coverage. However, the strength of the relationship between Black isolation and health-care coverage is unaffected by the educational opportunities in the metropolitan area. The measures of social and family breakdown in Model 4 also have a modest influence (10%) on the magnitude of the Black isolation coefficient, but neither variable has a significant direct effect on health-care coverage. In Model 5, we add the five measures of economic opportunities. The results indicate that metropolitan areas with higher rates of managerial/professional employment have a higher average odds of health-care coverage. Conversely, metropolitan areas with higher poverty rates have a lower average odds of health-care coverage. Additionally, economic opportunities explain a modest portion (10%) of the relationship between segregation and health-care coverage. Finally, the Black isolation effect increases somewhat

Table 2. Coefficients (Standard Errors), X-Standardized Odds Ratios, and Discrete Change Coefficients for Level 2 Variables from Multilevel Binary Logistic Regression Models of Health Insurance for Black Respondents.

Variable Name	Model 1		Model 2		Model 3		Model 4		Model 5		Model 6		
	β	OR	β	OR	β	OR	β	OR	β	OR	β	OR	DC
Fixed effects													
Level 2 variables													
Black isolation	-0.007* (0.003)	0.849	-0.009** (0.003)	0.814	-0.010*** (0.003)	0.803	-0.008* (0.004)	0.828	-0.008** (0.003)	0.842	-0.013*** (0.004)	0.736	-0.036
Bachelor's degree					-0.003 (0.019)	0.989							
High school dropout					-0.062** (0.020)	0.840					-0.005 (0.022)	0.987	-0.002
Married couples							-0.003 (0.020)	0.990			-0.009 (0.021)	0.967	-0.004
Female-headed households							-0.012 (0.038)	0.972			0.087* (0.038)	1.223	0.024
Percent poverty									-0.063** (0.024)	0.807	-0.101*** (0.030)	0.708	-0.041
Unemployment									0.084 (0.066)	1.244	0.069 (0.066)	1.197	0.021
Percent managerial/ professional									0.063*** (0.015)	1.365	0.063*** (0.018)	1.365	0.037
Percent manufacturing									0.010 (0.010)	1.059	0.013 (0.010)	1.079	0.009

	M1 β	M2 β	M2 OR	M3 β	M3 OR	M4 β	M4 OR	M5 β	M5 OR	M6 β	M6 OR	M6 DC
Union density								0.017 (0.009)	1.112	0.016 (0.011)	1.102	0.012
Population size		0.088 (0.069)	1.096	0.132 (0.068)	1.149	0.086 (0.069)	1.094	0.039 (0.060)	1.041	0.065 (0.062)	1.070	0.008
Median income per capita		0.252 (0.382)	1.046	-0.003 (0.442)	0.999	0.197 (0.420)	1.035	-1.435** (0.489)	0.775	-1.554** (0.481)	0.759	-0.033
Population density		0.060[a] (0.060)[a]	1.048	0.042[a] (0.059)[a]	1.033	0.067[a] (0.069)[a]	1.054	0.096[a] (0.061)[a]	1.079	0.082[a] (0.058)[a]	1.067	0.008
Constant	2.168*** (0.137)	-1.608 (3.591)		1.098 (4.149)		-0.751 (4.460)		14.312** (4.806)		15.274** (4.855)		
Random Effects												
Intercept variance	0.199	0.166		0.141		0.165		0.089		0.073		
Deviance	11371.558	11363.094		11353.894		11362.988		11338.754		11333.648		
AIC	11405.560	11403.090		11397.890		11406.990		11388.750		11389.650		
BIC	11534.600	11554.920		11564.900		11573.990		11578.530		11602.200		
Level 2 R^2	0.078	0.232		0.344		0.235		0.585		0.659		

Note: Level 1 $N = 14,633$ and Level 2 $N = 136$.

β = Coefficient; OR = X-standardized odds ratio (factor change); DC = Discrete change coefficient.

For each discrete change coefficient, the remaining variables are held at their means. The discrete change coefficients reflect a change in the predicted probability associated with a standard deviation increase, centered around its mean.

* $p < 0.05$; ** $p < 0.01$; *** $p < 0.001$ (two-tailed).

[a] These coefficients and standard errors have been multiplied by 1,000 for ease of presentation.

in magnitude in Model 6, the full model, which suggests that the Black isolation effect is even stronger if one controls for all of these factors simultaneously. It is possible that changes in coefficients across models are due to changes in unobserved heterogeneity (Mood, 2010). We addressed this potential concern by calculating y-standardized coefficients (based on the latent Y) for Black isolation and found very similar changes across models.

Overall, the results in Table 2 provide support for Hypotheses 1 and 4 and partial support for Hypothesis 3, but do not support Hypothesis 2. Blacks living in metropolitan areas with higher rates of Black isolation (i.e., more racial segregation) are predicted to have significantly lower chances of having health insurance than Blacks living in metropolitan areas with lower rates of Black isolation. Part of this influence of segregation for Blacks is due to limited economic opportunities in racially segregated metropolitan areas.

In order to examine the effect of Black isolation on the racial gap in health-care coverage, we estimated the models from Table 2 for both Black and White residents and generated predicted probabilities based on the Full Model (6) for each group. We present the predicted probabilities for Blacks and Whites across the range of Black isolation in Fig. 1. As Black isolation increases from its minimum to maximum levels (i.e., 0–80), the predicted probability of health-care coverage decreases substantially for Black residents (0.90 to 0.77) but remains relatively unchanged for White residents

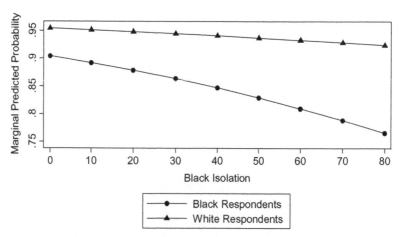

Fig. 1. The Effect of Black Isolation on the Predicted Probability of Having Health Insurance.

(0.95 to 0.92). At the lowest level of segregation, there is a very modest racial gap in the predicted probability of health-care coverage (0.05), but this grows to a very substantial gap at the highest level of segregation (0.15). In other words, as Black isolation increases the racial gap in health-care coverage increases as well, which provides support for Hypothesis 5.

DISCUSSION AND CONCLUSIONS

There are several main ways that people access health-care coverage, principally through their employment, through a family member, or through social assistance for those that qualify. Health insurance is a fundamental component of health-care access in the United States, especially for advanced and specialty care, which is usually unavailable through alternative forms of access such as free clinics, and too expensive to pay out of pocket. We hypothesized, drawing on Massey and colleagues' geographic concentration of poverty theory of segregation, that racial residential segregation could impact the ability of Black residents of segregated cities to access adequate health-care coverage (Krivo et al., 1998; Massey, 1990; Massey & Denton, 1993; Massey et al., 1994; Massey & Fischer, 2000). As segregation compounds poverty and social problems into one geographical area, these socioeconomic effects, which could impact one's access to health insurance, could lead to reduced access to health insurance. From the results, we found a substantial impact of Black isolation for working-age Black residents of 136 U.S. metropolitan areas on the likelihood of having health-care coverage. This effect was significant even when controlling for more obvious socioeconomic factors such as education, employment, and income at both the individual-level and the city-level. As Black residential segregation increased, Black residents of those cities were less likely, compared to Black residents of cities with lower levels of segregation, to have health-care coverage of any type. This result addresses our first research question, confirms our hypothesis, and confirms Massey and colleagues' theory that informs this study.

Related to our first research question, we also specified three hypotheses on the mechanisms by which segregation could impact access to health insurance. Using the effects of geographic concentration of poverty from Massey and colleagues' theory that we reasoned would be pertinent to the outcome of health-care coverage, we included the effects of educational opportunities, social breakdown, and economic opportunity in models predicting health-care coverage (Krivo et al., 1998; Massey, 1990; Massey & Denton, 1993; Massey et al., 1994; Massey & Fischer, 2000). However, when we tested these various negative impacts that segregation could have on access to health care at the metropolitan-area level, none of them substantially decreased the effect of Black isolation. Although a few of these measures were important indicators of either increased or decreased access to health insurance, none were able to account for the effect of residential segregation.

First, the educational factors that indicate the lack of educational achievement, by examining high school dropout rates, at the MSA-level did contribute to reduced access to health insurance. However, a high degree of achievement, a bachelor's degree, was not related to increased access to health insurance. Perhaps a variable for the percent of people in an MSA who have a bachelor's degree (versus more inclusive educational measures that would include associates degrees or vocational training programs) is not the best indicator of upward mobility and access to higher quality jobs that might provide benefits.

Second, social and family indicators did not have a significant effect on health-care access. Although none of the variables were significant, the model did slightly reduce the size of the coefficient for Black isolation. This facet of the negative consequences of segregation as a form of structural racism is emphasized in Massey and Denton's work (1993), as well as elsewhere in the literature, but does not appear to have a substantial effect. In the final, full model, percent of female-headed households was actually statistically significant and positively related to health-care coverage access. As this outcome specifies health-care coverage of any type, including social assistance, this effect may be significant as single mothers are often able to get coverage for their children and themselves through social assistance. Conversely, being married, as measured at the individual level, had a substantial positive effect on health insurance. Thus, these factors, as a structural, city-level effect were not important for understanding disparate access to health insurance and certainly did not diminish the effect of residential segregation.

Finally, the economic opportunity factors provided the best understanding of the outcome, but could still not completely account for the effect of segregation. An increased presence of professional or White collar jobs demonstrated an increased access to health-care coverage. Also, an increase in the percent of people in poverty decreased the likelihood of having health insurance. However, the effect of residential segregation remained strong in both of the models in which these measures were included. It is obvious, using both the measures at the individual-level and the metropolitan-level that socioeconomic factors play a role in obtaining health-care coverage, but these results demonstrate that segregation itself has a substantial effect on the outcome.

In sum, the results presented here only partially account for the causal mechanisms by which residential segregation can affect access to health-care coverage. We hypothesized, based on the geographic concentration of poverty theory, that segregation could affect health-care access by limiting educational opportunities, increasing the prevalence of family breakdown and social disorder, and limiting economic and occupational opportunities. However, none of these variables or even the combination of these variables could account for the effect of racial residential segregation. Although we included many measures for each of these different hypothesized effects, perhaps more variables or even a different operationalization of such variables could better account for the effect of segregation. Additionally, although the previous theory and research highlights these facets of segregation, perhaps racial residential segregation itself, as a form of institutionalized, structural racism, produces these effects and does not rely solely on the pathway of the three mechanisms hypothesized and tested here. These findings provide a framework for future research on the issue, which could assess more specifically how racial residential segregation can affect health-care access in a variety of ways.

Furthermore, when assessing our second research question, whether or not segregation contributes to the Black-White gap in health insurance, the results are quite noteworthy. While residential segregation demonstrates a strong decrease in the likelihood of having health-care coverage for Black respondents, there is no such effect for White respondents. While segregation for White respondents does actually slightly decrease their likelihood of having health insurance, the effect for White respondents was not substantial. Even without taking into account the effect of segregation, Blacks are less likely to have health insurance, but residential segregation further increases this gap, as evidenced in Fig. 1. These results affirm our expectations based on Massey and colleagues' theory. They argue that members of the dominant group not subject to segregation are spatially buffered from the negative effects of concentrated poverty resulting from segregation, which is what these results demonstrate.

Thus, these results present some evidence for applying Massey and colleagues' concentration of poverty theory to the outcome of health-care access. The results affirm the first implication of their theory, that segregation concentrates poverty, which produces certain negative social effects, in this case by limiting access to health-care coverage. Additionally, the results affirm the second implication of their theory, that by concentrating poverty in one racial group, the White dominant group is buffered from the negative effects of segregation, which was evidenced by showing that segregation contributes to the Black-White gap in health-care coverage. While the results conform to these aspects of the theory, the results fail to reveal some of the mechanisms brought forth by the concentration of poverty theory of segregation. The educational variables did not mitigate the effect of segregation at all. The social and economic opportunity variables provided some explanation for the effect of segregation on access to health insurance, but they could not account for much of this effect. Further work to understand the mechanisms of poverty concentration in segregated neighborhoods on the effect of reduced health-care access is an important consideration for future research to further build this argument and the evidence for concentration of poverty theory.

Overall, the findings presented here contribute to our understanding of the Black-White gap in health-care outcomes. The findings demonstrate that higher levels of segregation in cities limit access to health-care coverage for Black residents. Additionally, while segregation produces this effect for the Black community, White residents of these same areas are shielded from the effects of segregation. This study makes several major contributions to our understanding of these issues. First, while there has recently been a lot of literature demonstrating the effect of segregation on health outcomes, little is known about the impact of segregation on health care. While this study only examines one health-care outcome, health insurance, future studies on other facets of health-care access and use would be useful to further our understanding of this association. Second, this study uses a large, national sample and a multilevel statistical method, examining both individual and metropolitan-area levels of data. Other studies on the topic have either used a geographically limited area or methods that do not capture the full scope of the effect of segregation. Given these advantages, studies using a variety of methods and samples would be necessary to further our understanding of the impact of segregation on health-care outcomes.

Furthermore, these findings could contribute to our understanding of the Black-White health gap in the United States. Lack of access to health care, which has been shown to have detrimental health consequences, could have an intervening effect on health outcomes overall for the U.S. Black population. Previous studies as well as the descriptive statistics within this study have demonstrated that Black Americans in general are less likely to have health insurance compared to Whites (Hoffman & Paradise, 2008). The findings here demonstrate that residential segregation may play an important part in the perpetuation of both health and health-care racial inequities.

Since enforced segregation was made illegal by the Fair Housing Act of 1968, efforts to combat segregation and its effects for Black Americans have sharply declined. Although no longer legal, de facto segregation remains an important part of the social landscape of the United States. This study, among a growing body of literature on the subject, shows that the negative consequences of our failure to racially integrate as a society continue to produce deleterious effects for the Black community. The findings in this study indicate that in order to effectively address and combat the glaring health and health-care inequalities that persist in the United States, residential segregation must be a part of that discussion.

ACKNOWLEDGMENTS

The authors presented this paper at the annual meeting of the American Sociological Association in 2011 in Las Vegas, NV. The authors thank Tammy Mix for her comments on earlier drafts of the paper and Mike Wallace for sharing his metropolitan-area data.

REFERENCES

Andrulis, D. P. (1998). Access to care is the centerpiece in the elimination of socioeconomic disparities in health. *Annals of Internal Medicine, 129*, 412–416.

Bahr, P. R. (2007). Race and nutrition: An investigation of black-white differences in health-related nutritional behaviors. *Sociology of Health and Illness, 29*(6), 831–856. doi:10.1111/j.1467-9566.2007.01049.x

Bullard, R. D. (2005). Environmental justice in the twenty-first century. In R. D. Bullard (Ed.), *The quest for environmental justice: Human rights and the politics of pollution* (pp. 19–42). San Francisco, CA: Sierra Club Books.

Byrd, W. M., & Clayton, L. A. (2001). Race, medicine and health care in the United States: A historical survey. *Journal of the National Medical Association, 93*(3), 11S–34S.

Byrd, W. M., & Clayton, L. A. (2002). *An American health dilemma: Race, medicine, and health care in the United States 1900-2000*. New York, NY: Routledge.

Chang, V. W. (2006). Racial residential segregation and weight status among U.S. adults. *Social Science and Medicine, 63*, 1289–1303. doi:10.1016/j.socscimed.2006.03.049

Chang, V. W., Hillier, A. E., & Mehta, N. K. (2009). Neighborhood isolation, disorder and obesity. *Social Forces, 87*(4), 2063–2092.

Clarke, S. P., Davis, B. L., & Nailon, R. E. (2007). Racial segregation and differential outcomes in hospital care. *Western Journal of Nursing Research, 29*(6), 739–757. doi:10.1177/0193945907303167

Collins, C. A. (1999). Racism and health: Segregation and causes of death amenable to medical intervention in major U.S. cities. *Annals New York Academy of Sciences, 986*, 396–398. doi:10.1111/j.1749-6632.1999.tb08152.x

Collins, C. A., & Williams, D. R. (1999). Segregation and mortality: The deadly effects of racism? *Sociological Forum, 14*(3), 495–523. doi:10.1023/A:1021403820451

Ellen, I. G., Cutler, D. M., & Dickens, W. (2000). Is segregation bad for your health? The case of low birth weight. *Brookings-Wharton Papers on Urban Affairs*, 203–238.

Farley, J. (2005). Residential interracial exposure and isolation indices: Mean versus median indices, and the difference it makes. *The Sociological Quarterly, 46*, 19–45.

Farley, J. (2008). Even whiter than we thought: What median residential exposure indices reveal about white neighborhood contact with African Americans in U.S. metropolitan areas. *Social Science Research, 37*, 604–623. doi:10.1016/j.ssresearch.2007.10.004

Gaskin, D. J., Price, A., Brandon, D. T., & LaVeist, T. A. (2009). Segregation and disparities in health services use. *Medical Care Research and Review, 66*, 578–589. doi:10.1177/1077558709336445

Grady, S. C. (2006). Racial disparities in low birthweight and the contribution of residential segregation: A multilevel analysis. *Social Science and Medicine, 63*, 3013–3029. doi:10.1016/j.socscimed.2006.08.017

Greenberg, M., & Schneider, D. (1994). Violence in American cities: Young black males is the answer, but what was the question?. *Social Science and Medicine, 39*(3), 179–187. doi:10.1016/0277-9536(94)90326-3

Grier, S. A., & Kumanyika, S. K. (2008). The context for choice: Health implications of targeted food and beverage marketing to African Americans. *American Journal of Public Health, 98*(9), 1616–1629. doi:10.2105/AJPH.2007.115626

Haas, J. S., Phillips, K. A., Sonneborn, D., McCulloch, C. E., Baker, L. C., Kaplan, C. P., et al. (2004). Variation in access to health care for different racial/ethnic groups by the racial/ethnic composition of an individual's county of residence. *Medical Care, 42*(7), 707–714. doi:10.1097/01.mlr.0000129906.95881.83

Hart, K. D., Kunitz, S. J., Sell, R. R., & Mukamel, D. B. (1998). Metropolitan governance, residential segregation, and mortality among African Americans. *American Journal of Public Health, 88*(3), 434–438. doi:10.2105/AJPH.88.3.434

Hayanga, A. J., Kaiser, H. E., Sinha, R., Berenholtz, S. M., Makary, M., & Chang, D. (2009). Residential segregation and access to surgical care by minority populations in US counties. *Journal of the American College of Surgeons, 208*, 1017–1022. doi:10.1016/j.jamcollsurg.2009.01.047

Hayanga, A. J., Waljee, A. K., Kaiser, H. E., Chang, D. C., & Morris, A. M. (2009). Racial clustering and access to colorectal surgeons, gastroenterologists, and radiation oncologists by African Americans and Asian Americans in the United States. *Archives of Surgery, 144*(6), 532–535.

Hearst, M. O., Oakes, J. M., & Johnson, P. J. (2008). The effect of racial residential segregation on black infant mortality. *American Journal of Epidemiology, 168*(11), 1247–1254. doi:10.1093/aje/kwn291

Hoffman, C., & Paradise, J. (2008). Health insurance and access to health care in the United States. *Annals of the New York Academy of Sciences, 1136*, 149–160. doi:10.1196/annals.1425.007

Hummer, R. A. (1996). Black-white differences in health and mortality: A review and conceptual model. *The Sociological Quarterly, 37*(1), 105–125.

Iceland, J., & Wilkes, R. (2006). Does socioeconomic status matter? Race, class, and residential segregation. *Social Problems, 53*(2), 248–273. doi:10.1525/sp.2006.53.2.248

Kposowa, A. J. (2007). Is there a racial/ethnic hierarchy in health status and care. *The Western Journal of Black Studies, 31*(1), 17–32.

Krivo, L. J., Peterson, R. D., Rizzo, H., & Reynolds, J. R. (1998). Race, segregation, and the concentration of disadvantage: 1980-1990. *Social Problems, 45*(1), 61–80. doi:10.1525/sp.1998.45.1.03 × 0157a

Kwate, N. O. A. (2008). Fried chicken and fresh apples: Racial segregation as a fundamental cause of fast food density in black neighborhoods. *Health and Place, 14*, 32–44. doi:10.1016/j.healthplace.2007.04.001

Larson, N. I., Story, M. T., & Nelson, M. (2009). Neighborhood environments: Disparities in access to healthy foods in the U.S. *American Journal of Preventative Medicine, 36*(1), 74–81. doi:10.1016/j.amepre.2008.09.025

LaVeist, T. A., & Wallace, J. M., Jr. (2000). Health risk and inequitable distribution of liquor stores in African American neighborhood. *Social Science and Medicine, 51*, 613–617. doi:10.1016/S0277-9536(00)00004-6

LeClere, F. B., Rogers, R. G., & Peters, K. D. (1997). Ethnicity and morality in the United States: Individual and community correlates. *Social Forces, 76*(1), 169–198. doi:10.2307/2580322

Lewis Mumford Center for Comparative Urban and Regional Research. (2002). *Metropolitan racial and ethnic change – Census 2000.* Retrieved from http://mumford.albany.edu/census/WholePop/WPdownload.html. Accessed on July 1, 2010.

Massey, D. S. (1990). American apartheid: Segregation and the making of the underclass. *The American Journal of Sociology, 96*(2), 329–357. doi:10.1086/229532

Massey, D. S., & Denton, N. A. (1988). The dimensions of residential segregation. *Social Forces, 67*(2), 281–315. doi:10.2307/2579183

Massey, D. S., & Denton, N. A. (1989). Hypersegregation in U.S. metropolitan areas: Black and Hispanic segregation along five dimensions. *Demography, 26*(3), 373–391. doi:10.2307/2061599

Massey, D. S., & Denton, N. A. (1993). *American apartheid: Segregation and the making of the underclass.* Cambridge, MA: Harvard University Press.

Massey, D. S., & Fischer, M. J. (2000). How segregation concentrates poverty. *Ethnic and Racial Studies, 23*(4), 670–691.

Massey, D. S., Gross, A. B., & Shibuya, K. (1994). Migration, segregation, and the geographic concentration of poverty. *American Sociological Review, 59*(3), 425–445. doi:10.2307/2095942

Mood, C. (2010). Logistic regression: Why we cannot do what we think we can do, and what we can do about it. *European Sociological Review, 26*(1), 67–82. doi:10.1093/esr/jcp006

Patterson, A. (2009). Germs and Jim Crow: The impact of microbiology on public health policies in progressive era American south. *Journal of the History of Biology, 42*, 529–559. doi:10.1007/s10739-008-9164-x

Polednak, A. P. (1991). Black-White differences in infant mortality in 38 standard metropolitan statistical areas. *American Journal of Public Health, 81*(11), 1480–1482. doi:10.2105/AJPH.81.11.1480

Polednak, A. P. (1997). *Segregation, poverty, and mortality in urban African Americans.* New York, NY: Oxford University Press.

Raudenbush, S. W., & Bryk, A. S. (2002). *Hierarchical linear models: Applications and data analysis methods.* Thousand Oaks, CA: Sage.

Rodriguez, R. A., Sen, S., Mehta, K., Moody-Ayers, S., Bacchetti, P., & O'Hare, A. M. (2007). Geography matters: Relationships among urban residential segregation, dialysis facilities, and patient outcomes. *Annals of Internal Medicine, 146,* 493–501.

Sarrazin, M. S. V., Campbell, M. E., Richardson, K. K., & Rosenthal, G. E. (2009). Racial segregation and disparities in health care delivery: Conceptual model and empirical assessment. *Health Services Research, 44*(4), 1424–1443. doi:10.1111/j.1475-6773.2009.00977.x

Shavers, V. L., & Shavers, B. S. (2006). Racism and health inequity among Americans. *Journal of the National Medical Association, 98*(3), 386–396.

Shihadeh, E. S., & Flynn, N. (1996). Segregation and crime: The effect of black social isolation on the rates of black urban violence. *Social Forces, 74*(4), 1325–1352. doi:10.2307/2580353

Smith, D. B., Feng, Z., Fennel, M. L., Zinn, J. S., & Mor, V. (2007). Separate and unequal: Racial segregation and disparities in quality across U.S. nursing homes. *Health Affairs, 26*(5), 1448–1458. doi:10.1377/hlthaff.26.5.14481

Subramanian, S. V., Acevedo-Garcia, D., & Osypuk, T. L. (2004). Racial residential segregation and geographic heterogeneity in black/white disparity in poor self-rated health in the US: A multilevel statistical analysis. *Social Science and Medicine, 60,* 1667–1679. doi:10.1016/j.socscimed.2004.08.040

Testa, M., Astone, N. M., Krogh, M., & Neckerman, K. M. (1993). Employment and marriage among inner-city fathers. In W. J. Wilson (Ed.), *The Ghetto Underclass* (pp. 96–108). Newberry Park, CA: Sage.

U.S. Department of Health and Human Services. (2000). *Healthy People 2010.* 2nd ed. With Understanding and Improving Health and Objectives for Improving Health. 2 vols. Washington, DC: U.S. Government Printing Office.

Williams, D. R. (1999). Race, socioeconomic status, and health: The added effects of racism and discrimination. *Annals New York Academy of Sciences, 896,* 173–188. doi:10.1111/j.1749-6632.1999.tb08114.x

Williams, D. R., & Collins, C. (2001). Racial residential segregation: A fundamental cause of racial disparities in health. *Public Health Reports, 116,* 404–416. doi:10.1016/S0033-3549(04)50068-7

Williams, D. R., & Jackson, P. B. (2005). Social sources of racial disparities in health. *Health Affairs, 24*(2), 325–334. doi:10.1377/hlthaff.24.2.325

Wilson, W. J. (1987). *The truly disadvantaged: The inner city, the underclass, and public policy.* Chicago, IL: University of Chicago.

Wilson, W. J. (1996). *When work disappears: The world of the new urban poor.* New York, NY: Random House.

SECTION III
GENDER

GENDERING AFFECTIVE DISORDERS IN DIRECT-TO-CONSUMER ADVERTISEMENTS

Jennifer Arney and Rose Weitz

ABSTRACT

This chapter explores how direct-to-consumer advertisements (DTCA) for major depression and anxiety disorders use contemporary gender scripts to sell medications and disease definitions to consumers, and in the process reflect and reinforce those scripts for both men and women. Between 1997 and 2006, antidepressant DTCA in popular magazines overwhelmingly depicted depression as a (white) female disorder, as did anti-anxiety DTCA, although not to such an extreme extent. In addition, DTCA often alerted men to the benefits they might reap if the women in their lives sought treatment, while suggesting that women had a responsibility *to seek such treatment for the sake of their loved ones. Moreover, DTCA disproportionately encouraged women to monitor their emotions while encouraging men to monitor their physical sensations. Finally, DTCA suggested that medication would yield benefits for women primarily in their close relationships and for men primarily in their work lives, thus reinforcing the binary sex divisions implicit in hegemonic masculinity and emphasized femininity. At a broader level, DTCA studied for this article suggest to both women and men that individuals should*

Issues in Health and Health Care Related to Race/Ethnicity, Immigration, SES and Gender
Research in the Sociology of Health Care, Volume 30, 161–180
Copyright © 2012 by Emerald Group Publishing Limited
ISSN: 0275-4959/doi:10.1108/S0275-4959(2012)0000030010

monitor themselves and others for a wide variety of common emotions, behaviors, and physical sensations, thus individualizing social problems and encouraging the expansion of medical authority over everyday life.

Keywords: Direct-to-consumer advertisements; depression; anxiety; antidepressant DTCA; gender

INTRODUCTION

Recent years have seen growing concern about the impact of direct-to-consumer advertisements (DTCA) of psychotropic drugs and, especially, the ways in which such advertising may contribute to the medicalization of a wide range of everyday emotions, behaviors, and conditions (Arney & Rafalovich, 2007; Conrad, 2005; Conrad & Leiter, 2008; Emmons, 2010; Horwitz & Wakefield, 2007). Given the long history of medical surveillance of women's lives and bodies (e.g., Ehrenreich & English, 2005; Leavitt, 1999; Riessman, 1983; Wertz & Wertz, 1989), it is perhaps not surprising that research in this area has focused largely on advertising directed at women (Chananie, 2005; Emmons, 2010; Greenslit, 2005; Horwitz & Wakefield, 2007; Woodlock, 2005). Yet the rise of DTCA for products such as Viagra and Rogaine reflects the increasing medicalization of men's bodies as well (Conrad, 2007; Conrad & Leiter, 2004; Loe, 2004; Rosenfeld & Faircloth, 2006). To date, however, little research has systematically compared to the medicalization of women's and men's lives and bodies or analyzed the role of gender ideologies in this process (Riska, 2003; Rosenfeld & Faircloth, 2006). In this article, we apply a social constructionist perspective (Brown, 1995) to explore how contemporary DTCA for two types of affective disorders – major depression and anxiety disorders (social anxiety disorder, generalized anxiety disorder, and persistent anxiety) – use contemporary gender scripts to sell medications and disease definitions to consumers, and in the process reflect and reinforce those scripts for both men and women.

DTCA has a long – and gendered – history. Beginning in the mid- to late-1800s, patent medicines (proprietary drugs with secret formulas) were widely advertised in consumer publications as cure-alls for ailments including indigestion, fatigue, sleeplessness, and headaches (Conrad & Leiter, 2008). Reflecting age-old beliefs that women were especially susceptible to emotional problems, many of these early advertisements targeted women consumers. The 1909 *Sears Roebuck and Company Consumer Guide*, for example, advertised Brown's vegetable cure for "female weakness…, nausea, bad taste in the mouth…, feelings of languor…, hysterics…, dizziness, morbid feeling…, spirits depressed…, pain in the back upon exertion, fainting spells," and other problems (*Sears Roebuck and Company Consumer Guide*, 1979, p. 379). Although some of these symptoms were sex-neutral, "female weakness" obviously was not, and both hysterics and fainting spells were also understood at the time as "female complaints."

The use of DTCA has exploded since the 1980s, when the FDA began loosening strict rules first imposed on the pharmaceutical industry in the early 1900s (Pines, 1999). Current guidelines (issued in 1997) retain earlier requirements that advertising claims be substantiated and that ads provide a balanced description of risks and benefits, but no longer require that ads state all major risks associated with product use (62 Fed. Reg. 43171). Instead, advertisers need to only provide access to risk information via a toll-free telephone number, printed fact sheet, web page, or the like.

Adoption of the 1997 regulations generated a torrent of DTCA in all media outlets. Advertising expenditures have increased sixfold since then, rising between 13% and 20% almost yearly (IMS Health, 2002, 2010a). Similarly, between 1997 and 2009 Americans' prescription drug expenditures tripled, to $300.3 billion (IMS Health, 2009, 2010b). The increase has been particularly notable for antidepressants, which are used to treat both depression and anxiety. These drugs are now ranked fourth in dispensed prescriptions in the United States, with 164.2 million prescriptions dispensed and $9.9 billion spent on those prescriptions in 2009 alone (IMS Health, 2010b).

Despite these changes, however, now as in the past women receive twice as many antidepressant prescriptions as do men (Ashton, 1991; Beidel, Bulik, & Stanley, 2010; Nolen-Hoeksema, 2001). Given that community surveys consistently conclude that women are two to three times more likely than men to have depressive or anxiety disorders (Beidel et al., 2010; Nolen-Hoeksema, 2001), higher rates of antidepressant use among women are not surprising. However, such surveys may fail to distinguish between ordinary emotions and diagnosable psychiatric disease, and so women's higher rates of diagnosis and treatment do not necessarily indicate that women have higher rates of disease (Mirowsky & Ross, 2005). Instead, both doctors and consumers may be more likely to "read" women's experiences and feelings through a framework of psychopathology. To the extent that DTCA adopts a similar lens, it may both reflect and reinforce this pattern.

Previous research on DTCA for depression has found that marketing campaigns do indeed tend to associate women with this disease, potentially leading to under-diagnosis among men and over-diagnosis among women. Woodlock (2005) examined web-based DTCA during four months in 2003 and found that women are depicted in antidepressant ads more than twice as often as men. In addition, those ads were frequently linked to web searches for problems that more often plague women, such as rape and sexual abuse. Similarly, Grow, Park, and Han (2006) analyzed seven years of antidepressant DTCA in *Reader's Digest* and *Time* and found that advertisements for Paxil, Prozac, and Zoloft often depicted depression sufferers as women. Neither of these articles, however, explored further how gender operates within these advertisements.

Research on other psychiatric disorders also suggests that DTCA may disproportionately target women. Chananie (2005) examined 13 televised advertisements for a variety of disorders and found that the ads encourage women to medicalize their emotional and physical experiences by reinforcing medical authority, blaming and shaming women who don't seek medical treatment, framing medicalization in feminist and 12-step movement rhetoric, validating women's experiences and emotions, and promising women greater control over their "disordered" lives via medicalization. Through so doing, Chananie argues, these advertisements reconstruct "disempowering notions of feminine fragility and biological restrictions" (2005, p. 487). Similarly, Greenslit (2005) found that online DTCA for Sarafem – Prozac rebranded in a pink and lavender pill and marketed for the treatment of premenstrual dysphoric disorder – suggest that premenstrual symptoms hinder women's personal and social functioning, that women are responsible for treating those symptoms, and that using Sarafem "empowers" women.

As these examples suggest, most research on the medicalization of emotionality (as on gender and medicalization overall) has focused on women (Chananie, 2005; Emmons, 2010; Greenslit, 2005; Horwitz & Wakefield, 2007; Woodlock, 2005). Indeed, to the best of our knowledge no research has looked at the impact of DTCA on the medicalization of men's emotionality.

Our study aims to more fully flesh out the gendered nature of the medicalization of both men's and women's emotionality, using a broader and deeper sample than in previous research. We examine a full decade of print DTCA (from the FDA's liberalization of its DTCA policy in 1997 to 2006), using a wide variety of print sources, comparing marketing messages regarding and directed toward both women and men, and comparing DTCA for both social anxiety and depression.

METHODS

Study Design and Data Collection

For this research, we used content analysis to explore the gendered portrayal of affective disorders in print DTCA. We focused specifically on magazines because they are a common and effective advertising outlet, which facilitates scanning by consumers and thus can lead consumers to unintentionally absorb advertising messages even when they are not seeking information on a topic (Niederdeppe et al., 2007).

Advertisements were collected from the 1997 to 2006 issues of 10 magazines: four addressed to both men and women (*People, Time, Newsweek, Reader's Digest*), three addressed to women (*Cosmopolitan, Redbook, Ladies' Home Journal*), and three addressed to men (*Esquire, Gentlemen's Quarterly, Men's Health*). We chose these magazines because of their high advertising content and circulation revenues and because they target a wide variety of age groups, socioeconomic statuses, and education levels.

Dataset

Our search yielded a total of 320 DTCA for depressive and anxiety disorders. Of the 205 ads that discuss depressive disorder, we identified 27 unique advertisements (4 Prozac, 1 Paxil, 11 Zoloft, 3 Effexor, 4 Wellbutrin, and 4 Cymbalta). Of the 115 ads that discuss anxiety disorder, we identified 14 unique advertisements (5 BuSpar, 6 Paxil, 2 Zoloft, and 1 Effexor). Paxil, Zoloft, and Effexor are promoted for the treatment of both disorders, but never in the same advertisement. For this analysis, we calculate percentages based on the total sample of 320 DTCA, rather than on the 41 unique ads, because our focus is on how frequently each image (and its associated messages) was presented to magazine readers.

In the first two years covered by this study, beginning with the FDA's liberalization of its DTCA policy in 1997, DTCA for depression appeared four times more often than DTCA for social anxiety. Curiously, from 1999 to 2001 anxiety ads appeared six times more often than did depression ads, but for the remainder of our study period depression ads once again became more common, with anxiety ads completely disappearing in 2005–2006. We do not have an explanation for these changes, but certainly they indicate the ways in which marketing – and the medicalization of given behaviors, emotions, and social groups – responds quickly to prevailing conditions, whatever they may be.

Analysis

Analysis of advertisements was guided by principles of grounded theory (Charmaz, 2006; Glaser, 1978; Glaser & Strauss, 1967; Strauss & Corbin, 1990). We began our analysis of DTCA by examining the content of each advertisement and noting emergent themes in the dataset. The preliminary themes identified in this initial open coding procedure (Glaser, 1978) focused on whom the advertisements targeted, how ads portrayed symptomatology in men and women, and how ads medicalized or otherwise framed common complaints. Both authors reviewed all advertisements, and any disagreements in coding were discussed and resolved. This open coding procedure was followed by selective coding (Glaser, 1978), in which we examined each advertisement for specific examples of the preliminary themes. Our final coding centered on six themes, and the ways in which those themes intersected with gender. The themes were:

1. *Advertisement placement.* This includes the rates at which DTCA appears in men's, women's, and mixed audience magazines.
2. *Depiction of sufferers.* This includes the number and depiction of men, women, and characters that could not be coded by sex. Characters were further divided into those portrayed as suffering from the disorder or as witnesses to such individuals.
3. *Discussion of responsibility.* This includes ways in which ads indicate responsibility for the disorder and for seeking treatment.
4. *Encouragement to monitor self or others.* This includes messages that advise viewers why and how they should assess their emotional condition or that of others.
5. *Impact of affective disorders.* This includes messages concerning how affective disorders can affect individuals presumed to suffer from depression or anxiety as well as how these disorders can affect those around them.

6. *Locus of treatment benefits:* This includes messages pertaining to life arenas where individuals may experience improvement if they use medications.

RESULTS

In the following sections we explore how gender scripts are used, presented, and reinforced in DTCA for depression and social anxiety. Strikingly, *every* advertisement showed only white people (or no people at all), and so we cannot analyze any intersectional effects of race or ethnicity.

Feminizing Depression

Our findings demonstrate that antidepressant DTCA heavily target women, depict depression as a female disease, suggest to men that they will benefit if the women in their lives seek treatment, suggest to women that they owe it to others to do so and that their relationships will improve if they do so, and instruct women to self-monitor for any symptoms of depression.

Sexing DTCA Placement
Our most striking (if perhaps not unexpected) finding is the extent to which antidepressant DTCA target women. DTCA for antidepressants appear in women's magazines *fifteen* times more often than in men's magazines: 37% of antidepressant DTCA ($N = 75$) appeared in women's magazines and only 2% ($N = 5$) in men's magazines. The remaining 61% of antidepressant DTCA ($N = 125$) were found in magazines with mixed gender audiences. However, half of these appeared in *People Magazine*. Although *People* is not explicitly targeted toward women, 72% of its audience is female (People Media Kit, 2011). Women comprise approximately half of readers for *Time* and *Newsweek* and 63% of readers for *Readers Digest* (Newsweek Media Kit, 2011; Reader's Digest Online Media Kit, 2011; Time Media Kit, 2011). Thus, the percentage of antidepressant DTCA directed at women is even higher than it seems at first glance.

Sexing Depression Sufferers
The feminization of depression is also evident in advertisers' decisions regarding which sex to depict as suffering from depression. (All but 13% of the ads in our dataset – 27 ads – could be coded by sex.)

None of the advertisements – including those in men's magazines – explicitly or implicitly depicted men with depression. In contrast, 61% of antidepressant DTCA ($N = 125$) *explicitly* depict depression sufferers as female, as do *all* ads in the most recent years, 2005 and 2006. In addition, another 26% of the ads ($N = 53$) *implicitly* depict sufferers as women (cf. Emmons, 2010). For instance, one early Prozac ad contrasted a child-like cartoon drawing of a small, leafless tree on the left side of the ad with a drawing of a bird nesting in a large tree in full bloom on the right side, accompanied by the captions, "Depression isolates" and "Prozac helps." Another ad from the same series contrasted rain clouds with a bright sun ornamented with curly sunbeams, above the caption, "Chances are someone you know is feeling sunny again." Others in the series used images of broken vases versus a vase with a daisy in it and the like. In each of these instances, the ads use images (flowers in vases, curly sunbeams) and descriptors (sunny, blossoming) – that play on social expectations for female interests and emotions and so implicitly identify women as most likely to suffer from depression (cf. Emmons, 2010).

Alerting Men...About Women
As noted earlier, only 2% of the depression ads (5 ads) appeared in men's magazines, and all of these depicted only women as depression sufferers. These ads consistently encourage male readers to consider how their lives could be improved if their wives or girlfriends used antidepressants. For example, a 2002 Paxil advertisement in *Esquire* depicts a depressed woman – furrowed brow, downward gaze, arms folded, standing by herself – on the left side of the page, with her concerned husband and son gazing at her from the right side of the page. In the center of the page, separating the wife from her family, is a list of symptoms: depressed mood, loss of interest, sleep problems, difficulty concentrating, agitation, restlessness. The headline reads "What's standing between you and your life?" Although this headline could be directed at either the man or the woman, its placement in Esquire suggests that the man is the target audience. In any case, it is clear that the woman is the one troubled by the symptoms and that it is *her* depressed mood, loss of interest, and sleep problems causing – and not resulting from – her family's troubles. Thus, the ad suggests that men would benefit if only the women in their lives would get treatment.

Similarly, a 2006 Wellbutrin ad in *Men's Health* features a man and woman camping. Although the happy couple is pictured together, the ad depicts the woman's full face and the man in profile, making the woman the subject and the man the viewer. The headline reads "Wellbutrin XL works for my depression with a low risk of weight gain and sexual side effects." Given its placement in a men's magazine, the ad appears to suggest to men the benefits of getting their wives and girlfriends to use this drug: she'll be a happier and better companion, won't gain weight, and will regain interest in sex.

Blaming Women

Suggesting that men would benefit if their wives or girlfriends sought treatment implicitly suggests that women are to blame for men's suffering should they *not* do so. This message appears explicitly in 34% of anti-depressant DTCA ($N = 69$), including a 2005 Zoloft advertisement featuring Kathy, a 41-year-old wife and mother. In the first frame, Kathy – depicted as a cartoon bubble with sketched in eyes, nose, and lipsticked frown – recalls her daughter saying, "Mommy, you're no fun anymore." In the next frame, Kathy says, "It hit me. It was time to get help." She "went on the web and found that Zoloft is the number one prescribed brand of its kind," and then got a prescription for it from her doctor. In the subsequent frame, Kathy is shown with a lipsticked smile shopping for her family's groceries and declaring, "I soon noticed a difference. And so did my family." In the final frame, Kathy is perched on a couch with her husband, with the caption, "You get one chance to raise your kids. Why do it with depression?" While Kathy is drawn facing the reader, her husband's gaze is on Kathy; he appears pleased with his wife's medication use, implying his prior suffering from her depression. Through Kathy's story, readers are taught that women's untreated depression is a burden on their families, that a good woman will realize this and immediately seek treatment (and, by implication, a bad woman will "selfishly" ignore her own need for treatment), and that pharmaceutical products are the cure not only for depression but for an unhappy family.

Similarly, another 2005 Zoloft cartoon ad features 28-year-old Molly, who decided to seek help after her boyfriend noticed her "down mood." Molly reports, "I told him that it wasn't his fault. It was my problem." In the next frame, Molly realizes she has a medical problem, discovers Zoloft, and visits her (male) doctor. The caption for the ad reads, "Molly knew she had to do something about her depression." The message that *Molly* had to change allocates blame for the problems to Molly alone.

Encouraging Women's Self-Surveillance

Along with blaming women for not addressing their emotional problems, women are encouraged to engage in self-surveillance to identify those pro-blems early. Sixty-two percent of antidepressant DTCA ($N = 128$) suggest that women are responsible for monitoring their emotions, behaviors, and "symptoms" that fall on the border between emotional and physical conditions (appetite loss, difficulty concentrating, or sleep troubles). For instance, 17 Effexor ads feature only a woman and ask, "Are depression symptoms keeping you from where you want to be?" These ads then provide readers with a list of questions to use in assessing their emotional state, including, "Not involved with family and friends the way you used to be?" "Low on energy?" "Not motivated to do the things you once looked forward to doing?" and "Not feeling as good as you used to?" Because these ads feature women, they are especially likely to encourage women (rather than men) readers to unfavorably compare their present emotions with their past emotions and to define any changes as evidence of treatable depression.

Similarly, 13 Cymbalta ads feature only a woman and encourage readers to reinterpret their feelings and bodily experiences as signs of depression. The ads say, "You might feel sad or hopeless. You could have vague aches and pains, or even a backache. Many people wouldn't think of these as symptoms of depression." They then encourage readers to "Visit depressionhurts.com. You'll find a simple checklist of symptoms [of depression]. Compare it to what you're feeling. Then tell your doctor or healthcare professional what you're feeling." Thus, these facilitate and encourage women to evaluate their experiences, emotions, and physical troubles within a medicalized framework; these 13 ads are the only antidepressant DTCA that warn readers to watch for aches and pains that most would likely interpret purely as physical troubles.

Gendering the Benefits of Treatment: Emphasizing Close Relationships
One consistent finding in the literature on gender norms and femininities is the extent to which girls and women learn to focus their energies on maintaining interpersonal relationships (e.g., Beal, 1994; Chodorow, 1978; Martin & Kazyak, 2009; Rosenfield, Vertefeuille, & McAlpine, 2000; Thorne, 1993). Pharmaceutical manufacturers both reinforce and rely on this expectation in selling antidepressant medications. Almost three-quarters of the ads (73% or 150 ads) paint depression as a barrier between women and their friends or loved ones and portray antidepressant usage as a cure for social isolation. Ad after ad portrays women's isolation before antidepressant use and then shows them happily engaging with friends and loved ones after antidepressant use. For example, a 2003 Effexor advertisement pictures a woman in three scenes: first alone and sad, forehead resting on her hand; then sitting with another woman but neither looking at nor talking with her; and finally facing the woman, smiling, and engaged in

conversation. Advertisers encourage women to "Talk to your doctor about your symptoms, and ask if EFFEXOR XR is right for you." Thus, this ad depicts social isolation as pathological, social engagement as health, and antidepressants as the cure. Similarly, a 2006 Cymbalta advertisement shows an active, healthy, young mother playing in the fall leaves with her two young sons, and another shows a woman resting her head against a man's, both under the caption "Depression hurts emotionally and physically. But you don't have to."

Numerous other ads show women happily ensconced in romantic relationships now that they are taking antidepressants. For example, Wellbutrin published a series of advertisements showing happy couples camping, rowing a boat, or the like. In each advertisement, the woman is shown full face and foreground and the man in profile or on the side, smiling at the woman, suggesting once again that the woman is the subject of the ad and the one targeted for antidepressant usage.

In contrast, only 3% of the ads ($N = 7$) refer to women's productivity at work or in the public domain, and some of these also reference women's interpersonal relationships. For instance, in a 2005 Zoloft ad Denise, a choir director, confesses, "I felt like I was an octave lower before Zoloft. I was depressed. I had to do something." She decides to take Zoloft after learning from her doctor that the drug has "helped millions like me." Denise subsequently declares, "Before long, I realized that Zoloft was helping me *at work and at home.*" (emphasis added).

Gendering Anxiety

Here we focus on ways in which anti-anxiety DTCA utilizes different strategies to target men and women, and the gendered forms of anxiety that are portrayed in ads.

Sexing DTCA Placement

Whereas antidepressant DTCA appeared 15 times more often in women's magazines than in men's magazines, DTCA for anti-anxiety medications appear "only" twice as often in women's magazines: 30% of anti-anxiety medication ads ($N = 34$) were found in women's magazines and only 12% ($N = 14$) were found in men's magazines. The remaining 58% of anti-anxiety medication advertisements ($N = 67$) were found in mixed gender readership magazines, with the majority of these in *People Magazine*. As discussed above, though, *People Magazine* predominantly attracts a female audience

and so DTCA for anti-anxiety medications targets women to a greater
extent than is immediately apparent.

Sexing Anxiety Sufferers
In 1999, when anti-anxiety DTCA first began depicting individuals suffering
from anxiety, ten ads featured women and only one featured a man. During
2000 and 2001, however, men were featured less often than women, and
from 2002 on *no* men were depicted as anxiety sufferers.

Overall from 1997 to 2006, only 23% ($N = 26$) of anti-anxiety DTCA
depict men as suffering from anxiety. In contrast, 59% ($N = 68$) explicitly
depict sufferers as female. Eighteen percent ($N = 25$) depict the androgynous
Zoloft bubble or do not show any anxiety sufferers.

Alerting Men and Women, Mostly About Women
As was true for antidepressant DTCA, anti-anxiety DTCA in men's
magazines primarily alert men to *women's* anxiety: 71% of such ads
($N = 10$) depict female anxiety sufferers, whereas only 29% ($N = 4$) depict
male sufferers. Similarly, 53% of anti-anxiety DTCA in women's magazines
($N = 18$) depict female sufferers, compared to 29% ($N = 10$) that depict male
sufferers. Thus, like antidepressant ads, anti-anxiety ads primarily depict
women sufferers, regardless of whether ads appear in men's or women's
magazines. (The remaining ads could not be coded by sex.) Common
readership magazines show a similar pattern: 56% ($N = 39$) of anti-anxiety
DTCA depict women sufferers, 17% ($N = 12$) depict male sufferers, and 27%
cannot be coded by sex. Thus, although anti-anxiety ads occasionally alert
readers to men's anxiety, like antidepressant ads, most depict anxiety
disorders as female problems.

Blaming Anxiety Sufferers
As was true for antidepressant DTCA, anti-anxiety DTCA sometimes
suggest that drugs offer an easy solution for irritability, restlessness,
isolation, or anxiety, and, by extension, blame those who do not seek such
solutions. And as with anti-depressant DTCA, such messages more often
appear in ads featuring women. Twenty-six percent of all anti-anxiety
DTCA ($N = 30$) both convey such messages and feature women, compared
to 8% ($N = 9$) that feature men. For example, BuSpar ads depict cartoon
women crouched beneath and struggling to lift written phrases such as "I'm
worried. Why am I so irritable? I'm so restless." The ad asks, "Is that you,
feeling crushed by an onslaught of excessive worry? Good thing there's
something you can do about it. A medication called BuSpar can help."

Similarly, a Paxil ad that depicts a woman wearing a nametag, reads, "If you feel intense and persistent fear, anxiety, even panic from social situations with unfamiliar people, it could be social anxiety disorder." The headline, "Let the world say hello to the real you," implies that the sufferer has chosen to keep the world at bay rather than "letting" it in, and thus suggests that she is to blame for her social problems.

Gendering Self-Surveillance

Almost all anti-anxiety DTCA (91%, $N = 105$ ads) encourage readers to self-examine for signs of anxiety disorder. However, men and women are instructed to be alert for somewhat different sets of symptoms.

Forty-four percent of DTCA in women's magazines focus almost entirely on readers' *feelings*, and all of these depict female sufferers. For instance, BuSpar ads that feature cartoon drawings of women encourage readers to identify with statements such as, "I'm worried," "Why am I so irritable?" "I can't concentrate," and "I'm so restless." Similarly, Zoloft ads suggest treatment for any readers who identify with the statements "You may feel embarrassed when you are in a group. You may worry that you are being judged. You just feel so isolated." All of these ads present lists of emotional problems that are thought to be symptomatic of anxiety disorder and only briefly mention physical manifestations of anxiety. In fact, muscle tension is the only physical sign of anxiety included in ads that depict female sufferers. The remaining 56% of the anti-anxiety DTCA in women's magazines – over half of which feature male anxiety sufferers – present a more balanced list of emotional and physical symptoms of anxiety.

In contrast, 57% of anti-anxiety ads in men's magazines focus on *physical* sensations or behaviors. For instance, Paxil ads for men describe social anxiety disorder as "an intense, persistent fear" (a feeling) but go on to describe it in behavioral terms, including "avoidance of social situations" sometimes leading to heavy alcohol use or suicide and in physical terms, noting that sufferers "may blush, sweat, shake, or even experience a pounding heart." The remaining 43% of the anti-anxiety ads in men's magazines all feature *women* sufferers and present a balanced mix of physical and emotional symptoms of anxiety.

Gendering the Benefits of Treatment

Whereas antidepressant DTCA (which essentially target only women) solely promise stronger bonds with friends and family, anti-anxiety DTCA promise benefits in both close relationships and in the work world. However, these depictions vary along gendered lines.

Although 34% of anti-anxiety DTCA that depict women mentions work in text, none are set in a work context. Ten percent ($N = 7$) do show women wearing clothes that can be interpreted as work attire (suit jackets and dark skirts or slacks), but none of these ads mention work in the text. Instead, they depict women bombarded by phrases such as "I can't sleep," "I'm worried," "I'm always tired," and "I can't concentrate." The reader can only assume, based on the women's attire, that anxiety is affecting their work productivity.

In contrast, *all* anti-anxiety ads that depict men mention work in the text and 35% show them in work settings. For example, the first panel of one Paxil ad shows a business man sitting with a group of colleagues around a conference table, accompanied by the caption "What it is." The second panel shows the same man sitting under an interrogation light, with the caption "What it feels like." The ad's caption warns that persons with untreated social anxiety disorder may "drop out of school…, turn down job promotions or choose unsatisfying jobs beneath their skill level."

Conversely, 29% of ads that depict women show them in close relationships, and 38% include textual references to such relationships. For example, one Effexor ad depicts a woman playing with a small child, accompanied by the caption "Effexor XR helps you…enjoy the company of the people you love."

In contrast, no anti-anxiety DTCA that depict men show them experiencing anxiety in relationships with friends of family. However, all briefly mention dates, as part of a list of life arenas that can be affected by social anxiety disorder. These ads (all from Paxil) state that anxiety sufferers may "drop out of school. Some refuse to date. Some turn down job promotions or choose unsatisfying jobs beneath their skill level. Their anxiety can affect the decisions they make every day. Who they see, what they do, where they go."

CONCLUSIONS

From 1997 to 2006, antidepressant DTCA analyzed for this research overwhelmingly targeted women and depicted depression as a (white) female disorder (cf. Grow et al., 2006; Woodlock, 2005). Anti-anxiety DTCA followed the same pattern, although not to such an extreme extent. In both cases, the portrayal of depression and anxiety disorders as "female" conditions far exceeded sex differences in the prevalence of these disorders found in population surveys (Beidel et al., 2010; Nolen-Hoeksema, 2001).

The portrayal of these affective disorders in DTCA as primarily female problems reflects long-standing Western cultural ideas that define the female body and mind as weak, inferior, and in need of medicalized control (Tuana 1993; Weitz, 2009). Although American doctors no longer label women "hysterical" (at least not publicly), the frequent equation of depression and dysfunctional anxiety with femaleness in DTCA – like the increasing medicalization of menstruation, menopause, post-partum disorder, sexual sensations, and other female experiences – continues the tradition of portraying the female body and mind as fragile and best left to doctors' supervision and control (cf. Barker, 1998; Hartley, 2003; Padamsee, 2011). Moreover, repeated exposure to these ideas in DTCA may not only reflect but also *reinforce* the idea that women are physically and mentally deficient and thus, naturally more at risk than men for affective as well as other disorders (Bandura, 1994; Munce, Robertson, Sansom, & Stewart, 2004).

Ironically, the total absence of nonwhites in the DTCA analyzed in this article may also be problematic, if for opposite reasons. This absence may *reduce* the chances that nonwhite consumers might seek, or doctors might prescribe, potentially beneficial psychotherapeutic drugs. Similarly, DTCA's tendency to link affective disorders to womanhood may *reduce* the chances that men might seek or be offered relief from affective disorders. In addition, the absence of nonwhite characters in DTCA for affective disorders may both reflect and reinforce the disproportionate labeling of nonwhites as either severely mentally ill ("he's not anxious, he's schizophrenic") or lacking in moral character ("she's not depressed, she's just lazy").

Along with framing depression and anxiety disorders as primarily female, both the antidepressant DTCA and, to a lesser extent, the anti-anxiety DTCA analyzed in this study often alerted men to the benefits they might reap if the women in their lives sought treatment. Such advertisements not only *invite* men to critique women (by providing justification for so doing) but also *instruct* men in how to do so. At the same time, these advertisements shift the focus away from both men's behaviors and women's circumstances, and instead locate women's troubles wholly within their own emotional (and biological) constitution.

Meanwhile, the ads often suggested that women had a *responsibility* to seek such treatment for the sake of their loved ones; no such message appeared in ads depicting male sufferers. These ads reflect and reinforce highly traditional expectations of emphasized femininity that require women to comply with and satisfy men's needs and desires (Connell, 2005). In much the same way that advertisements for diet pills or Spanx may teach women to discipline their bodies (cf. Bartky, 1988; Bordo, 1993), these DTCA may teach women to blame themselves for any troubles with their loved ones (no matter the cost to their self-respect) and thus to sacrifice time, money, and energy to change themselves and ameliorate the troubles they have caused.

Moreover, antidepressant DTCA *solely* encouraged women and anti-anxiety DTCA *disproportionately* encouraged women to monitor their *emotions* while encouraging men to monitor their physical *sensations*. These differences cannot be explained on medical grounds, given that diagnostic criteria for depression and anxiety disorders in the American Psychiatric Association's *Diagnostic and Statistical Manual* (2000) indicate sex differences for other disorders but not for these. Instead, the different monitoring strategies presented to men and women in antidepressant and anti-anxiety DTCA appear to reflect marketing strategies based on an awareness of gendered norms. As Connell (2005) describes, hegemonic masculinity requires men to present an aura of "toughness" and competence and to squash any emotions (such as sadness or anxiety) that suggest weakness or, by extension, femininity. In contrast, emotional sensitivity is to some extent inherent in the expectations for emphasized femininity (Connell, 2005).

Finally, both antidepressant and anti-anxiety DTCA suggested that medication would yield benefits for women primarily in their close relationships and for men primarily in their work lives. Thus, these ads reinforce the binary sex divisions implicit in hegemonic masculinity and emphasized femininity, while deemphasizing women's work in the public sphere and men's lives outside of that sphere. This finding contrasts with one previous study on the portrayal of Prozac (Blum & Stracuzzi, 2004) which found that Prozac was disproportionately promoted to women (in popular magazine articles) as a way to overcome their inherent "female weaknesses" and thus, to reach presumed "masculine" levels of productivity and success. Both that study and ours, however, found that discourse surrounding pharmaceutical therapies implicitly reinforces binary sex divisions.

At a broader level, DTCA studied for this article suggest to both women and men that individuals should monitor themselves and others for a wide variety of common emotions, behaviors, and physical sensations – far beyond the diagnostic criteria for affective disorders presented in the *Diagnostic and Statistical Manual* (2000). Similarly, these DTCA urge consumers to seek medical treatment if any such "symptoms" are observed, thus potentially encouraging a dramatic expansion of medical authority over everyday life. For this reason, many have argued that (not surprisingly) DTCA appears designed more to sell products than to educate or otherwise help consumers (Bell, Wilkes, & Kravitz, 2000; Hollon, 2005; Kravitz et al., 2005; Lexchin & Mintzes, 2002).

Finally, DTCA may facilitate the "individualization of social problems": the process of locating the source of troubles within individual personalities or behaviors, while ignoring potential social sources of the problem (Conrad, 2007, p. 152). As Horwitz and Wakefield (2007) note, psychiatric practices tend to attribute many social problems to individuals' mental disorders, although sadness "is much more likely to be the result rather than the cause of social problems" (p. 20). None of the DTCA we analyzed portrayed any of the common social factors – such as poverty, abuse, job loss, discrimination – that often affect both men's and women's mental and physical well-being. Instead, they framed affective disorder purely as individual illnesses requiring treatment, thus, obscuring any social underpinnings of the problem and impeding other approaches to the problem.

Our study is limited in its focus on print advertisements for antidepressants and anti-anxiety medications. Future research might evaluate the use of similar techniques in advertisements for other medication categories and other media. That said, our study has several strengths. First, the longitudinal design allowed us to view gendering in DTCA as it occurred in the first 10 years after the 1997 liberalization of the advertising policy, and involves analysis of a broader range of DTCA than in previous studies. Second, we went beyond descriptive data about advertisement placement, and analyzed corresponding messages to more fully understand advertisers' aims and techniques. Third, our design allowed us to compare marketing messages regarding women and men, and regarding both depression and anxiety disorders. Thus, our study provides more depth than previous research and allows for a more thorough examination of medicalization as a gendered phenomenon. Our findings offer insight into the role social phenomena, such as media, play in shaping both patterns of health and illness and cultural ideas about women and men within society.

REFERENCES

American Psychiatric Association (2000). *Diagnostic and Statistical Manual of Mental Disorders* (Revised 4th ed.). Washington, DC: Task Force.

Arney, J., & Rafalovich, A. (2007). Incomplete syllogisms as techniques of medicalization: The case of direct-to-consumer advertising in popular magazines, 1997–2003. *Qualitative Health Research, 17*, 47–60.

Ashton, H. (1991). Psychotropic drug prescribing for women. *British Journal of Psychiatry, 158*, 30–35.

Bandura, A. (1994). Social cognitive theory of mass communication. In J. Bryant & D. Zillman (Eds.), *Media effects: Advances in theory and research* (pp. 61–90). Hillsdale, NJ: Lawrence Erlbaum Associates, Inc.

Barker, K. (1998). A ship upon a stormy sea: The medicalization of pregnancy. *Social Science and Medicine, 47,* 1067–1076.

Bartky, S. (1988). Foucault, femininity and the modernization of patriarchal power. In L. Quinby & I. Diamond (Eds.), *Feminism and Foucault: Paths of resistance* (pp. 61–86). Boston, MA: Northeastern University Press.

Beal, C. R. (1994). *Boys and girls: The development of gender roles.* New York, NY: McGraw Hill.

Beidel, D. C., Bulik, C. M., & Stanley, M. A. (2010). *Abnormal psychology: A scientist-practitioner approach.* New York, NY: Prentice Hall.

Bell, R. A., Wilkes, M. S., & Kravitz, R. L. (2000). The educational value of consumer-targeted prescription drug print advertising. *Journal of Family Practice, 49,* 1092–1098.

Blum, L. M., & Stracuzzi, N. F. (2004). Gender in the Prozac nation: Popular discourse and productive femininity. *Gender & Society, 18,* 269–286.

Bordo, S. (1993). *Unbearable weight: Feminism, western culture and the body.* Berkeley, CA: University of California Press.

Brown, P. (1995). Naming and framing: The social construction of diagnosis and illness. *Journal of Health and Social Behavior, 35,* Extra Issue: Forty Years of Medical Sociology: The State of the Art and Directions for the Future, pp. 34–52.

Chananie, R. A. (2005). Psychopharmaceutical advertising strategies: Empowerment in a pill? *Sociological Spectrum, 25,* 487–518.

Charmaz, K. (2006). *Constructing grounded theory: A practical guide through qualitative analysis.* Los Angeles, CA: Sage.

Chodorow, N. (1978). *The reproduction of mothering: Psychoanalysis and the sociology of gender.* Berkeley, CA: University of California Press.

Connell, R. (2005). *Masculinities* (2nd ed.). Cambridge: Polity Press.

Conrad, P. (2005). The shifting engines of medicalization. *Journal of Health and Social Behavior, 46,* 3–14.

Conrad, P. (2007). *The medicalization of society: On the transformation of human conditions into treatable disorders.* Baltimore, MD: The Johns Hopkins University Press.

Conrad, P., & Leiter, V. (2004). Medicalization, markets, and consumers. *Journal of Health and Social Behavior, 45,* 158–176.

Conrad, P., & Leiter, V. (2008). From Lydia Pinkham to Queen Levitra: Direct-to-consumer advertising and medicalization. *Sociology of Health and Illness, 30,* 825–838.

Ehrenreich, B., & English, D. (2005). *For her own good: Two centuries of the experts' advice to women.* New York, NY: Anchor.

Emmons, K. K. (2010). *Black dogs and blue words: Depression and gender in the age of self-care.* New Brunswick, NJ: Rutgers University Press.

Feinman, J. (Ed.). (1979). *Sears Roebuck and Company Incorporated 1909 Catalog.* New York, NY: Ventura Books, Inc.

Glaser, B. G. (1978). *Theoretical sensitivity: Advances in the methodology of grounded theory.* Mill Valley, CA: Sociology Press.

Glaser, B. G., & Strauss, A. L. (1967). *The discovery of grounded theory: Strategies for qualitative research.* Chicago, IL: Aldine.

Greenslit, N. (2005). Depression and consumption: Psychopharmaceuticals, branding, and new identity practices. *Culture, Medicine and Psychiatry, 29*, 477–501.

Grow, J. M., Park, J. S., & Han, X. (2006). Your life is waiting!" Symbolic meanings in direct-to-consumer antidepressant advertising. *Journal of Communication Inquiry, 30*, 163–188.

Hartley, H. (2003). "Big Pharma" in our bedrooms: An analysis of the medicalization of women's sexual problems. *Advances in Gender Research, 7*, 89–129.

Hollon, M. F. (2005). Direct-to-consumer advertising: A haphazard approach to health promotion. *Journal of the American Medical Association, 293*, 2030–2033.

Horwitz, A. V., & Wakefield, J. C. (2007). *The loss of sadness: How psychiatry transformed normal sorrow into depressive disorder.* Oxford: Oxford University Press.

IMS Health. (2002). *Doctors and DTC.* Retrieved from http://www.imshealth.com/portal/site/imshealth/menuitem.a46c6d4df3db4b3d88f611019418c22a/?vgnextoid = a4b68 ede1ca19110VgnVCM10000071812ca2RCRD&vgnextfmt = default. Accessed on January 5, 2012.

IMS Health. (2009). *U.S. pharmaceutical market trends: Tremendous slowdown.* Retrieved from http://www.imshealth.com/portal/site/imshealth/menuitem.a46c6d4df3db4b3d88f61101 9418c22a/?vgnextoid = bd34c71e81a32210VgnVCM100000ed152ca2RCRD&vgnextfmt = default. Accessed on January 5, 2012.

IMS Health. (2010a). *2009 U.S. sales and prescription information.* Retrieved from http:// www.imshealth.com/deployedfiles/imshealth/Global/Content/StaticFile/Top_Line_Data/ PromoUpdate2009.pdf. Accessed on January 5, 2012.

IMS Health. (2010b). *IMS Health reports U.S. prescription drug sales grew 5.1 percent in 2009, to $300.3 billion.* Retrieved from http://www.imshealth.com/portal/site/imshealth/ menuitem.a46c6d4df3db4b3d88f611019418c22a/?vgnextoid = d690a27e9d5b7210Vgn VCM100000ed152ca2RCRD&vgnextfmt = default. Accessed on January 5, 2012.

Kravitz, R. L., Epstein, R. M., Feldman, M. D., Franz, C. E., Azari, R., Wilkes, M. S., et al. (2005). Influence of patients' requests for direct-to-consumer advertised antidepressants. *Journal of the American Medical Association, 293*, 1995–2002.

Leavitt, J. W. (Ed.). (1999). *Women and health in America* (2nd ed.). Madison, WI: University of Wisconsin Press.

Lexchin, J., & Mintzes, B. (2002). Direct-to-consumer advertising of prescription drugs: The evidence says no. *Journal of Public Policy and Marketing, 21*, 194–202.

Loe, M. (2004). *The rise of Viagra: How the little blue pill changed sex in America.* New York, NY: New York University Press.

Martin, K. A., & Kazyak, E. (2009). Hetero-romantic love and heterosexiness in children's G-rated films. *Gender and Society, 23*, 315–336.

Mirowsky, J., & Ross, C. E. (2005). Measurement for a human science. *Journal of Health and Social Behavior, 43*, 152–170.

Munce, S. E. P., Robertson, E. K., Sansom, S. N., & Stewart, D. E. (2004). Who is portrayed in psychotropic drug advertisements? *The Journal of Nervous and Mental Disease, 192*, 284–288.

Newsweek Media Kit. (2011). *The audience every marketer seeks.* Retrieved from http:// mediakit.newsweekdailybeast.com/combined.html. Accessed on January 4, 2012.

Niederdeppe, J., Hornik, R. C., Kelly, B. J., Frosch, D. L., Romantan, A., Stevens, R. S., et al. (2007). Examining the dimensions of cancer-related information seeking and scanning behavior. *Health Communication, 22*, 153–167.

Nolen-Hoeksema, S. (2001). Gender differences in depression. *Current Directions in Psychological Science, 10,* 173–176.

Padamsee, T. J. (2011). The pharmaceutical corporation and the 'good work' of managing women's bodies. *Social Science & Medicine, 72,* 1342–1350.

People Media Kit. (2011). *People: 2011 Rate Card.* Retrieved from http://www.people.com/people/static/mediakit/media/pdf/ratecard.pdf. Accessed on January 4, 2012.

Pines, W. L. (1999). A history and perspective on direct-to-consumer promotion. *Food and Drug Law Journal, 54,* 489–518.

Reader's Digest Online Media Kit. (2011). *Demographic profile – Adults.* Retrieved from www.blueskyagency.com/ClientApprovals/RD/OMK/fullSite/demographics.html. Accessed on January 4, 2012.

Riessman, C. K. (Summer 1983). Women and medicalization: A new perspective. *Social Policy, 14,* 3–18.

Riska, E. (2003). Gendering the medicalization thesis. In M. T. Segal, V. Demos & J. J. Kronenfeld (Eds.), *Advances in gender research series, Vol 7: Gender Perspectives on Health and Medicine* (pp. 59–87). Bingley: Emerald Group Publishing, Ltd.

Rosenfeld, D., & Faircloth, C. A. (Eds.). (2006). *Medicalized masculinities.* Philadelphia, PA: Temple University Press.

Rosenfield, S., Vertefeuille, J., & McAlpine, D. D. (2000). Gender stratification and mental health: An exploration of dimensions of the self. *Social Psychology Quarterly, 63,* 208–223.

Strauss, A., & Corbin, J. (1990). *Basics of qualitative research: Grounded theory procedures and techniques.* Newbury Park, CA: Sage.

Thorne, B. (1993). *Gender play: Girls and boys in school.* New Brunswick, NJ: Rutgers University Press.

Time Media Kit. (2011) *U.S. Audience Profile.* Retrieved from www.timemediakit.com/us/index.html. Accessed on January 4, 2012.

Tuana, N. (1993). *The less noble sex: Scientific, religious, and philosophical conceptions of woman's nature.* Bloomington, IN: Indiana University Press.

Weitz, R. (2009). A history of women's bodies. In R. Weitz (Ed.), *The politics of women's bodies* (3rd Ed., pp. 3–12). New York, NY: Oxford University Press.

Wertz, R., & Wertz, D. (1989). *Lying-in: A history of childbirth in America.* New Haven, CT: Yale University Press.

Woodlock, D. (2005). Virtual pushers: Antidepressant internet marketing and women. *Women's Studies International Forum, 28,* 304–314.

"MORE THAN BOOBS AND OVARIES": BRCA POSITIVE YOUNG WOMEN AND THE NEGOTIATION OF MEDICALIZATION IN AN ONLINE MESSAGE BOARD

Elena Frank

ABSTRACT

The discovery of the BRCA1 and BRCA2 genes has facilitated the construction of a new group of women referred to as "previvors" – individuals who are survivors of a predisposition to cancer but who are not presently ill. These "previvors" constitute the first generation of women faced with the option to make preventative health choices based on this kind of genetic information. Therefore, this research examines how young BRCA positive women negotiate the medicalization of their bodies based on their new "potentially ill" status. Analyzing the posts in an online forum specifically for "young previvors," the findings indicate that the majority share an "anything's better than cancer" mantra, suggesting that fear of death largely outweighs all other fears or concerns. Consequently, asserting control by taking preventative action is considered a mechanism for quelling the fear, uncertainty, and stress associated with being a BRCA gene carrier. Constructed as a medical

Issues in Health and Health Care Related to Race/Ethnicity, Immigration, SES and Gender
Research in the Sociology of Health Care, Volume 30, 181–199
Copyright © 2012 by Emerald Group Publishing Limited
All rights of reproduction in any form reserved
ISSN: 0275-4959/doi:10.1108/S0275-4959(2012)0000030011

diagnosis, carrying the BRCA mutation is consequently perceived as requiring a corresponding medical treatment. As such, despite the connection these women describe feeling with the "parts that make them a woman," they appear to believe that they must undergo prophylactic surgery and disassociate from their bodies in order to save their lives. Ultimately, they convince themselves to view their breasts and ovaries simply as nonessential organs, rather than as core components of their feminine, sexual, and reproductive identities.

Keywords: Gender; women; BRCA; previvors; cancer

The discovery of the BRCA1 and BRCA2 genes at the end of the twentieth century facilitated the construction of a new group of women sometimes referred to as "previvors" – individuals who are survivors of a predisposition to cancer but who have not actually had the disease ("Cancer Previvors," n.d.). According to the National Cancer Institute, carriers of either BRCA gene are approximately five times more likely to develop breast cancer and approximately seven to seventy times more likely to develop ovarian cancer in their lifetime than the general population. These estimates are based on previous research which indicates that carriers of the BRCA1 or BRCA2 gene have anywhere from a 50% to 80% lifetime risk of developing breast cancer and anywhere from a 15% to 40% lifetime risk of developing ovarian cancer ("BRCA1 and BRCA2", 2009).

BRCA gene "previvors" constitute the first generation of women faced with the option to make preventative health choices based on this kind of genetic information. As a result, these choices are not easy ones to make. Moreover, none of these options completely eliminate the risk of cancer, and all of them are accompanied by side effects or increases in noncancer health risks (Happe, 2006). Women who carry a BRCA gene are generally presented with a variety of medical options to decrease or delay their risk of getting cancer. As the least invasive preventative option, surveillance generally consists of regular cancer screening in the form of such procedures as mammography, clinical breast exams, magnetic resonance imaging (MRI), transvaginal ultrasound, or blood tests for specific antigens. Chemoprevention consists of taking a drug, such as Tamoxifen or Raloxifene, which is intended to reduce the risk of developing cancer in the future. The most invasive option, prophylactic surgery usually consists of a bilateral mastectomy, which is the removal of both breasts, or an oophorectomy, which is the removal of the fallopian tubes and ovaries ("BRCA1 and BRCA2", 2009).

There have been many critiques of genetic testing for the BRCA gene, with some researchers concluding that the benefits are quite limited. Brédart, Autier, Riccardo, Audisio, and Geraghty (2001) summarize some of these critiques, explaining that routine testing for the BRCA gene would be wasteful since research indicates that over 90% of those tested would be negative. They also argue that the role of other genetic factors, or those that may be hormonal, dietary, or environmental, are not considered in determining whether the BRCA mutation will cause cancer in a given individual. Moreover, since the BRCA genes were discovered only a little over a decade ago, there is no conclusive data regarding the effectiveness of the various preventative strategies. Finally, because some BRCA gene carriers will never develop cancer, many individuals will undergo unnecessary procedures with no benefits.

MEDICALIZATION AND COMMERCIALIZATION

Despite these critiques, BRCA testing continues to increase as the cancer establishment pushes screening, corporations benefit, and the news media promotes an overgeneticized image of cancer. The "fear [they create] ... increases demand for services" (Zones, 2000). According to Conrad (1997), individuals utilize news media and public discourses as significant resources for making meaning of various social phenomena and their own lives. In the case of genetic predictors of cancer, not only do these discourses generate fear, but Conrad argues that they tend to present an "overgeneticized" image (p. 149). As a result, individuals are convinced that their genetic status is the most primary or only factor in determining their risk for cancer, so they consequently seek out genetic testing. Conrad (2005) contends that this promotion of genetic testing contributes to medicalization today.

As a result, whereas previously an individual's family history of cancer served as the primary predictor for future illness, at present any carrier of the BRCA mutation is considered at risk, regardless of family history. According to Happe (2006), "... what counts as ... 'actionable' risk has shifted ... . A consensus is slowly emerging regarding prophylactic surgery as a rational, commonsense option for all women with inherited genetic mutations" (p. 172). Many doctors and researchers now suggest that BRCA positive women reprioritize their family and reproductive goals in order to *possibly* reduce their potential cancer risk by undergoing prophylactic surgery.

In essence, then, designation as a BRCA mutation carrier is now seen not simply as a risk, but as a *diagnosis* that requires a corresponding *treatment*.

Moreover, an *actionable* treatment such as prophylactic surgery is frequently recommended over a more *passive* treatment such as surveillance. In this cancer discourse "potentially ill" status is synonymous with illness itself, with the BRCA mutation "… functioning essentially as a trope for a disease" that often necessitates surgery (Happe, 2006, p. 174). Ultimately, "heredity … and risk [define] the disease" (pp. 179–180).

THE EXPERIENCE OF (POTENTIAL) ILLNESS

This research examines how BRCA mutation carriers represent their experience of potential illness on an online message board. While much research exists on women's experiences of breast cancer, only a handful of studies examine women's experiences as BRCA gene carriers. Much of this research has been conducted from a psychological perspective, with the goal of determining stress and distress levels related to the testing process itself. One study by Croyle, Smith, Botkin, Baty, and Nash (1997) specifically examines predictors of psychological distress following BRCA testing for female carriers and noncarriers. The results indicate that mutation carriers possess more symptoms of distress than noncarriers, and that the women who experience the greatest distress are those who never have experienced cancer or cancer-related surgery previously, but tested positive for the BRCA gene. However, Croyle, Smith, Botkin, Baty, and Nash also found that distress tends to decline by approximately 20% one to two weeks after the test regardless of carrier status, suggesting that some anxiety may be relieved simply by finding out the test results. While useful for understanding the psychological effects of the genetic testing process on the individual, studies like these do not capture the experience of living over time with the BRCA gene.

Previous research suggests that most individuals conceive of knowledge gained from genetic testing as beneficial. A study by Bradbury et al. (2009) on the experiences and impact of a parent's genetic status to his or her offspring in communication of genetic risk confirms this idea, in that findings indicate that offspring "… identified the potential to engage in preventative health behaviors as a general benefit to learning of a familial risk at an early age" (p. 205). However, Mahowald et al. (1996) suggest that this same information may increase pressures and evoke additional burdens for some women. Press, Fishman, and Koenig (2000) relate our society's underlying obsession with obtaining knowledge about risk with the concept of uncertainty. Many women may seek out genetic testing in order to mitigate their uncertainty about when or if they will develop cancer;

however, in this case they may often find that these risk statistics raise more questions for them than produce answers.

Previous research on how individuals cope with the uncertainty of illness suggests that for many individuals the primary mechanism for managing this uncertainty may revolve around "... finding ways at least to *feel* that they [are] in control of their lives" (Weitz, 1989, p. 272). In the case of BRCA gene carriers, this suggests that many women might seek a feeling of control by choosing an *actionable* treatment method such as prophylactic surgery in order to quell their feelings of uncertainty regarding when or if they will develop cancer. In the case of AIDS, research also indicates that some individuals fear the knowledge that could be gained by getting tested. They prefer ignorance based on their fear of how the knowledge of testing positive might affect their psychological health (Weitz, 1989). This concept could likely apply to testing for the BRCA gene as well, in that some women may prefer not to be faced with the questions and choices that arise from learning of a positive carrier status.

There are only a few studies that have specifically focused on examining the lived experience of being a BRCA mutation carrier. In a 2007 qualitative study of young women living with the BRCA gene who do not have cancer, Werner-Lin asserts that "... family experiences with cancer, genetic testing, and interactions with medical professionals,... [as well as] issues around partnering, sexuality, various pathways to parenthood, and career development" are important themes that become particularly salient as these women consider the possibility of undergoing prophylactic surgery (p. 339). Werner-Lin's findings also indicate the identification of "danger zones" by participants, meaning "... specific ages at which cancer risk was believed to increase dramatically" (p. 341). In a follow-up study, Werner-Lin (2008) also notes the importance of coming from a "cancer family" for a young woman in terms of thinking of family planning and development because of the looming genetic threat of illness (p. 427). Other significant findings relate to how the meaning of genetic testing and choosing treatment options changes depending on the individuals partner status, in that those women with long-term life partners may be more likely to choose to undergo surgery, as well as how the meaning of being a BRCA gene carrier and having undergone prophylactic surgery may inhibit a woman's sexuality (pp. 427–428). The results of this study suggest that there are many factors at every level of the testing and decision-making processes that may change the meaning and experience of illness for these young women, which certainly warrant further investigation.

Babb et al. (2002) conducted a qualitative study comparing BRCA positive women who underwent a prophylactic oophorectomy with women who were currently undergoing ovarian cancer surveillance. They found that more than 90% of the participants in both groups reported being satisfied with their decision. Also significant was that both groups reported obtaining medical information as being central to their decision-making process. In addition, the researchers identified four specific categories that had a noteworthy impact on the participants' decision-making process that varied for individuals depending on their personal perceptions and attitudes as follows: (1) risk perception and fear; (2) perceived impact of surgery; (3) personal perceptions of sexuality, fertility, and femininity; and (4) personal relationships with individuals with cancer and personal experiences with death (p. 91). These findings are important for understanding the wide array of considerations that women identified as BRCA gene carriers must take into account in deciding how to proceed with their lives and whether or not to pursue preventative health options.

THE INTERNET AND EXPERIENCE OF ILLNESS

Increasingly, individuals living with illness have turned to cyber-message boards for support and information, especially people with stigmatizing or rare disorders (White & Dorman, 2001). Because of the high level of anonymity provided by these groups, many individuals may be more likely to express themselves more frequently and honestly than otherwise. Moreover, participation in an online support group is not as physically demanding as attending one in person, and the benefits of having access to individuals with similar problems around the world are substantial. These online groups also encourage more participation than in-person support groups because they are accessible 24 hours a day. Despite technically being a public forum, moreover, these message boards provide an illusion of privacy that encourages full disclosure from its participants. Consequently, an analysis of online message boards reflects the way ill, or in this case, potentially ill individuals speak to *each other*, rather than how they respond to researchers' or doctors' inquiries. Indeed, the internet may be the most frequently utilized source for seeking additional information on the BRCA gene and cancer risk for offspring after being told of their parent's positive carrier status (Bradbury et al., 2009). This finding, in conjunction with the relative rareness of encountering another BRCA positive individual in day-to-day life and the potential stigma involved with having breast or ovarian cancer, suggests that young BRCA mutation carriers may be particularly likely to seek out information and support on the internet.

Recent research on the experience of illness as expressed on online support groups may be relevant to studying the experience of living with the BRCA gene. One study of an HIV/AIDS online support group found that there are five common types of social support that are generally expressed, including informational, emotional, tangible, esteem, and social network support (Phoenix & Coulson, 2008). These forms of social support are likely applicable to BRCA positive women seeking social support online as well. Other research indicates that men with prostate cancer primarily seek informational support, while women with breast cancer prefer social and emotional support in an online setting (Seale, Ziebland, & Charteris-Black, 2006). Women also appear to be more likely to use language associated with emotions, people, and appearance. One particularly interesting finding is that both sexes appear to express themselves more openly, honestly, and comfortably in the more "private" online forum than in interviews with researchers. This finding suggests that examination of an online message board as the primary sampling frame may yield more accurate data than through other methods when it comes to studying the experience of illness.

Other research indicates that there may be waves in which breast cancer patients' communication needs occur, starting with concern, prediagnosis, and postdiagnosis, and then concluding with postsurgery, recovery and follow-up treatment, and end-of-life issues (Radin, 2006). In addition, Kenen, Shapiro, Friedman, and Coyne's (2007) research on a message board specifically for women at risk for breast and ovarian cancer indicates that "while the provision of emotional support was a key element, the women were also eager to learn about the latest scientific and medical data," often citing information from professional journals as well as contact information for medical facilities and relevant organizations in their posts (p. 765). This plays into the idea that the Internet's role as a "massive expert database...a global broker...[and] a global collective memory" can be a promoter of change in how cancer is experienced as an illness (Radin, 2006, p. 593). This is important to think about in terms of the role that this Internet communication may have on the possibilities for how individual women may manage their status as BRCA gene carriers.

METHOD

The main goal of this research was to gain an understanding of women's experience living with the BRCA gene through the analysis of an online support group. The primary research question for this project was as follows: How do young BRCA positive women negotiate the medicalization of their bodies based on their new status as "potentially ill" individuals? A passive content analysis of a message board located on the *Facing Our Risk of Cancer Empowered (FORCE)* website (http://www.facingourrisk.org) was conducted. FORCE is an organization dedicated to improving the lives of individuals and families affected by hereditary breast and ovarian cancer. This research specifically examined the posts initiated by BRCA positive women who were not currently diagnosed with cancer. The "Young Previvor's Forum" was specifically for "young women who are facing issues specific to being high-risk and without cancer to discuss their experiences and support one another," so this message board occupied the primary site of analysis ([6]"FORCE Message Board Forum Index", n.d.). The majority of the women starting threads in this forum identified themselves to be in their twenties or early thirties and were recently informed of their BRCA carrier status. Most also appeared to be very interested in and strongly considering undergoing a prophylactic bilateral mastectomy or oophorectomy.

An initial reading of the message board was conducted in order to identify specific themes related to the primary research question. The sample from the "Young Previvors Forum" included in this analysis consisted of all topics and the corresponding response threads posted between July 19, 2008 and September 30, 2008. This included 35 topic threads and a total of 198 individual posts. This date range only applies to when the initial topic thread was started. Consequently, the sample contained individual posts past these date ranges as responses within these topic threads. Because this particular group did not require a subscription to view or post messages, this forum could be considered a public domain. As a result, informed consent was not required. Pseudonyms were used for all screen names to preserve the posters' anonymity.

There are several important limitations relating to the sample in this study that are important to note. First, because women are generally not tested for the BRCA gene unless they become ill or are aware of a relatives' BRCA positive status, it makes sense that the majority of the women posting on the FORCE website share this aspect of the experience. This is not necessarily a problem, however, because this is more or less reflective of those in the general population who have been notified of their BRCA status. Second, this analysis does not account for female BRCA mutation carriers who may read the posts on the FORCE messages boards, but not initiate posts themselves. Consequently, it is possible that those women who do choose to ask questions and share their experiences are a self-selected group who are particularly interested in pursuing prophylactic surgery. Third, it is essential to remember that this analysis is based on how these women identify and represent themselves in an online forum. While it seems unlikely that many posters would purposively misrepresent themselves in this type of forum, it is important to consider that misrepresentation is possible.

RESULTS

Poster Characteristics

The FORCE message board allows for posters to register as users and create a unique personalized screen name, post as a guest and provide a temporary screen name, or post solely as "guest." Within the time frame analyzed, in the "Young Previvors Forum" the posts can be broken down as follows: 49 registered users and 47 guests. It is important to note that the guest postings may include multiple postings by the same person, but there is no way to measure this because they did not choose a unique identifier. Of the registered users and guests who provided a temporary screen name, 54 only posted one time, with 30 posting more than once. The average number of posts for those who posted multiple times was 4.5. Based on the 52 posters in this forum who identified their age, the average was 30 years old, and ranged from 21 to 44.

Two main groups of women started threads in this forum: (1) women who were recently informed of their BRCA positive status and were seeking general information about their preventative options, as well as emotional support, and (2) women who were recently informed of their BRCA positive status and were seeking specific medical information. Many of these posts follow a similar format in that they generally consist of discussion of the following components: (1) the illness or death of one or more close female relative(s) from breast or ovarian cancer, (2) own age and experience of finding out BRCA positive carrier status, (3) current family status or future plans for family, and (4) request for advice or statement of uncertainty about how to proceed with this knowledge. Many of the response posts follow an abbreviated version of this format as well, appearing to seek to provide a sense of solidarity and emotional support for their fellow "young previvors" by demonstrating that they have undergone similar experiences.

Content and Themes

Rejecting Medicalization
Discussion of the consequences of undergoing a prophylactic bilateral mastectomy or oophorectomy, or hysterectomy, largely dominated in the "Young Previvors Forum," with 87 distinct posts referring to prophylactic

bilateral mastectomy and 34 posts referring to oophorectomy or hysterectomy in some way. In the course of engaging with this topic with other BRCA gene carriers these women express both rejection and acceptance of the medicalization model. They appear to reject medicalization in two primary ways: (1) by expressing their concerns about choosing to make themselves ill and hurt their own body knowing that they are currently healthy young women, and (2) expressing a sense of loss with regard to what "makes them a woman" – their femininity, sexuality, and reproductive potential.

Many women reject the potential medicalization of their bodies by expressing their apprehension about having to "become sick" in order to decrease the risk of future illness.

The thought of having to mutilate [my body] was devastating to me. *Jackie*

We have a son who is 16 months old ... and the thought of becoming sick, leaving him and my husband, etc. makes me extremely upset. *Mgreen*

I'm still not convinced that removing a healthy body part will prevent cancer from appearing elsewhere, if I'm already predisposed. Seeing my mother go through a lifetime of repeated painful surgeries (and her related emotional trauma) makes me unwilling to subject myself to it if I don't have to. *Steinfriend*

These women also appear to be preoccupied with normalcy, expressing concerns about feeling both internally and visibly deviant as a result of the medicalization of their bodies.

I feel like I'm different and damaged. *NancyT*

Not only am I vain about the way I look, but I feel somewhat vain about who I am. I don't want everyone to know for the rest of my life that something is wrong with me. That I am defective in some way. *Jnfr82*

While a number of women posting in this forum express concerns about becoming ill, many more appear to be overcome by a sense of loss with regard to their femininity, sexuality, and reproductive potential. They fear that the medicalization of their bodies will strip them of both the physical, and subsequently emotional, aspects that comprise their identity as women. Consequently, some women assert a newfound connection with and love for what they view as the physical manifestations of their femininity – their breasts and ovaries.

I'm 23 and BRCA2 + and just don't think that I am at a point in my life (unmarried, no kids) when I am willing to lose all those parts that make me feel female. *Apding04*

I'm so afraid of losing all that makes me a woman. It sounds so vain ... but I can't help it. *Guest*

[I'm] worried about viewing my body as deformed and not feeling at home in my body as well as having to say goodbye to my breasts. However I find that part strange as well. I've never really been attached to my small A cups until finding out my BRCA 1 + status. Now, all of a sudden I've become fiercely attached to them when before I complained of their small size ... Odd how that works. *Jackie*

Some of these young women also express concerns regarding the effect that the medicalization of their bodies may have on future romantic and sexual interactions. They frequently use the term "foobs" to describe their future "fake boobs."

One of the reasons that I sought to have this done earlier was because I felt like that if I make this decision before I have my family and get married then I wouldn't have to deal with issues of being in a marriage where I knew my husband would know how I looked before and after ... personally I felt that if I were to do this before I got married that my husband would already be aware and 'really' know what he is going to marry into. *Teeny22*

Yes I have a wonderful BF who supports my decision and told me I'm going to be beautiful but if when he sees my 'foobs' and he's repulsed ... or what if we break up and I have to explain to other men about my 'situation'? *Jackie*

One final way that some of these women reject the medicalization model is by expressing a desire for "natural" motherhood – something that they cannot achieve after undergoing a mastectomy or oophorectomy. They emphasize the importance of physically carrying and birthing a child themselves, as well as breast feeding, to their role as "mother."

I want to be 'whole' when I am having children. *Mgreen*

Both me and my fiancé want kids, and probably at least two of them. Though I read a lot about women deciding very early to have mastectomies, my bigger concern is the ovarian cancer. My tentative plan is to have kids ... ideally ... a few of them at the same time because I would like to have my ovaries removed shortly thereafter. *Sweetiepie123*

Accepting Medicalization

While a number of women express concerns in their message board posts that suggest a rejection of the medicalization model, the majority of the posters in the "Young Previvors Forum" overwhelmingly indicate an ultimate acceptance of medicalization; with many encouraging each other to accept and embrace this medicalization of their bodies. The women appear to accept and advocate for the medicalization model in three primary ways: (1) expressing the belief that cancer is inevitable for all BRCA gene carriers, (2) constructing the BRCA mutation as a medical diagnosis that requires a corresponding preventative medical treatment, and (3) choosing surgery over the "all the parts that make them a woman."

When, Not If
Regardless of individual women's circumstances or risk factors, the posters on this message board overwhelmingly appear to believe that cancer is inevitable for all BRCA gene carriers. They seem to buy into the "cancer panic" spread by the medical industry and the media, and consequently the medicalization model, by conceiving that their genes override all other risk factors.

> I have always felt it wasn't a matter of IF I got cancer, but when. *Rachel1982*

> I can't live my life waiting for the other shoe to drop. I know I'll stop living and start waiting and stressing. Plus ... I'll be SO angry at myself if I don't do the PBM [prophylactic bilateral mastectomy] and end up w/ BC [breast cancer] anyway. *Jackie*

These women further support the medicalization model by expressing their support for genetic testing in general, in that the information gained can and should be utilized to plan for the future.

> I think the best thing about knowing our gene status is that we can plan (for the most part) appropriately. It allows us the opportunity to really research options and not make a hasty decision. We are lucky because of this; unlucky because of watching close family members fight what we hope we never will have to. *Megan C*

> Knowledge is power and unlike many of our family members before us we did have the gift of knowledge. *Andrea*

The BRCA Gene "Diagnosis"
It becomes apparent by the way that these women talk about themselves as being "cancer time bombs," that they consider notification of their BRCA gene carrier status to be a sort of medical diagnosis rather than simply a genetic fact. Consequently, they appear to support medicalization by constructing prophylactic surgery as an active treatment option, with nonsurgical surveillance options positioned as more passive. Exerting control by taking preventative action becomes constructed as a mechanism for quelling the fear, uncertainty, and stress associated with being a BRCA gene carrier.

> I want to take control; I don't want to feel like a cancer time bomb waiting to go off. *Jackie*

> For me it is a sence [sic] of control ... instead of being scarred [sic] and waiting for the cancer to find me ... I'm going to GET IT!! Cancer sucks, and if I can do something to avoid it altogether I will. *Diane*

> The stress was too much for me so I decided to have surgery. *Mercedes*

These women do not appear to view themselves as overmedicalized individuals, nor do they perceive the concept of overtreatment as problematic, as long as it reduces their risk or even their stress about their future risk of getting cancer. Their posts suggest that they view the additional risks and pain associated with surgery as better than the only perceived alternative – cancer.

> Just seems weird to face menopause before I've even hit thirty! Oh well, it's better than cancer! *Rel898*

> I totally understand ... about not doing the surgery until I am comfortable w/ it and know it's what I really want. But I don't think it will ever be what I really want. However I don't want breast cancer more! *Jackie*

Some women further express their acceptance of the medicalization model with their assertion that they feel a newfound alienation from their bodies after notification of their BRCA "diagnosis." They use this idea that their body has turned against them in order to rationalize the need to "take action" and regain control of their bodies by undergoing prophylactic surgery.

> I have to admit, at 26 I love the way I look. I love my boobs. I love that they are mine. And I hate that they have turned against me. *Jnfr82*

> I'm sure there will be small imperfections but at least my new tatas won't kill me. Right? *Jackie*

> I have fantastic breasts now (if I do say so myself) and they are part of me, but they are part of me that is 'dangerous.' I guess I have detached from them ... I don't fool myself into thinking [foobs] will feel the same or even look the same ... but they'll be safe. They won't try to kill me. *Diane*

In addition to expressing their own acceptance of the medicalization of their bodies, many of the women in this forum who have already undergone prophylactic surgery encourage others to accept the medicalization model by focusing on the potential benefits of surgery, such as bigger (or smaller) breasts or a flatter stomach.

> I have to say that my breasts look better than before! I spared my nipples and I think that helped me (mentally) keep thinking they were mine. I was a B before and now I am a C. I am 9 weeks out ... and a couple weekends ago I went out and was able to go braless. It ... was ... AWESOME! *JenCT*

> It seems awful, but if I can find a positive to my surgery (like my flat tummy) I'm going to focus on that. *GrinningGal*

Those who have already undergone surgery also further encourage acceptance of the medicalization model by attempting to reassure those considering surgery that the stress they are currently experiencing will diminish greatly postsurgery.

> The anxiety sucks going in but it really is better on the other side. I had surgery in May, turned out great. *SpecRin*

> I know it's hard knowing that the gene is with you but I have to say that my peace of mind has increased since I had the surgery as now my risk of cancer has decreased so much. *LaurenJoy*

Choosing Medicalization over Gender

The final way in which many of these "young previvors" appear to accept and advocate for medicalization is by choosing to undergo surgery despite the fact that they will lose the body parts that are so vital to their identity as women. Their willingness to remove both the internal and external organs that they view as being so essential to their sense of femininity, sexual pleasure, and capacity for "natural" motherhood indicates their ultimate acceptance of the medical model. One way that some of these women attempt to rationalize this seeming degendering of their bodies for the sake of science is by suggesting that it is not these body parts that necessarily define a woman.

> My boobs defined me. They always did. Now, I feel empowered by having my PBM [prophylactic bilateral mastectomy]. *JessyN*

> There is a lot more to a woman than boobs and ovaries ... there are a whole lot of us here to tell you we're still women and most of us still have active sex lives and enjoy our femininity. *Kathy*

In addition, many of these young women further express the idea that they can still fulfill their role and identity as women with the help of medicalized reproduction, through such mediums as in vitro fertilization or surrogacy. Furthermore, many of these women emphasize the importance of having "BRCA free" children.

> My OBGYN has recommended me to go to a reproduction center ... and consider having eggs froze because I'm not in any situation right now where kids are an option. *Meliss11*

> I want to make sure my kids DO NOT have this gene, and therefore I would want the eggs screened. *Sweetiepie123*

I am on the fence in regards to invitro and 'selecting' non-mutated embryos. When I first heard of it I was like, 'well of course,' but then I think ... how much can I really prevent? Suppose I take all of these precautions and my child develops another cancer or disease or disorder unrelated to BRCA's risks? Yet at the same time, it would be nice to know if my future children are BRCA 'free.' *ABY*

DISCUSSION

The primary objective of this study was to examine how young women with the BRCA gene accept or reject the medicalization of their bodies based on their new "potentially ill" status. While the women posting on this message board expressed a diversity of experiences and emotions, there also appears to be a "shared chronicle" of illness for women who carry the BRCA gene mutation (Barker, 2005, p. 64). This is evident by the fact that many of the women shared parallel stories that started with the cancer and often death of a close female relative, led to the "diagnosis" of their own BRCA status, caused them to rethink their reproductive plans, and ultimately resulted in taking some kind of preventative action. Consistent with Radin's (2006) research suggesting that breast cancer patients' communication needs occur in waves, it appears that each forum on the FORCE message board may be aimed at women at different stages in their decision-making process who have varying communication needs. The "Young Previvors Forum" looks to serve primarily as a place for young women who recently discovered their BRCA status to discuss their emotions, find solidarity, and seek help in determining the next step. After getting over their initial uncertainty and fear about their BRCA positive status, some women may move on to some of the more specialized forums. The fact that this online message board captures the way these women speak to each other, rather than to a researcher, their doctor, or their family is crucial for gaining an increased understanding of the lived experience of illness or potential illness for these individuals.

The data presented clearly indicates that one of the primary functions the "Young Previvors" message board serves is to provide a forum for young BRCA gene carriers to debate and negotiate the medicalization of their bodies. Some of the women express a rejection of this medicalization by discussing their discomfort with making themselves sick, as well as by conveying a sense of loss with regard to the body parts that they consider to be at the core of their gender identity. However, the theme that emerges and appears to be the most consistent between posts is in support of medicalization – the women overwhelmingly appear to believe that cancer is inevitable for all BRCA gene carriers. It appears that many of these women may be making this conclusion based on their own family medical history, information disseminated by medical professionals or the medical industry, popular media, and other BRCA positive women. Most of these posters appear to conceive of knowledge gained by genetic testing as an opportunity to plan for the future. They do not view themselves as overmedicalized individuals, and they appear to be comfortable with the concept of over-treatment, as long as it reduces their risk of cancer or even their stress about their future risk of getting cancer. The majority of these women also buy into the "cancer panic" spread by the medical industry and media, and consequently an "over-geneticized" image where they feel that their genes override all other risk factors (Conrad, 1997, p. 140).

As a consequence of this idea that cancer is a matter of "when, not if" for these BRCA positive women, another theme materializes – where asserting control by taking preventative action is constructed as a mechanism for quelling the fear, uncertainty, and stress associated with being a BRCA gene carrier. In this case, action is associated with surgery. As a result, numerous women in their twenties and early thirties appear to be reprioritizing their family and reproductive goals by seriously considering or actually under-going prophylactic surgery far earlier than necessary, not only to reduce their risk of cancer but also to reduce their stress regarding what they perceive to be a genetic inevitability. The fact that discovery of their BRCA status is so closely associated with taking medical action for these women suggests that possessing the BRCA mutation is being constructed as a medical diagnosis, rather than simply a genetic fact, and consequently perceived as requiring a corresponding preventative medical treatment. In addition, the discussion threads primarily indicate that surgery is considered to be the ultimate form of "taking control" or action; whereas nonsurgical forms of monitoring or risk management are constructed as more passive options that are accompanied by exorbitant levels of stress and anxiety. When framed in this way, prophylactic surgery is viewed as the strongest and most reasonable option for all BRCA positive women, regardless of their individual risk factors or life circumstances.

Finally, it becomes apparent that for these women medicalization essentially trumps gender. Despite the connection many of them describe feeling with the "parts that make them a woman," they appear to believe that they must disassociate from these parts in order to save their lives. They must convince themselves to view their breasts and ovaries simply as nonessential organs, rather than as core components of their feminine, sexual, and reproductive identities. The fact that these healthy young women would choose not only to purposefully submit to a series of potentially life-threatening medical procedures but also to strip themselves of the body parts that they deem so vital to their womanhood, suggests that they are imbuing biomedicine with an enormous amount of power. This point where a woman believes that she must essentially deny herself of the physical embodiment of gender in order to preserve her own life is particularly disconcerting, because conceiving of more or less degendering women in order to preserve their health suggests that there may be something inherently damaged or deviant with women's bodies; a concept that could largely be used to repress and subjugate women.

CONCLUSION

Regardless of the actual statistics on breast and ovarian cancer risk, it appears that cancer is conceived as an inevitable genetic reality by many female BRCA mutation carriers. Personal experience with the illness or death of a close family member with breast or ovarian cancer appears to manifest itself as evidence of the power of the BRCA gene to unfailingly cause illness. The "anything's better than cancer" mantra shared by the majority of the posters on this message board suggests that for these women fear of death largely outweighs all other potential fears or concerns, including that of "choosing" to become ill while still a healthy individual or losing "all the parts that make them a woman."

While it might be obvious to academics that the medical industry has purposefully manipulated women's fears about their reproductive potential and mortality by creating a culture of fear around women's cancers in order to bring in patients and consequently increase profits, it appears that most of these women just do not care. As long as they believe that "knowledge is power," they will continue to pursue genetic testing and subsequent preventative medical treatment. The promise that prophylactic surgery *might* reduce the risk or delay the onset of breast or ovarian cancer appears to be enough to allow these women to feel happy and satisfied with their decision to take a proactive preventative health measure. However, it is important to consider the potential dangers in advocating preventative health treatments that remove what for many women can be considered the primary physical markers of their gender.

As further medical and technological advancements are made in the future, it is almost certain that similar types of genetic markers will be found and be associated with higher risk for specific conditions or illnesses. Based on this, it is important to understand how individual's identified as carriers of these genetic mutations may negotiate the medicalization of their bodies and navigate their preventative health options in order to be able to determine how to best guide and assist them through this process. Until data on the ultimate benefits of undergoing these various risk management procedures in terms of reducing the probability of or delaying illness become available, or the potential dangers of physically degendering healthy women become more apparent, these women must rely on themselves and each other to make difficult choices with the minimal knowledge they do possess; with the hope that one day their children will not have to endure the same journey.

REFERENCES

Babb, S., Swisher, E. M., Heller, H. N., Whelan, A. J., Mutch, D. G., Herzong, T. J., & Rader, J. S. (2002). Qualitative evaluation of medical information processing needs of 60 women choosing ovarian cancer surveillance or prophylactic oophorectomy. *Journal of Genetic Counseling, 11*, 81–96.

Barker, K. K. (2005). *The fibromyalgia story: Medical authority and women's worlds of pain.* Philadelphia, PA: Temple University Press.

Bradbury, A. R., Patrick-Miller, L., Pawlowski, K., Ibe, C. N., Cummings, S. A., Hlubocky, F., ... Daugherty, C. K. (2009). Learning of your parent's BRCA mutation during adolescence or early adulthood: A study of offspring experiences. *Psycho-Oncology, 18*, 200–208.

BRCA1 and BRCA2: Cancer Risk and Genetic Testing. (2009). *National Cancer Institute.* Retrieved from http://www.cancer.gov/cancertopics/factsheet/risk/brca

Brédart, A., Autier, P., Riccardo, A., Audisio, A., & Geraghty, G. (2001). Psychosocial dimensions of BRCA testing: An overshadowed issue. *European Journal of Cancer Care, 10*, 96–99.

Cancer Previvors. (n.d.). *FORCE: Facing Our Risk of Cancer Empowered.* Retrieved from http://www.facingourrisk.org/pre-vivors_and_survivors/cancer_pre-vivors.html?PHPSESSID=7f584414dbdca523ac6635993bcb932f

Conrad, P. (1997). Public eyes and private genes: Historical frames, new constructions, and social problems. *Social Problems, 44*, 139–154.

Conrad, P. (2005). The shifting engines of medicalization. *Journal of Health and Social Behavior, 46*, 3–14.

Croyle, R. T., Smith, K. R., Botkin, J. R., Baty, B., & Nash, J. (1997). Psychological responses to BRCA1 mutation testing: Preliminary findings. *Health Psychology, 16*, 63–72.

Happe, K. (2006). Heredity, gender and the discourse of ovarian cancer. *New Genetics and Society, 25*, 171–196.

Kenen, R. H., Shapiro, Friedman, & Coyne. (2007). Peer-support in coping with medical uncertainty: Discussion of oophorectomy and hormone replacement therapy on a web-based message board. *Psycho-Oncology, 16*, 763–771.

Mahowald, M.B., Levinson, D., Cassel, C., Lemke, A., Ober, C., Bowman, J., ... Times, M. (1996). The new genetics and women. *The Milbank Quarterly, 74,* 239–283.

Phoenix, K. H. M., & Coulson, N. S. (2008). Exploring the communication of social support within virtual communities: A content analysis of messages posted to an online HIV/AIDS support group. *CyberPsychology & Behavior, 11,* 371–374.

Press, N., Fishman, J. R., & Koenig, B. A. (2000). Collective fear, individualized risk: The social and cultural context of genetic testing for breast cancer. *Nursing Ethics, 7,* 237–249.

Radin, P. (2006). To me, it's my life: Medical communication, trust, and activism in cyberspace. *Social Science & Medicine, 62,* 591–601.

Seale, C., Ziebland, S., & Charteris-Black, J. (2006). Gender, cancer experience and internet use: A comparative keyword analysis of interviews and online cancer support groups. *Social Science & Medicine, 62,* 2577–2590.

Weitz, R. (1989). Uncertainty and the lives of persons with AIDS. *Journal of Health and Social Behavior, 30,* 270–281.

Werner-Lin, A. V. (2007). Danger zones: risk perceptions of young women from families with hereditary breast and ovarian cancer. *Family Process, 46,* 335–349.

Werner-Lin, A. V. (2008). Beating the biological clock: The compressed family life cycle of young women with BRCA gene alterations. *Social Work in Health Care, 47,* 416–437.

White, M., & Dorman, S. M. (2001). Receiving social support online: Implications for health education. *Health Education Research, 16,* 693–707.

Zones, J. (2000). Profits from pain: The political economy of breast cancer. In A. S. Kasper & S. Ferguson (Eds.), *Breast cancer: Society shapes an epidemic.* New York, NY: St. Martins.

CLOSE-CALLS THAT OLDER HOMEBOUND WOMEN HANDLED WITHOUT HELP WHILE ALONE AT HOME

Eileen J. Porter and Melinda S. Markham

ABSTRACT

Although competence to live alone is typically associated with measures of activities of daily living, such measures fail to capture problematic situations that older people face in daily life. In particular, little is known about how older homebound women handle potentially harmful incidents. During a descriptive phenomenological study of the experience of reaching help quickly (RHQ) with 40 older homebound women, 33 women spontaneously reported 139 incidents (falls, "tight spots," near-falls, health problems, and unwanted visitors) that they managed alone. The purpose of this secondary phenomenological analysis of RHQ project data was to describe the experience of those women with handling "close-calls." Data yielded a typology of close-call incidents and five components of the phenomenon, managing a close-call. *In addition to self-directed intentions to lessen the impact of each incident, there were four component phenomena relative to help-seeking, ranging from no mention of need for help (70% of incidents) to managing without desired or*

Issues in Health and Health Care Related to Race/Ethnicity, Immigration, SES and Gender
Research in the Sociology of Health Care, Volume 30, 201–232
ISSN: 0275-4959/doi:10.1108/S0275-4959(2012)0000030012

solicited help (6% of incidents). Contextual factors, including avail-ability of potential helpers and access to help-seeking devices, influenced intentions in close-calls. Findings are springboards for further research and stimuli for new approaches to practice. Researchers should broaden the focus of competence assessment to take in empirical situations. Further work should be done to explore how older people appraise their status following close-calls and how they move from self-management to consideration of help-seeking and in some cases, on to active help-seeking. Because few close-calls were reported, practitioners could use our typology as an assessment protocol during routine visits. Practitioners can elicit self-management intentions relative to a particular close-call and build dialogue around those intentions, thereby bolstering ability of older women to manage close-calls effectively.

Keywords: Older women; help-seeking; homebound; close-calls; phenomenology

Community-dwelling older women who live alone at home are at-risk for various "adverse health events and injuries" (Lau, Scandrett, Jarzebowski, Holman, & Emanuel, 2007, p. 831). In contrast to the usual focus on help-seeking during such situations, we describe potentially harmful situations that older homebound women managed without help while they were at home alone. The topic has an important public health impact, in part because the number of women aged 85 and older is projected to double between 2010 and 2050 (Vincent & Velkoff, 2010). During a descriptive phenomenological study of the experience of reaching help quickly (RHQ), older homebound women spontaneously reported near-falls, falls, health problems, intrusions by unwelcome visitors, and other unusual incidents that they managed alone instead of seeking help or after failing to reach help. During interviews, we began to refer to such situations as *close-calls*, in keeping with the phenomenological imperative to use vernacular phrases to describe experiences (Husserl, 1913/1962). After completing RHQ project interviews, we found that the term close-call had been used to refer to near-errors in health-care delivery (Coyle, 2005) and health-care decisions that involve "no 'single' best choice" (O'Connor et al., 2009, p. 3). In the epidemiological literature, the term has been used to mean "near-injury" in studies with children (Morrongiello, 1997, p. 500) and "narrow escape from danger" (Davidson, Hughes, Blazer, & George, 1991, p. 715) in research on factors associated with post-traumatic stress disorder. Our perspective is akin to that of Davidson et al. (1991). We view the close-call as a type of *emergent situation* (Porter, Markham, Kinman, & Ganong, 2011), one that "arises unexpectedly [and] calls for prompt action" (Mish, 2005, p. 407) to preclude physical or psychological harm. Because there are few descriptions of close-call experiences of older women, those data from the RHQ project warranted a secondary analysis, which we report here.

BACKGROUND

Community-dwelling older women are vulnerable to a variety of emergent situations. They are at-risk for unintentional injuries, especially falls (Mack, 2004) due to factors such as compromised mobility and the prevalence of home hazards (Wyman et al., 2007). Furthermore, compared to men, women are more likely to have multiple chronic health problems and the attendant complications of comorbidity (Wolff, Starfield, & Anderson, 2002). Of noninstitutionalized women aged 85 and older, about 60% live alone (U.S. Department of Health and Human Services, 2006). Of that group, about 50% are homebound; they are unable to leave home without help (Smith & Longino, 1995). In an emergency while at home alone, older women are at great risk for complications that could prevent them from fulfilling their chief intention – to continue living at home for as long as possible (Porter, 1994a).

For older persons who live alone, help-seeking has long been viewed as a critical ability (Butler & Lewis, 1973). Researchers have emphasized the importance of seeking and obtaining help as soon as possible in emergency situations (Johnston, Grimmer-Sommers, & Sutherland, 2010). Devices such as the personal emergency response system (PERS) were designed to enable quick help-seeking (Dibner, 1992). However, it has long been recognized that some older people with potentially grave symptoms do not seek help (Stoller, Forster, Pollow, & Tisdale, 1993). Little is known about the intentions of older people who experience potentially harmful situations or when they consider help-seeking in lieu of handling such situations alone.

The ability to decide whether to seek help or to manage a close-call alone could be seen as relevant to the construct of competence. Competence in everyday activities is a basic issue for older people (Horgas, Wilms, & Baltes, 1998). The construct of competence "addresses what the individual can do, not what he or she actually does" and captures the "mental ability to make critical decisions regarding care of self" (Willis, 1996, p. 600). However, "self-report assessment of everyday competence [has been] of limited usefulness" (Diehl, 1998, p. 426), possibly because researchers have asked older persons to "solve tasks of daily living [cited on] printed material associated with each IADL [instrumental activities of daily living] domain" (Willis, 1996, p. 597). Such a test fails to meet a standard of empirical relevance. During daily life, older adults do not face the challenge of completing a paper-and-pencil test of self-care potential; instead, they can face out-of-the-ordinary situations like close-calls.

There has been limited qualitative work related to how older adults manage problematic situations in daily life. One team of psychologists sought "to examine the phenomenological experience of everyday problems actually encountered" (Berg, Strough, Calderone, Sansone, & Weir, 1998, p. 30). They asked about 500 persons, classified into 4 age-based cohorts, to write about or describe any everyday problem they had experienced as well as a particular problem in each of six domains, including health. Berg et al. (1998) did not specify a method beyond using an "open-ended approach method of assessment" (p. 31). However, they categorized problem domains and goals according to a broad, preconceived set of codes, because "more fine-grained distinctions would have hampered formal statistical analysis" (p. 32).

Nonetheless, some findings of Berg et al. (1998) about everyday problems are an impetus for more definitive, descriptive phenomenological study of the problematic experiences of older persons. Because the oldest adults (aged 60–85) expressed more variability in goals than did younger subjects, Berg et al. saw the need to "reorient research on everyday problem solving toward understanding what [older] individuals are trying to accomplish from their own perspective" (p. 42). One way to effect that reorientation is to seek to understand experiences such as close-calls through in-depth qualitative studies with a series of interviews over time.

Descriptive phenomenological studies are designed to enable understanding of persons' intentions with regard to particular experiences (Porter, 1998). Furthermore, understanding the context of an experience is basic to descriptive phenomenology (Porter, 1995a, 1998). Although Berg et al. (1998) observed that reports of daily problems reflect "the larger context in which individuals find themselves in daily life" (p. 39), they did not elaborate or define context. Context can be defined as the personal and sociocultural factors in which experience is nested (Hinds, Chaves, & Cypess, 1992). Context can be understood in terms of *lifeworld* – "the taken-for-granted frame in which all the problems which I must overcome are placed" (Schutz & Luckmann, 1973, p. 4). For older women, contextual factors could influence decisions about how to handle problematic situations we characterize as close-calls, including availability of potential helpers and access to help-seeking devices.

For older homebound women who live alone, the experience of close-calls and its personal–social context remain unexplored. That research problem has implications for practice. Practitioners need to understand the intention of older women to "take care of it myself" in situations when they might have advised help-seeking instead. To address unmet safety needs of older persons, practitioners need protocols for assessing types of close-calls and basic information about strategies older women use to manage various close-calls. The purpose of this study was to describe the experience of self-managing close-calls and its context.

METHOD

We did a secondary descriptive phenomenological analysis of an extensive database of in-person and telephone interviews obtained during a prior project, a study of the experience of RHQ. We briefly explain the design, sampling, recruitment, and data-gathering for the RHQ project. Then we describe the secondary analysis, addressing the rationale and framework, data pertaining to close-calls, and analytical activities.

Data Source: The RHQ Project

This was an in-depth, longitudinal investigation of the experience of RHQ for older homebound women, approved by the University of Missouri Health Sciences Institutional Review Board (IRB) as a minimal-risk project requiring informed consent. Women from six counties in central Missouri were recruited through contacts with social service agencies and media advertisements. Project staff visited volunteers to explain the study, read the informed consent aloud, and answer questions; volunteers were encouraged to invite a trusted person to attend that session. Forty volunteers gave informed written consent to participate in the RHQ project. Participants met these inclusion criteria: (a) being a woman 85 years of age or older, (b) living alone in a residential setting (a home or an apartment without services), and (c) being homebound or reporting "a condition that prevents them from leaving their home . . . without help" (Smith & Longino, 1995, p. 31). On enrollment, the 40 participants ranged in age from 85 to 98 years ($M = 89.6$). Each woman was to have 4 interviews over 18 months. The number of in-person interviews ranged from 1 to 5 ($M = 3.4$). The duration of participation ranged from 1 to 18 months ($M = 13$ months), and 23 women (57%) were retained for all 18 months of the project.

Data were obtained in lengthy open-ended interviews in the women's homes and monthly telephone calls when interviews were not scheduled. The team developed a protocol of questions for telephone calls and an Interview Guide for each in-home interview in the series. The first author was lead interviewer, conducting or coconducting all but one interview. The second author coconducted several interviews. Most questions were open-ended; we used probes to follow up on interesting points the women raised about RHQ and their lives alone at home, viewing such information as contextual to the RHQ experience. Data obtained during 134 in-person interviews and 307 telephone calls were tape-recorded, transcribed, and entered into QSR N6 qualitative software (QSR International Qualitative Solutions and Research Pty Ltd., 2002).

The Secondary Analysis

Rationale and Framework

The RHQ project dataset included data about incidents when women sought quick help (Porter, Markham, & Ganong, in press) and incidents when they had help-on-the-scene (Porter et al., 2011), as well as unexpected data about close-call incidents. As the primary interviewer, the first author found it necessary to set aside the preconceived notion that all useful data would pertain to incidents when women tried to RHQ. Participants were at least as interested in explaining how they had managed close-calls alone, revealing that they perceived those incidents as worthy of our interest. However, because RHQ project aims did not encompass analysis of close-call data, there was rationale for a secondary analysis of close-call reports. It is consistent with Husserl's (1913/1962) philosophy to use a phenomenological method for a secondary analysis of data from a prior phenomenological study. The University of Missouri Health Sciences IRB deemed the close-call project as human subjects' research but exempt from review, as it involved study of extant, de-identified data.

The first author's particular perspective on secondary analysis was informed by the methodological work of Fielding (2004), Hinds, Vogel, and Clarke-Steffan (1997), and Thorne (1994). We did a "retrospective interpretation" (Thorne, p. 266) of a "sub-set of the original data" (Fielding, p. 98) to answer a new research question about a "concept that seemed to be present but was not specifically addressed in the primary analysis" (Hinds et al., p. 410). We used Porter's (1998) descriptive phenomenological method to conduct the secondary analysis.

Database

These questions from the RHQ project telephone-call protocol stimulated close-call narratives: (a) "Tell me what has been happening in your life since we last saw you," (b) "Have you taken a fall?", and (c) "Have you had any other kind of emergency at home?" These questions from the in-person Interview Guide were fruitful in eliciting narratives about close-calls: (a) "Has a situation come up when you wondered if you should get help quickly?" and (b) "Have you tried to reach help quickly since we were last here?" Such questions stimulate reporting of "real-life, respondent-generated dilemmas" (Marshall & Rossman, 2011, p. 191). After denying a recent attempt to RHQ, Ms. F said, "Oh, but I did have one thing happen" and related an incident we viewed as a close-call. We sought validation of our views that situations could be considered close-calls. Ms. T forgot to turn on a light before walking into the living room one night. She walked about 10 feet in the dark, fearful of falling. "[So that was kind of a close-call, really?] Well, yes, because I was afraid, really. I had to just walk really slow."

To establish the database for the secondary analysis, we reviewed all in-person and telephone interviews to identify close-calls that occurred when women were alone "in or around the home" (Nachreiner, Findorff, Wyman, & McCarthy, 2007, p. 1440). We found no evidence of close-calls in data of 7 women who had only one or two interviews; a coinvestigator verified that conclusion. Thus, the sample for this secondary analysis consisted of 33 women, 3 Black women and 30 White women who were 85 to 97 years old ($M = 89.4$). With regard to the PERS, 18 were subscribers, and 15 were nonsubscribers. All 33 women needed to use (a) personal help, a walking device, or both to get to a vehicle ($n = 25$) or (b) a walking device to get to a car that they drove to a few local destinations ($n = 8$). Of the 33 women, 23 (66%) were retained for the 18-month RHQ project. The other 10 women moved to a more supervised setting ($n = 6$), had deteriorating health ($n = 2$), lost interest in the project ($n = 1$), or died ($n = 1$).

Analysis

All close-call narratives of the 33 women were the focus of the secondary analysis. We started by characterizing the nature of each close-call (such as a fall). If a woman said that while falling, she deliberately maneuvered to avoid landing on the floor, we labeled it as preventing a fall. We did not label an "accidental landing" on a bed or a sofa as either a fall or preventing a fall. However, when Ms. E reported a "lucky landing" in a chair but had trouble getting out of that chair, we classified it as an example of "getting out of a tight spot." Next, we counted close-calls; most reports were so specific that we could easily count distinct episodes. Others were not so clear-cut, so we adopted decision rules to improve accuracy. For instance, Ms. J said she had "at least five or six other falls" after a major fall, but we counted only the four incidents about which she could report details. We also had to decide how to count multiple occurrences. One woman had a close-call with atrial fibrillation most nights for months; we counted each report of multiple episodes during an interview as one incident. Finally, we categorized each close-call as occurring before or during the project. When a woman reported incidents of the same health problem before and during, we counted it in both categories.

Having established a database of close-calls, we used Porter's phenomenological method (1994a, 1998) to describe the essence of the experience of self-managing close-calls. By exploring details about what it is like to live an experience, specific intentions can be discerned. Activities of "describing, comparing, distinguishing, and inferring" (Husserl, 1913/1962, p. 93) are involved in comparing experiences of persons in the sample. As similarities and differences in intentions emerge, the structure of the experience is discerned, with broader intentions subsuming more specific ones. That structure is presented as a leveled taxonomy, with a group of similar intentions specified as a broader component phenomenon, and a group of similar component phenomena specified as a phenomenon (Porter, 1994a, 1998). According to Kohak (1978), a phenomenon is "something like what a thing is in principle" (p. 9). Credibility of analysis was enhanced in that most insights about close-calls were confirmed with women during the interview when data were reported or at a later interview. To discern intentions, we reviewed data for each close-call, focusing on what the woman was trying to do at the time and labeling that intention in vernacular terms, such as *increasing my availability to a helper just in case.*

While working to describe the experience of self-managing close-calls, we characterized its context. The first author views context as *lifeworld* (Porter, 1995a) – "the taken-for-granted frame in which all the problems which I must overcome are placed" (Schutz & Luckmann, 1973, p. 4). Older women share lifeworld data as they explain reasons for their intentions (Porter, 1995a). Relevant lifeworld data included availability of helpers and prior experience with a close-call. Because lifeworld is to be detailed in "objectivated categories" (Schutz & Luckmann, 1973, p. 180), Porter (1995a) had earlier devised labels for levels of a lifeworld taxonomy. An *element* can evoke the singularity of a person's context; a *descriptor* captures similarities among elements (Porter, 1995a), and a lifeworld *feature* captures similarities among descriptors.

Finally, in the discussion, we linked findings about the close-call experience to those of a prior study of the broader experience of living alone at home (Porter, 1994a). That strategy was informed by Husserl (1913/1962). Findings of phenomenological studies of related experiences are to be interlaced whenever possible to reflect the complexity of experience (Porter, 1998).

FINDINGS

Findings are in four sections. We begin with a close-call exemplar. After presenting a close-call typology, we describe intentions with regard to close-calls – intentions concerned with depending on oneself and a range of possibilities relative to help-seeking. Finally, we consider the context of the unique intentions captured in the broad phenomenon, *managing a close-call.*

Exemplar of a Close-Call

After denying a recent need to RHQ, Ms. A reported this "palpitation" exemplar:

> The only thing I had that was quite scary was these rapid heartbeats or palpitations. My son and his wife had the flu, and that was kind of heart-rending, because I knew they couldn't come to help me, that I would have to seek the ambulance people. But I didn't have to do that, because they weren't that bad. They were sort of like the panic attacks I'd been having, more or less caused from a build-up of gas on my stomach. See, I have that acid reflux. [Yes. Tell us about this situation then. You had rapid heartbeats?] Yes. It would come on in the night. After I would take my night medication and go to bed, I would get up and take my Rolaids. I had my Thorazipam tablet I could take later; it has a calming effect and slows your heart down. That's what helped it. And I would make it through the night until time to take my morning medications. I would be alright if I could make it through the night 'til that time. [There were nights when you wondered what you might have to do?] Yes, but I wouldn't have hesitated to call 911 if I'd needed it. [How would you have decided that you needed it?] Well, if I wasn't having any chest pains. I was not in a great deal of pain. If I had been, I would have. [That would have been your signal.] That would have been my signal. Yes.

Types of Close-Calls

We classified the 139 close-calls in five categories shown in Table 1. Each category is phrased as an intention to capture what women were trying to do in that situation. Table 1 also reports the timeline of reported occurrence of close-calls. Of the 139 close-calls, 57 (41.0%) occurred prior and 82 (59.0%) occurred during the project. The 23 women who were retained for the full 18-month project reported 116 (83.5%) incidents; in contrast, the 10 women who were not retained reported only 23 (16.5%) close-calls. Next we describe each type of close-call and report exemplars, with interviewer remarks in brackets and explanatory material in parentheses.

Getting Up After Falling to the Floor
These 56 close-calls involved falls to the floor from a standing position, after which women got up from the floor. In some cases women fell close enough to a sturdy piece of furniture that they could maneuver to it and pull up.

Table 1. Types of Close-Call Incidents Managed Alone.

Type of Incident and Frequencies Prior to and During the Project	Total
Getting up after falling to the floor	
Prior to the project	37
During the project	19
Subtotal	56 (40.3%)
Getting out of a tight spot	
Prior to the project	10
During the project	23
Subtotal	33 (23.7%)
Preventing a fall here and now	
Prior to the project	4
During the project	21
Subtotal	25 (18.0%)
Managing a sudden health problem	
Prior to the project	2
During the project	15
Subtotal	17 (12.20%)
Getting rid of an unwanted visitor	
Prior to the project	4
During the project	4
Subtotal	8 (5.8%)
Total	139

Ms. C said, "I started across the floor, and I had my feet tangled up in this rug. So down I went. I was just between the bed and the door that goes out in the hallway. [What did you do next?] I just turned around and went over to the bed and got up." In other cases, getting back into an upright position involved artful use of a handy device to access a sturdy piece of furniture. Ms. D explained how she got up after a fall. "I was hurting so, my back was, and I kept trying to turn over, and I couldn't. I took my cane and reached over to the chair and pulled the chair by the leg over here where I could get up." Most women, including Ms. C and Ms. D, were able to get up fairly soon after they fell. However, that was not the case for Ms. B, who fell in her kitchen prior to enrollment in the project. "Once I fell in the kitchen, and it took me 3 hours to scoot from the kitchen to my bed and get in my bed. I just I couldn't turn over to crawl."

Getting Out of a Tight Spot
The metaphorical notion of finding oneself in a "tight spot" and working out of it was evoked in 33 diverse, unusual close-calls, such as the one reported by Ms. E, who had severe peripheral neuropathy.

> Now this morning, for example, I had dressed myself in the bathroom after I had my sponge bath. I thought I got dressed alright. When I got into the bedroom, I discovered I had my pants on backwards. So I had to take the darn things off. I started to sit on the bed, and I decided this (she points to the walker) is a little lower; it might be safer to sit on the seat, so I sat down on it. I got them off, and then I had quite a time getting my legs into them. I finally got one foot in and then the other one in, and I got them pulled up. After I got them on, I had kind of a difficult time getting myself up on my feet, 'cause I didn't really have anything to grab hold of very well. I couldn't seem to manage getting up anyway, but I finally did. [By pushing on these walker handlebars?] Well, I took hold of them, and finally I pushed forward enough. When I get up, I have to lean forward.

Ms. F reported another unusual tight-spot incident. She had fallen repeatedly indoors, so she was very concerned about reducing her risk of falling. She always used a walker indoors and to walk the 20 feet on the sidewalk to her car on the street. One day she stepped out of the car and hit the automatic lock before closing the door. The walker was still in the locked car.

> [What did you do?] Well, I walked on in the house with nothing. I thought, 'Oh, no.' There wasn't a neighbor around here. There never is when you want one, and I didn't have my cell phone. Everything was against me all the way, so I think it was a test. I think I was being tested: 'Can you do it or not?' And I said, 'I can do it.' I walked in this house by myself with no assistance, and I did fine.

When we asked how she felt at the time, she said: "Very, very frightened. Very scared. I didn't know how I was even going to make it. I was afraid to get caught in the middle. Actually, it's like being in the water and not knowing how to swim. That's the way you feel."

Ms. G reported a different sort of fear of "being caught in the middle." When she tried to get up from her recliner, she got her leg caught between the chair and the extension ("the leg").

> I was in this chair, and I had the leg up. I forgot it (was up). The phone rang, and I didn't have my portable phone. I wanted to get over to this phone (She points to a landline phone on a Table 2 feet from her chair). I tried to get out of there. Boy, that was something for me! The phone just went on ringing, 'cause I couldn't get up, but I finally got out of it. [You got your leg caught?] I got it caught in there. And I thought, 'Why can't I move from here?' But I got up without any injury.

Ms. G had to make a difficult change in position to avoid remaining in an undesirable position, a descriptor that captured several other close-calls. Other women had to make a quick position change to avoid landing on the floor. While napping, several women realized they were too close to the edge of the bed; they had to move back quickly to the center of the bed to avoid rolling off.

Some women thought or knew that if they were on the floor they would have trouble getting up. When they deliberately or spontaneously got on the floor (kneeling to scrub) or close to it (bending to pick up something), they had to extricate themselves from that position. Ms. H wanted to scrub and wax her floor before going to the hospital for hip replacement surgery. She got down on hands and knees in her customary fashion. After having "a hard time getting off the floor," she managed to do so by crawling to a sturdy stepstool. "I could get up from there, but it wasn't easy. I don't have a lot of strength in my legs, which made it difficult to get up, but I made it. I knew I would have hard trouble getting up, but I wanted to get it done." Ms. I, a PERS subscriber, was putting quarters into her collection when several "rolled down" to the floor.

> I was sitting on the side of the bed and reaching, and I kind of slipped. But I picked up a back scratcher and pulled 'em toward me. But I told my daughter, 'Boy, I was within an inch of having my page.' (She refers to pressing her help-button.) She said, 'Oh yeah? You quit fiddling with quarters.' I says, 'If there's money on the floor, I'm gonna pick it up.' (laughter) [Did you feel that you might have trouble getting up?] Well, if I'm down on the floor, I can't get up.

Ms. J found herself in a tight spot when she sat on a footstool, as she had done routinely in the past, to pick up some things off the floor in her den.

Here awhile back, I thought, 'Well, I believe I can get up off of that.' I sat down on it, and I thought I wasn't ever going to get off of it. It's kind of high, but it wasn't high enough. I just can't get my rear up. [How did you go about getting up then?] I just kept a-going like that (She rocks forward). Finally, I thought, 'I've got to get up from here.' I gave a great effort, and then I made it. [Were you hanging on to anything?] Just my cane. [Were you pushing down on it?] Yeah.

Other women slid off of chairs or sofas onto the floor and had to pull up to a seated position. During the project Ms. K reported three incidents of slipping off of a chair. "I just nodded off like old people do." She took this recurrent situation in stride, because she pulled herself up and "was not hurt." However, Ms. L was troubled about an incident that happened as she answered her daughter's routine evening phone call. She missed the sofa and hit the floor before dropping the phone. Having previously pulled up using the footboard of her bed, she scooted about 20 feet into the bedroom. "I believe if I had really tried, I could have got up without going in there, 'cause, I got up really easy. Yeah. I think if I'd tried, I could have got up without going in there." She was upset about her decision to scoot to the bedroom and to do so without "taking my phone along." After she pulled up, she walked back to the living room and spoke to her daughter. "She was waiting to see what all happened. She kind of got worried."

As is evident, anxiety accompanied some tight spots involving awkward physical positions. However, several women managed tight spots of a strictly psychosocial nature, when they felt quite "blue" or anxious. Ms. M felt "very down" while recovering from major surgery. "There were days I wished I had someone here for moral support." Yet rather than calling someone, she waited, expecting another friend or neighbor to drop by for a visit. When asked if she had recently wondered whether she might need help right away, Ms. G said:

Yes, I came close to calling my neighbors. Let's see. When was it? (She ponders this briefly.) Oh, I realized there was something wrong with the phone. I said to myself, 'I've got to call them and ask them to call in and get the phone fixed.' I was going to call them, but then I realized, 'I can't call them. There is something wrong with the phone.' I was kind of going around, and I thought, 'Well, I will go over there and tell them.' Then I came back to check, and the phone was alright. So I don't know. Maybe I didn't get the thing on there right, but there wasn't any dial tone. That kind of panics me, to not have a phone.

Preventing a Fall Here and Now
In another 25 close-calls, women recognized an imminent risk of falling. They were aiming to prevent a fall by maintaining balance, selectively maneuvering to achieve a "soft landing," or relying on a walking device.

We provide an example of each scenario. First, Ms. N sought to maintain her balance by waving her arms around and "doing fancy steps" to avoid falling. Ms. G had "never fallen onto the floor ... [but] I've come awfully close," including an incident while she was making up the bed. "I don't know what happened, but I did fall over, fell backwards, but I caught myself on the bed. ... I did not fall bad." During a telephone interview with Ms. F, we asked if she sought quick help recently.

> I just haven't had any occasion to do so. But I thought I was going to. [Tell me the story.] I hopped out of bed, and my left leg absolutely would not work. It was just like putty. Oh, it was terrible. Finally I just leaned over my walker; I just stood there and stood there. And pretty soon, it just seemed to come back to life again. I'd never had anything like it. It was awful, one of those scary things.

Managing a Sudden Health Problem
Participants reported 17 close-calls involving self-management of health-related problems, such as leg cramps, chest pain, vomiting, injuries unrelated to falls, and cardiac problems like Ms. A's "palpitations." Ms. M had vertigo attacks "without warning." "I have had an attack of vertigo when I was in bed, and my medicine was in the kitchen. And I've had to crawl to the kitchen, because you cannot stand up when you have a vertigo spell." For months, Ms. O dealt with episodes of atrial fibrillation every night.

> I got up last night about 1 o'clock. My heart started pounding, and it went on for awhile. I wanted to go to sleep. I keep the medicine right there in the bathroom. So I took the medicine and went back to bed, and it settled down. It's transient, has been most of the time, anyway. I didn't call anybody, because there was no use bothering anybody. [You were trying not to bother anyone?] Right. I took care of it myself.

Other women dealt with recurrent health problems although the pattern was unpredictable. Ms. P had "this, it's supposed to be congestive heart failure ... and also this fibrillation."

> It doesn't scare me. I know just what to do, and it hasn't ever been bad enough that I've had to call for help. [What do you do when it comes?] Well, I just try to take deep breaths and try to relax and try to talk myself out of it, that I'm okay, that I'm gonna be fine. And after a little bit, it'll pass over. Maybe it won't always do that, but so far, I haven't had to call for help in that line.

Rather than undertaking active strategies to manage a health problem, some women used more passive approaches, waiting it out or "riding it out," as Ms. M did after a major surgery.

> There was one time recently that I did feel like I might need help quickly during this deal. I just felt terrible. I had pain in my stomach; the tube was bothering me, and the diarrhea

had not been controlled. I was very light-headed, and I was being afraid to move. And I began to consider, well, maybe I needed some help. But I rode out the situation. I didn't get any worse, and I did feel somewhat better.

Getting Rid of an Unwanted Visitor
The last group of 8 close-calls occurred when women confronted intruders or unwanted visitors. Six involved a confrontation with a troublesome person when women were home alone. Ms. Q lived in a four-plex, single-story apartment unit in a rural housing project for older persons and persons with disabilities.

One day, along toward evening, a man that lived over here in this apartment, who I know, he's about 45, came to the door, and I opened the door. He was wanting to use my telephone. I told him no, and he said, 'Well, I got a credit card.' I said, 'I don't care if you've got a credit card. I don't want you using my phone.' So he turned around, and walked out then. And I got up and locked the door again.

Two other women dealt with "would-be intruders" in incidents that troubled them greatly. Late one evening, Ms. R heard running water. She got up to check the toilets and realized water was running outdoors. She opened the front door without turning off the home-security alarm, setting it off. Someone had stolen a garden hose and left the water running. Meanwhile, the security alarm had "lured the police," who she said, insisted that they "search the whole house." She "finally" convinced them that it was she, not the thieves, who had triggered the alarm. At two ensuing interviews, she voiced chagrin over the potential police intrusion, not the vandalism.

Ms. K had repeated encounters with another type of "intruder." At her first interview, she said she began having hallucinations during a hospitalization about a year earlier.

It was grown people from foreign countries, a lot of them, but it was bad at night. The doctors couldn't tell me what was doing it; through the process of elimination, I finally found out it was caffeine in tea. I quit that. But now at home, I still imagine people are here. So, if I can't sleep and think somebody's around, I just get up and go through every room. And I have my doors locked, and if they're all still locked, and I can't see anybody, then I go back to bed and go to sleep.

During a telephone call a year later, when we asked how she was, she said:

Oh, not doing too well. I'm not sleeping right. I have all kinds of, sort of hallucinations. I tend to imagine things, of people being around that shouldn't be. They kind of upset me, and I'm just not sleeping too well, so I sleep in the day some.

During our next monthly call, she said, "There's too many intruders coming in the house, all imaginary." We asked how she handled it. "Oh, I talk to them sometimes. It always turns out alright, but I still get up, go around. I seldom, if ever, sleep in my bed all night."

Intentions in Close-Call Incidents

Depending on Myself First In an Out-of-the-Ordinary Situation

Data about every close-call revealed very specific intentions about *limiting the impact* of the incident, such as these in the "palpitation" exemplar of Ms. A: *taking extra medications selectively and sequentially* and *making it through the night*. All close-call reports yielded data about a personalized post-incident appraisal – *figuring out how I was afterwards*. Two examples related to fall incidents included *deciding that I was not hurt* and *deciding that I was not really hurt, although I was really hurting*. The phrase *deciding that I was not that bad off* was consistent with postincident appraisals of some close-calls involving falls or health problems. Another postincident intention, especially associated with post-fall injuries and health problems, was *keeping my eye on the situation*. All of these intentions were parts of a broader component phenomenon, *depending on myself first in an out-of-the ordinary situation*.

Data also yielded variations in the degree to which women considered seeking help to manage the close-call, ranging from focusing solely on self-management to wanting or seeking help at the time. We captured those variations in four component phenomena that run parallel to the five close-call categories, as shown in Table 2. After presenting findings, we report variations in intentions to seek health-care, one day or more after a close-call, for sequelae like pain.

Managing by Myself

As shown in Table 2, most close-calls (70%) were characterized *only* by self-focused intentions, which we grouped into the component phenomenon, *managing by myself*. There were examples in all five close-call categories, such as (a) *pulling myself up onto something solid* (getting up after falling to the floor), (b) *getting that part of my body out of that trap* (getting out of a tight spot), (c) *turning enough that I can land on the sofa* (preventing a fall here and now), (d) *dealing with a vertigo attack* (managing a sudden health problem), and (e) *sending him packing when I realized what he wanted* (getting rid of an unwanted visitor). None of the women referred to help in these narratives. We asked Ms. K if she had needed to RHQ since the last interview. "No reason like that. I've had some falls, but I've always

Table 2. Frequencies of Close-Call Incidents for Each Component
Phenomenon Related to Help-Seeking.

Component Phenomena and Close-Call Types (subtotal, percentage)	Total
Managing this close-call by myself	(95, 68.4%)
Getting up after falling to the floor	44
Getting out of a tight spot	17
Preventing a fall here and now	20
Managing a sudden health problem	6
Getting rid of an unwanted visitor	8
Seeing no need for that help to manage this close-call	(12, 8.6%)
Getting up after falling to the floor	4
Getting out of a tight spot	2
Preventing a fall here and now	3
Managing a sudden health problem	3
Wondering if I might have to seek help to manage this close-call	(22, 15.8%)
Getting up after falling to the floor	3
Getting out of a tight spot	11
Preventing a fall here and now	2
Managing a sudden health problem	6
Managing this close-call without the help I wanted, needed, or had hoped to have	(10, 7.2%)
Getting up after falling to the floor	5
Getting out of a tight spot	3
Managing a sudden health problem	2
Total	139

managed to handle them." When we asked if she had thought of seeking help when she slipped out of a chair, she said, "No, because I thought I'd get up by myself, which I did."

In the other 30% of close-calls, self-directed intentions were accompanied by thoughts of potential helpers, by speculation as to whether help might be needed or by efforts to obtain help. Some intentions evoked the passage of time; as noted earlier, women were *keeping an eye on the situation,* and some did so while contemplating help-seeking. In the "palpitation" exemplar, Ms. A was *holding off on seeking help unless I get that signal.* Other key intentions were *deciding how serious it is before deciding whether to seek help, waiting to see if I might need to RHQ right now,* and *deciding whether I can get by without help.* Such intentions coalesced into one of other three component phenomena, which we present sequentially to represent progression from seeing no need for particular help, to wondering if help would be needed, to hoping for help to manage the close-call or seeking it without success.

Seeing no Need for That Help
In reports of 10 close-calls, women expressly stated that they felt no need to contact particular people from whom they could have sought help. For instance, in "palpitation" exemplar, Ms. A, a nonsubscriber to PERS, said she decided not to contact "the ambulance people." Several PERS subscribers who intended to manage a close-call without help stated that they saw "no need" to press the help-button. Ms. O explained, "I had a fall last week in my driveway ... I didn't call for help; it wasn't that serious. But I had my (PERS trade name) button on, and I could have called help if I had needed it." Likewise, she said this about her recurrent palpitations. "When these episodes are happening with my heart, I think, 'Do I need to call?' And I think, 'No, I know that this'll settle down in about 20 minutes if I take the medication. There's no use bothering my daughter.'"

Wondering If I Might Have to Seek Help
Reports of 20 close-calls were characterized by uncertainty about the potential need to contact help during the incident. Ms. P said:

> Once in awhile I've told my son (a respiratory therapist), 'Came very near calling you last night.' 'What about?' I says, 'I was kind of short of breath.' 'Why didn't you?' I said, 'Well, because I didn't have any chest pains or anything like that.'

Some women prepared for the possibility that they would have to contact help. Ms. B, who had recurring leg cramps at night, sought to ensure that helpers could get in. "Sometimes I get up and walk, because I feel if they get to the point where somebody had to come out, I would want to be able to let them in." Women used creative means to increase access to potential helpers. Ms. R, a nonsubscriber, got her bracelet chain caught in the screen door, with her arm behind her back.

> Fortunately, I was eventually able to get the bracelet open and get out of it. It was pretty crazy. [Did you think you might have to call for help then?] Well, I didn't know what I was going to do. But I put the garage door up, and the people were here mowing my yard, so I had help close if I needed it. But it was just so unexpected.

Some women, especially nonsubscribers to PERS, recalled contemplating their proximity to the nearest telephone while they were wondering if they would have to seek help. Ms. A was sitting on a chair, putting items under her bed, when one item "went way back under."

> I tried to get down there. I was trying to reach, and I got pretty well down on my knees. But I had a-hold of my chair and the bed, and I was able to pull myself back up again. When I was trying to reach, I was thinking, 'I've got to hang on to my bed. I've got to

hang on to my chair, so I can be able to get up. [So you were purposely saying to yourself, 'Hang on.'] Yes, because I know that I can't kneel down. When I fell once, flat on my back in the street, I could not get up. I know I would have to have help. But I was there close to the telephone where I could have summoned help. I could have reached the telephone.

Ms. S, a PERS subscriber, always put her PERS help-button on a table beside her bed at night.

[Tell me how you have been lately.] Not too good. I don't feel too good. I woke up this morning, and I ain't know whether I was going to get out of bed or not. And I got to the thing, in here, around my neck. And, all I got to do is call for the ambulance, and they come and get me and take me to the hospital.

She "got to the thing" by reaching for the help-button cord and putting it on again.

Women who wondered if they might have to seek help nonetheless emphasized an intention to take initial steps to manage the problem. Ms. J, who had fallen repeatedly and used either a cane or walker at all times, spent "at least 10 minutes" trying to get off the footstool.

[What would you have done if you decided that you couldn't get up without help?] I had thought that I would scoot off the stool onto the floor, over to the basement door, and get my feet a couple of steps down and get a-hold of those railings. I think I could pull myself up. [Were you concerned about what might happen if put your feet on the basement steps and tried to stand up?] Yes, I thought about that, but I believe I could do it. [So you feel you could do that safely?] I have done it before, but then I was more able to handle myself than I am now, but I think I could have done it. I was gonna try that before I called anybody. [And your reason for thinking of trying that first?] I thought how stupid I would feel if I had to call somebody to get me off that footstool. I just didn't want to call.

Ms. J was a PERS subscriber who always wore her help-button. Although she would not hesitate to use it for "something sensible ... [like] "if I fell in the house," she hesitated to use it for "something stupid," like getting up from a footstool. Instead, she would have tried to manage alone, engendering a risk of falling down the basement stairs to stand.

Managing Without the Help I Wanted, Needed, or Had Hoped to Have
In 8 close-calls, women either directly sought help or hoped to have spontaneous help with a close-call – help that did not materialize. Some incidents occurred in places around the home with public access, such as an open porch, from where they called out to passers-by. Ms. T fell in her driveway. "Nobody had come by at that time. I pulled myself over to the fire hydrant and pulled up by that. [If someone had come by, would you have

called?] I would have motioned or something." Ms. B had episodes of vomiting at night. Before the project, she had called a friend to be with her at such times. One night during the project, she "managed to make it to the bathroom to throw up twice," but she did not call for help. "I hate calling people in the middle of the night." When we asked if she was taking precautions as a person living alone, she said. "I try to be careful about what I eat, because when you get sick in the night, and you are alone, you feel like you need somebody." She wanted someone with her, but she managed alone rather than bothering anyone.

Summary of Intentions Associated with Self-Managing Close-Calls
We viewed the five component phenomena (depending on myself first in an out-of-the ordinary situation; managing by myself; seeing no need for that help; wondering if I might have to seek help; and managing without the help I wanted, needed, or had hoped to have) as parts of a larger phenomenon, *managing a close-call*. That phenomenon characterized the essence of the experience of the 33 women. These data from Ms. B, a PERS subscriber, are an exemplar:

> [Have you needed to reach help quickly for any reason?] No. Oh, at night I have awful cramps in my feets and legs, but I didn't press my button, because I figured it would soon go away. Sometimes at 2 and 3 in the night, I get up and walk when my limbs start cramping. I walk until they straighten out and go back to bed.

Variations in Seeking Health-Care for Sequelae After a Close-Call
Because we routinely asked if any problems resulted from a close-call, we had data about physical sequelae (including pain, bleeding, swelling, and bruising) and the psychosocial sequela of ongoing worry about the incident. We discerned three intentions related to seeking postincident care for close-calls with sequelae: (a) *electing not to contact a provider*, 11 close-calls; (b) *notifying provider via telephone or a previously scheduled appointment*, 8 close-calls; and (c) *seeking health care one day or more after the incident*, 10 close-calls. PERS subscribers reported 19 of the 29 close-calls with sequelae (8 incidents before they subscribed to PERS and 11 afterwards), and nonsubscribers reported 10 such incidents. Although sequelae resulted from all five types of close-calls, most sequelae resulted from a fall to the floor. Six women who sustained "bumps" on the head did not notify a provider. For example, Ms. V fell, hit her head on the refrigerator and the floor, and broke her glasses. Ms. W reported that she fell in the bedroom, hit her head, and had a "goose egg" and a black eye for days. Neither woman contacted a provider after the incidents. Other women elected to notify a

provider by telephone or during their next scheduled appointment. Ms. H fell, hitting her head on the door and her hip, which had been surgically replaced a few months earlier, on the floor. When her "nurse-friend" came the next day, she told her about it. "I have a pocket of blood there, I'm putting an ice pack on it. That part is painful, but my hip don't hurt. She said I should tell my doctor at my next appointment (in four days); otherwise, I wouldn't." Her physician ordered an X-ray of the hip and "It was okay." Women who sought care a day or more after a fall typically "felt okay" after getting up off the floor, only to experience pain later. Although most sequelae apparently had no major consequences, several were very serious. While in pain with a broken arm, Ms. C stayed alone at home one winter night. Ms. U fell in her bedroom and reported, "I didn't feel any pain when I got up." The next morning, she was in pain and visited the doctor, who hospitalized her. Ms. X waited "about a week" after she fractured her pelvis before seeing her physician because "I could walk."

Lifeworld as Context for Managing a Close-Call

All 33 women were in the position of *finding myself in a close-call situation here at home alone*. That lifeworld descriptor conveys the vulnerability of being in circumstances that were "quite scary" (according to Ms. A, a non-subscriber to PERS) or "out-of-the-ordinary" (according to Ms. B, a PERS subscriber). Lifeworld is "the arena, as well as what sets the limits, of action" (Schutz & Luckmann, 1973, p. 6). The arena in which each close-call played out affected the woman's intentions and accordingly, the actions that she viewed as possible relative to managing the close-call. We address personal–social factors before considering how having a device for RHQ influenced self-management of close-calls. Finally, we address participants' reflections about close-calls and comment on project participation as a stimulus of reflections.

Personal-Social Factors

With regard to self-managing health problems, a key personal factor was prior experience with managing that problem, which for Ms. P, was coupled with prior experience as a medic. She typically managed her severe nose-bleeds without help. However, an important social factor diminished her concern; she could call her son and his wife, "trained health professionals" who lived a few minutes away, for advice or on-the-spot help.

Other women who wondered if they might have to seek help were considering accessibility of providers and availability of persons who might provide transportation to a health-care facility. Ms. M, a PERS subscriber, explained the factors she considered while wondering if she might have to seek help during the episode of postsurgical pain and diarrhea.

> I considered the day and the time of day and who was going to be available to help me, if I needed to go to the emergency room. If it's close to night, you don't wait too late, 'cause it's hard to get in. If it's a weekend coming up, I might wait 3 or 4 days for my doctor to give some advice. This was a Friday, and I was thinking, 'If this doesn't let up, I'm gonna have to make a call.' [Who would you have called?] I would probably have called my neighbors, because I know that they can drop whatever they're doing and do it. My grandson has the baby, and my son's 60 miles away, so that would not help me much in an emergency.

Having a Device for Reaching Help Quickly

Most women who were wondering if they would have to seek help considered (a) their proximity to a device they could use to reach help quickly and (b) which device they might use if more than one was available. Ms. M was a PERS subscriber, but she would have used the phone she carried with her to call her neighbors instead of "going directly to the (trade name for PERS) to ask for an emergency vehicle." The neighbors had taken her to the emergency room several times before she subscribed to a PERS; they were more available to help than her family. In part because she thought of them first, the telephone was her device of choice for RHQ, rather than the PERS help-button.

With regard to managing close-calls, most PERS subscribers considered the help-button as a fall-back option. Like nonsubscribers, they emphasized their overall intention to handle such incidents without seeking help. On average, each woman reported 4.1 close-calls. Of the 139 close-calls managed alone, the 18 PERS subscribers reported 77 (55.4%) incidents (an average of 4.3/person), whereas the 15 nonsubscribers reported 62 (44.6%) incidents (an average of 4.0/person). Having access to a PERS, a device designed to reach help quickly, was no guarantee that subscribers would voice an intention to use it when they could manage alone.

Several PERS subscribers managed close-calls alone with great difficulty, although they could have pressed the help-button to obtain aid. These situations were of three types. Ms. B was not wearing the help-button when she fell in the kitchen and had to scoot 20 feet to her bed. Ms. C fell outside on her back steps in the late afternoon, forgot she was wearing the PERS button, and with great difficulty, crawled into the house and went to bed. "I forgot all about having that thing. I just wanted to get into the house before dark." Other women were wearing the help-button but did not realize that they could have used it in the situation. Ms. F, who had walked into the house from her car without a walker, was a PERS subscriber who routinely wore the help-button even when she went out. She was interested in having help or she would not have planned to ask for help "if one had been out." She knew that the PERS would work outside the house; once she had "hit it by accident and the police came running in." But before walking into the house unaided, she did not think of pressing her help-button. The PERS dispatcher would have contacted her first-responders or sent other help. Ms. F had successfully used the PERS to reach help when she fell inside the house, but she did not think of using it to possibly prevent a fall outside. Yet each time we asked how she would RHQ if necessary, her response was akin to this: "If I had to reach help, I would reach up and push my button. Right there it is." However, she routinely tempered that response, continuing in this manner. "If I can't handle it myself, I push the button. I first would evaluate whether I could handle it myself or not."

Reflections on Close-Call Experiences
Most of these women emphasized a very positive view of their abilities to do what needed to be done to manage these close-calls. Some were minimizing the potential significance of certain incidents – a viewpoint that was likely warranted in some cases. However, others recognized that if circumstances had been different, they might have needed to RHQ in those situations. If so, some said that they would have been "helpless" in such situations, and they affirmed a stronger sense of concern about having ready access to a device for RHQ. Ms. R, a former PERS subscriber, had a home-security system with a portable help-button "on a chain." She fell in the kitchen and got up with difficulty. When we asked if she had contacted help, she said, "No. I wished I'd had that chain on, but I didn't have it. Since then, I have it on, day and night." Soon thereafter, she fell again and chose to re-subscribe to the PERS. "I need it for peace of mind." Furthermore, women typically concluded close-call stories by relating intentions to prevent such situations in the future. Due to her bouts with acid reflux, Ms. A said, "I have to be careful. For supper I just have soup and sandwich most of the time, because I don't want to get upset during the nighttime." After Ms. T took that "scary" walk across her living room in the dark, she said, "I'll never turn out all the lights again."

Taking Part in Project Interviews

There were indications that for some women, being interviewed was a lifeworld influence on reflections about self-managing close-calls. First, women tended to repeat stories about close-calls that were especially troubling to them. The chance to express feelings about these "signal" close-calls might have served a therapeutic purpose; some women said that they had not told anyone else about some close-calls or that they had "kept secrets" from family or friends to avoid upsetting them. Finally, our questions about close-calls enabled women to think aloud about how they would have sought help if necessary. After Ms. E told us how she had struggled to get up from her walker seat, she said:

> For awhile I thought I was gonna have to call for my daughter (who lived next door).
> I didn't have any idea whether she was indoors or outdoors. [Did you have some thought
> about how you would do that?] Well, I thought she probably was outdoors. She was, but
> whether she would have heard me? She might have heard that bell (pointing to a school
> bell she rang to call her night-aide), although it's not very loud. But if necessary,
> I could've punched this thing. (She points to her PERS help-button.) They would have
> called her; they have her number.

Summary of Findings

The 33 older homebound women who were living alone managed various close-calls alone, including falls, intrusions, and health-related problems. Unique personal and social factors interfaced to influence intentions of managing each close-call. Potential helpers available to each woman (and the degree to which such helpers were available) varied widely, as did the extent to which each woman had a RHQ device available. More than two-thirds of close-calls featured only self-focused intentions. Some women saw no need to contact a particular helper, whereas others wondered if they might need to seek help. Relatively few women wanted help to manage a close-call or sought help that did not materialize. Most women sought to manage close-calls on their own, whether or not they were PERS subscribers. Having a PERS did not mean that women remembered they had it or realized that they could use it. Several PERS subscribers were so opposed to seeking help for particular incidents that they were willing to try risky strategies to manage alone if their initial efforts failed. Essentially, these women were trying to carry on without contacting help. Only about 10% of close-calls were reported to providers in some fashion. In several incidents with noteworthy sequelae such as painful fractures, women notified a physician more than a day afterwards.

DISCUSSION

This work begins to fill a knowledge gap by revealing that self-management of a variety of close-calls is part of daily life for older homebound women. The prevalence of close-calls in this small sample was noteworthy. The 33 women reported 4 close-calls on average with more than half occurring during a relatively brief window of 18 months. Researchers have focused on self-management of chronic diseases (Sevick et al., 2007; Thorne, Paterson, & Russell, 2003). That work has been ground-breaking, but findings of the present study are a rationale for expanding the self-care arena to include the full spectrum of close-calls managed alone.

For older adults, self-care responses to physical symptoms can "reflect and reinforce the meaning of social relations" (Dill, Brown, Ciambrone, & Rakowski, 1995, p. 8). In this study, intentions associated with some close-calls were influenced by social context and grounded in relationships with key persons, but this was not always the case, even with health-related close-calls. In 11 of those 17 situations, women referred to potential helpers, but in the other 6 health-related close-calls, women simply reported that they managed the situation alone.

Indeed, in about 70% of all close-calls, women emphasized their intention to manage alone. With regard to the emphasis on self-management rather than help-seeking, our findings are similar to those of Berg et al. (1998). More participants of all age groups, including "older adults 60-85 years" (Berg et al., p. 31), reported taking self-action rather than involving others with health-related concerns. However, Berg et al. concluded that participants who viewed a problem as interpersonal were more likely to involve others in solving it. Our data suggest a somewhat different conclusion; some women hesitated to seek help in part because they viewed the close-call as a personal problem. When they considered seeking help or did so, they viewed the resolution of the close-call, not the close-call itself, as interpersonal.

It could be argued that few close-calls reported here were life-threatening and that delays in seeking care for most close-calls with sequelae were likely inconsequential. Self-reported delays in care-seeking have failed to predict adverse health-related outcomes or mortality among older persons (Rupper, Konrad, Garrett, Miller, & Blazer, 2004). However, that epidemiological logic fails to consider the empirical and personal relevance of close-calls, based on recurrence of certain types of incidents, individual impact of a given incident, or both. Through an ongoing series of interviews, we invited women to share certain health-related dilemmas they had faced. As they did so, they revealed what they were thinking at the time the close-call occurred.

They recalled and shared the retrospective self-talk that respondent-generated dilemmas are designed to elicit (Marshall & Rossman, 2011). Ms. F recalled her thoughts when she found herself in a tight spot on the footstool. "I thought, 'I've got to get up from here.'" From compelling self-talk data of that sort, we discerned that self-management was central to their intentions in close-calls.

Furthermore, findings expand a developing understanding of the lifeworld of older women who live alone. The lifeworld descriptor, finding myself in a close-call situation here at home alone, is a cross-cutting exemplar of two lifeworld features, "being in the position" and "facing vulnerability" (Porter, 1995a, p. 36). Likewise, the phenomenon, managing a close-call, is at the interface of "going my own way" and "reducing my risks" (Porter, 1994a, p. 22), two phenomena of the experience of living alone. As well as contributing to a phenomenology of the lives of older women, findings are stimuli for new research directions and practice initiatives.

Research Directions

The self-management of close-calls could be viewed as consistent with a transactional model of everyday competence, in which person and environment are intertwined (Diehl & Willis, 2003). Competence "represents older adults' potential or capacity for making decisions necessary for care of themselves" (Willis, 1996, p. 600). As revealed in our data, older home-bound women confront actual, emergent situations that evoke that capacity. Indeed, Ms. F characterized her success with walking into the house without her walker as that of being faced with a "test" and "pass[ing] it." Competence is often tapped by measures of IADL, which are essentially a-contextual and a-situational (Porter, 1995b, 2007). Such measures are not designed to capture narratives about close-calls, even those related to a particular IADL task. Ms. F found herself in a tight spot, walking without her walker, but she could not take that situation into account if she were asked to rate her difficulty with the IADL task of moving about outdoors (Chipperfield, 1996). Compared to IADL tests, the ways in which older women handle close-calls are more accurate reflections of their ability to care for themselves. Researchers could broaden competence assessment to take in empirical situations by soliciting close-call narratives.

For older adults, indicators of need (including perceived and evaluated health status) have been the strongest predictors of emergency department use (McCusker, Karp, Cardin, Durand, & Morin, 2003). However, few scholars have explored how variations in perceived health status influence decisions to manage close-calls alone. In this study, women depended upon themselves to decide how a close-call had affected them initially and over time. After the immediate impact, they were keeping an eye on the situation, a metaphor that evokes the passage of time. In the "palpitation" exemplar, for instance, Ms. A was *holding off* on seeking help unless she got a certain signal and *waiting* to see if she might need to RHQ. We lack specific data about time intervals associated with intentions like holding off and waiting; such data should be obtained in future longitudinal studies. Further studies are needed to explain (a) how perceived health status is appraised and reappraised during a close-call and (b) how and why self-management of a close-call segues to consideration of help-seeking and, in some cases, on to active help-seeking.

Practice Implications

This study informs practice in a new, necessary direction, suggesting both a rationale for and an approach to incorporating routine assessment of close-calls in geriatric health care. Because physicians were rarely notified about close-call incidents, we advise that these questions from our Interview Guide be included in each encounter with a provider: (a) "Have you had any kind of emergency at home?" and (b) "Has a situation come up when you wondered if you should get help quickly?" When a client presents with a close-call narrative, practitioners can use the typology of self-managed close-calls as a framework for classifying the incident. That is, practitioners should inquire about the circumstances of the close-call, self-management intentions, and the nature of help-seeking intentions, if any. Practitioners can build upon the intentions of clients to prevent such close-calls in the future and offer supplemental guidance to enable them to expand the skill-set to manage close-calls effectively. In addition to explaining how to prevent falls, providers can emphasize the importance of seeking care postfall and explain when a provider should be notified. Providers should maintain a record of the close-calls reported by older women; an increasing incidence could be linked to other problems with sustaining oneself at home alone. Deterioration in ability to recall and relate circumstances of close-calls reported for the first time could be indicative of actual difficulty with managing close-calls alone. Because these indicators are far more relevant to daily life than a score on a mental status inventory, they could be useful elements of a safety assessment for women living alone.

Limitations

For various reasons, the number of close-calls reported for this sample is only an estimate. First, regardless of category, participants reported more close-calls during the project than they reported as having occurred prior to it. This trend was likely an artifact of project participation (and perhaps difficulty with recall about earlier events), rather than an indicator of increased incidence over time. Second, the relative percentages of some close-call categories raise questions about accuracy. For instance, compared to fall-prevention incidents, women reported more than twice as many close-call falls (56:25). This finding seems counter-intuitive, because older women tend to have difficulty with balance, gait, or both before experiencing a fall (Porter, 1994b). However, one can become so accustomed to correcting one's balance that such incidents are not viewed as instances of difficulty (Porter, 2007). Indeed, rather than reports of "simple" efforts to regain balance, most fall-prevention narratives invoked a sense of impending danger – the risk of "falling and breaking a hip." Some women repeated these narratives at multiple interviews. Therefore, fall-prevention close-calls were likely under-reported with only the most troublesome incidents shared. That conclusion is consistent with an observation of Peterson, Harbeck, and Moreno (1993) about the "near injuries" (p. 192) of children. "It seems likely that many such events occur without being noticed, and that only when serious injury is averted is the event recognized as a near injury" (p. 192).

Our data-gathering and analysis strategies could have affected validity of findings in some cases. Although we took care to use standardized questions to elicit information, our strategies might not have yielded all available data. Our monthly inquiries about risky situations probably stimulated recall of recent events, but women might not have recalled all close-calls, and some might have decided not to divulge a particular incident. We used decision rules for classifying close-call narratives to increase empirical validity of findings. However, we categorized close-calls in a manner that emerged from self-report data; the content of self-reports about incidents such as a "fall" (Zecevic, Salmoni, Speechley, & Vandervoort, 2006) or getting up from the floor (Bergland & Laake, 2005) can vary. Accordingly, the typology of close-calls is likely an incomplete classification of close-calls that older homebound women manage alone.

Furthermore, just as self-care activities cannot be neatly categorized (Dill et al., 1995), the five component phenomena of managing a close-call are not necessarily discrete. For instance, there are nebulous distinctions between managing alone and considering help-seeking. Women who considered help-seeking might have chosen not to mention that or to deny it when we asked, electing to focus on success with managing alone. Rather than a limitation, this is a by-product of the method. We did not "define" each component phenomenon; instead, we sought to reveal its essence relative to the experiences of our sample.

Conclusions

To explore similarities and differences in intentions associated with managing a close-call, further descriptive work is warranted with other samples of older homebound women. Yet beyond efforts to categorize types of close-calls, it is critical to emphasize that each incident occurs in a unique personal–social context. When older homebound women succeed in managing a close-call alone, this should be celebrated, but at the same time, the occurrence of a close-call sounds a cautionary note. As with any self-care activity (Dill et al., 1995), the circumstances associated with self-managing each close-call could exemplify lifelong patterns and reveal rapidly changing circumstances. Practitioners and researchers who try to understand intentions associated with self-managing close-calls must do so in recognition of the overall goal of older women – to sustain themselves at home for as long as possible (Porter, 1994a).

ACKNOWLEDGMENTS

The project described was supported by Grant Number 1 R03 AG032981-01 from the National Institute on Aging. The content is solely the responsibility of the authors and does not necessarily represent the official views of the National Institute on Aging or the National Institutes of Health. The authors acknowledge the contribution of Dr. Lawrence H. Ganong, Co-Investigator, with an initial phase of data analysis.

REFERENCES

Berg, C. A., Strough, J., Calderone, K. S., Sansone, C., & Weir, C. (1998). Role of problem definitions in understanding age and context effects on strategies for solving everyday problems. *Psychology and Aging, 13*(1), 29–44. doi:10.1037/0882-7974.13.1.29

Bergland, A., & Laake, K. (2005). Concurrent and predictive validity of 'getting up from lying on the floor'. *Aging-Clinical & Experimental Research, 17*(3), 181–185.

Butler, R. N., & Lewis, M. I. (1973). *Aging and mental health: Positive psychosocial approaches.* St. Louis, MO: C. V. Mosby.

Chipperfield, J. G. (1996). Perceived adequacy of instrumental assistance: Implications for well-being in later life. *Journal of Aging & Health, 8,* 72–95.

Coyle, G. (2005). Designing and implementing a close call reporting system. *Nursing Administration Quarterly, 29*(1), 57–62.

Davidson, J. R. T., Hughes, D., Blazer, D. G., & George, L. K. (1991). Post-traumatic stress disorder in the community: An epidemiological study. *Psychological Medicine, 21*(3), 713–721.

Dibner, A. S. (Ed.). (1992). *Personal response systems: An international report of a new home care service.* Binghamton, NY: Haworth Press.

Diehl, M. (1998). Everyday competence in later life: Current status and future directions. *The Gerontologist, 38*(4), 422–433. doi:10.1093/geront/38.4.422

Diehl, M., & Willis, S. L. (2003). Everyday competence and everyday problem solving in aging adults: The role of physical and social context. In H.-W. Wahl, R. J. Scheidt, & P. G. Windley (Eds.), K. W. Schaie (Series Ed.), *Annual Review of Gerontology and Geriatrics* (Vol. 23, pp. 130–166). New York, NY: Springer.

Dill, A., Brown, P., Ciambrone, D., & Rakowski, W. (1995). The meaning and practice of self-care by older adults: A qualitative assessment. *Research on Aging, 17*(1), 8–41. doi:10.1177/0164027595171002

Fielding, N. (2004). Getting the most from archived qualitative data: Epistemological, practical and professional obstacles. *International Journal of Social Research Methodology, 7*(1), 97–104. doi:10.1080/13645570310001640699

Hinds, P. S., Chaves, D. E., & Cypess, S. M. (1992). Context as a source of meaning and understanding. *Qualitative Health Research, 2*(1), 61–74. doi:10.1177/104973239 200200105

Hinds, P. S., Vogel, R. J., & Clarke-Steffan, L. (1997). Pearls, pith, and provocation: The possibilities and pitfalls of doing a secondary analysis of a qualitative data set. *Qualitative Health Research, 7*(3), 408–424. doi:10.1177/104973239700700306

Horgas, A. L., Wilms, H. U., & Baltes, M. M. (1998). Daily life in very old age: Everyday activities as expression of successful living. *The Gerontologist, 38*(5), 556–568. doi:10.1093/geront/38.5.556

Husserl, E. (1962). *Ideas: General introduction to pure phenomenology* (W. R. B. Gibson, Trans.). London: Collier-Macmillan. (Original work published 1913)

Johnston, K., Grimmer-Sommers, K., & Sutherland, M. (2010). Perspectives on use of personal alarms by older fallers. *International Journal of General Medicine, 3,* 231–237.

Kohak, E. (1978). *Idea & experience: Edmund Husserl's project of phenomenology in Ideas I.* Chicago, IL: The University of Chicago Press.

Lau, D. T., Scandrett, K. G., Jarzebowski, M., Holman, K., & Emanuel, L. (2007). Health-related safety: A framework to address barriers to aging in place. *The Gerontologist, 47*(6), 830–837. doi:10.1093/geront/47.6.830

Mack, K. A. (2004). Report from the CDC: Fatal and nonfatal unintentional injuries in adult women, United States. *Journal of Women's Health, 13*(7), 754–763. doi:10.1089/jwh.2004.13.754

Marshall, C., & Rossman, G. B. (2011). *Designing qualitative research* (5th ed.). Los Angeles, CA: Sage.

McCusker, J., Karp, I., Cardin, C., Durand, P., & Morin, J. (2003). Determinants of emergency department visits by older adults: A systematic review. *Academic Emergency Medicine, 10*(12), 1362–1370. doi:10.1197/S1069-6563(03)00539-6

Mish, F. (2005). *Merriam-Webster's collegiate dictionary* (11th ed.). Springfield, MA: Merriam-Webster, Inc.

Morrongiello, B. A. (1997). Children's perspectives on injury and close-call experiences: Sex difference in injury-outcome processes. *Journal of Pediatric Psychology, 22*(4), 499–512.

Nachreiner, N. M., Findorff, M. J., Wyman, J. F., & McCarthy, T. C. (2007). Circumstances and consequences of falls in community-dwelling older women. *Journal of Women's Health, 16*(10), 1437–1446. doi:10.1089/jwh.2006.0245

O'Connor, A. M., Bennett, C. L., Stacey, D., Barry, M., Col, N. F., Eden, K. B., ... Rovner, D. (2009). Decision aids for people facing health treatment or screening decisions (review). *The Cochrane Database of Systematic Reviews,* (3):1–113. doi: 10.1002/14651858. CD001431.pub2

Peterson, L., Harbeck, C., & Moreno, A. (1993). Measures of children's injuries: Self-reported versus maternal-reported events with temporally proximal versus delayed reporting. *Journal of Pediatric Psychology, 18*(1), 133–147. doi:10.1093/jpepsy/18.1.133

Porter, E. J. (1994a). Older widows' experience of living alone at home. *Image: Journal of Nursing Scholarship, 26*(1), 19–24. doi:10.1111/j.1547-5069.1994.tb00289.x

Porter, E. J. (1994b). "Reducing my risks": A phenomenon of older widows' lived experience. *Advances in Nursing Science, 17*(2), 54–65.

Porter, E. J. (1995a). The life-world of older widows: The context of lived experience. *Journal of Women & Aging, 7*(4), 31–46. doi:10.1300/J074v07n04_04

Porter, E. J. (1995b). A phenomenological alternative to the "ADL Research Tradition". *Journal of Aging and Health, 7*(1), 24–45.

Porter, E. J. (1998). On "being inspired" by Husserl's phenomenology: Reflections on Omery's exposition of phenomenology as a method for nursing research. *Advances in Nursing Science, 21*(1), 16–28.

Porter, E. J. (2007). Scales and tales: Older women's difficulty with daily tasks. *Journal of Gerontology: Social Sciences, 62B*(3), S153–S159.

Porter, E. J., Markham, M. S., & Ganong, L. H. (in press). Incidents when older homebound women tried to reach help quickly. *Research in Gerontological Nursing.*

Porter, E. J., Markham, M. S., Kinman, E. L., & Ganong, L. H. (2011). Emergent situations when older homebound women had fortuitous help and a typology of helpers who were involved. In J. J. Kronenfeld (Ed.), "Access to Care and Factors That Impact Access, Patients as Partners in Care and Changing Roles of Health Providers", *Research in the Sociology of Health Care* (Vol. 29, pp. 117–148). Bingley: Emerald Group Publishing Limited.

Qualitative Solutions and Research (QSR) International Pty Ltd. (2002). *QSR N6.* Melbourne, Australia: Qualitative Solutions and Research (QSR) International Pty Ltd.

Rupper, R. W., Konrad, T. R., Garrett, J. M., Miller, W., & Blazer, D. G. (2004). Self-reported delay in seeking care has poor validity for predicting adverse outcomes. *Journal of the American Geriatrics Society, 52*(12), 2104–2109. doi:10.1111/j.1532-5415.2004.52572.x

Schutz, A., & Luckmann, T. (1973). *The structures of the life-world* (R. M. Zaner & H. T. Engelhardt, Jr., Trans.) Evanston, IL: Northwestern University Press.

Sevick, M. A., Trauth, J. M., Ling, B. S., Anderson, R. T., Piatt, G. A., Kilbourne, A. M., &
    Goodman, R. M. (2007). Patients with complex chronic diseases: Perspectives
    on supporting self-management. *Journal of General Internal Medicine, 22*(Suppl 3),
    438–444. doi:10.1007/s11606-007-0316-z
Smith, M. H., & Longino, C. F. (1995). People using long-term care services. In Z. Harel &
    R. E. Dunkle (Eds.), *Matching people with services in long-term care* (pp. 25–48).
    New York, NY: Springer.
Stoller, E. P., Forster, L. E., Pollow, R., & Tisdale, W. A. (1993). Lay evaluation of symptoms
    by older people: An assessment of potential risk. *Health Education Quarterly, 20*(4),
    505–522.
Thorne, S. (1994). Secondary analysis in qualitative research. In J. M. Morse (Ed.), *Critical
    issues in qualitative research methods* (pp. 263–279). Thousand Oaks, CA: Sage.
Thorne, S., Paterson, B., & Russell, C. (2003). The structure of everyday self-care decision
    making in chronic illness. *Qualitative Health Research, 13*, 1337–1352.
U.S. Department of Health and Human Services (2006). *Beyond 20/20 WDS: Trends in Health
    and Aging.* Retrieved from http://209.217.72.34/aging/TableViewer/tableView.aspx
Vincent, G. K., & Velkoff, V. A. (2010). *The next four decades, The older population in the
    United States: 2010 to 2050 (Current Population Reports* No. P25-1138). Washington,
    D.C.: U.S. Census Bureau.
Willis, S. L. (1996). Everyday cognitive competence in elderly persons: Conceptual issues and
    empirical findings. *The Gerontologist, 36*(5), 595–601. doi:10.1093/geront/36.5.595
Wolff, J. L., Starfield, B. S., & Anderson, G. (2002). Prevalence, expenditures, and compli-
    cations of multiple chronic conditions in the elderly. *Archives of Internal Medicine,
    162*(20), 2269–2276.
Wyman, J. F., Croghan, C. F., Nachreiner, N. M., Gross, C. R., Stock, H. H., Talley, K., &
    Monigold, M. (2007). Effectiveness of education and individualized counseling in
    reducing environmental hazards in the homes of community-dwelling older women.
    Journal of the American Geriatrics Society, 55(10), 1548–1556. doi:10.1111/j.1532-5415.
    2007.01315.x
Zecevic, A. A., Salmoni, A. W., Speechley, M., & Vandervoort, A. A. (2006). Defining a fall and
    reasons for falling: Comparisons among the views of seniors, health care providers, and
    the research literature. *The Gerontologist, 46*(3), 367–376. doi:10.1093/geront/46.3.367

SECTION IV
POLICY ISSUES AND
RACE/ETHNICITY

COUNTERVAILING INFLUENCES OF BLACK AND WOMEN LEGISLATORS ON STATE AGE FRIENDLINESS

Jean Giles-Sims, Joanne Connor Green and Charles Lockhart

ABSTRACT

We examine the influences of African-American and female legislators on the supportiveness of states toward elders. Previous research shows complementary supportiveness among women and minority legislators on education policy and a range of social policies affecting families. Women legislators extend this support to various dimensions of "state age friendliness." We examine here whether African-American legislators extend their support similarly. We draw on a cross-sectional data set for the 50 American states around the year 2000 in conjunction with regression. We find that, controlling for the most prominent alternative factors generally shaping state orientations and policies, women legislators are selectively supportive of dimensions of state elderly friendliness, but African-American legislators do not share this support.

Issues in Health and Health Care Related to Race/Ethnicity, Immigration, SES and Gender
Research in the Sociology of Health Care, Volume 30, 235–259
ISSN: 0275-4959/doi:10.1108/S0275-4959(2012)0000030013

We attribute the discrepancy in the support of this area of social policy to women and minority legislators having specific divergent priorities with regard to elders as well as to how these priorities are conditioned by women and black legislators being concentrated in different states having distinctive cultures.

Keywords: Women's legislative influence; Blacks' legislative influence; state age friendliness; state public social policy; comparative state public policy

The baby boom generation has begun to retire and will continue to do so across the next two decades. Many baby boomers can reasonably anticipate living a quarter-century past the increasingly common early average retirement age of 62 (He, Sengupta, Verkoff, & DeBarros, 2005). This aging of American society poses challenges to a range of social institutions.

States will face growing challenges such as financing their Medicaid programs which, among other activities, currently fund about two-thirds of the expenses of nursing facility long-term care and growing proportions of Home and Community Based Services (HCBS) care provided in older citizens' homes as well as assisted-living complexes and other community venues. We focus on state-level challenges in confronting an aging society in this paper, particularly differences in cross-state achievements in various aspects of "state age friendliness" (Lockhart & Giles-Sims, 2010). States differ in the degree to which their social orientations and public policies support the varying aspirations and needs of older citizens, and we seek a more thorough explanation of how these differences relate to the sex and ethnicity of legislators.

The degree to which women and African-Americans are represented in state government may affect differential state success in supporting older citizens. Recent research (e.g., Reingold, 2008) finds women legislators are especially interested in women's rights as well as programs involving education, medical care, and the welfare of families with children, and others report that women legislators extend this support to policies focused on older citizens (Giles-Sims, Green, & Lockhart, 2012). Still other research (e.g., Barrett, 1995) suggests that women and persons of color are allies with respect to education, medical care, and the welfare of families with children so that African-Americans complement some of the influences of women in state legislatures. Controlling for other relevant variables, we examine the association between women and African-American legislators' presence and states' support for particular aspects of the welfare of family elders. We find that, likely because of factors we introduce in the following section, black state legislators do not follow their women colleagues in extending support in this manner.

The "value-added" of this study begins with describing how women and African-American legislators differ with regard to support of various aspects of state age friendliness. More importantly, we explain how these differences arise from the contrasting priorities of women and black legislators. But, these priorities are conditioned by the differing circumstances of states in which women and African-American legislators enjoy prominence. In what follows we (1) explain why women and African-American legislators might disagree on extending support to age-friendly programs, (2) briefly review other relevant literature, (3) explain our research design and data, (4) relate our results, and (5) discuss their meaning.

CONTRASTING PRIORITIES FOR ELDERS' WELFARE ACROSS SEX AND ETHNICITY

Women and Aging

Several factors likely underlie the support that women legislators extend to age-friendly state policies. Women tend to live longer than men and consequently are more likely to live alone (He et al., 2005; Howes, 2009). Living longer fosters higher rates of various disabilities and the need for medical care and assistance with activities of daily living (ADLs) (Salganicoff, Cubanski, Ranju, & Newman, 2009). But the income histories and net worth of women are characteristically lower than those for men (Folbre, Reimers, & Yoon, 2009; Hartmann & English, 2009), so paying for professional health and long-term care services is frequently difficult. Moreover, adult women often keep closer track and are more keenly aware of their parents' situations than men, and they routinely bear the lion's share of the caregiving provided by family members to elderly parents.

So, female legislators might be more sympathetic than male legislators to nursing facility residents and other elders because of personal experience with the stresses associated with family caregiving as well as their concern for older women. State age friendliness might even be considered, at least to some extent, a women's right and/or women's welfare issue meriting special efforts of support from women legislators. It seems reasonable that as women gain legislative influence, they will consider policies helping older citizens as integral aspects of the family-friendly policies of which they are recognized as supportive.

African-Americans and Aging

Several factors might suggest that African-American legislators would similarly extend support to age-friendly state policy. First, African-Americans 65-or-older (hereafter 65 +) exhibit cross-sex differences like those characterizing the American population overall, and their circumstances are generally less encouraging than those of white Americans (He et al., 2005). Black life expectancies are about six years less for both men and women in comparison to whites. Shorter life expectancies arise from a variety of health factors that may in turn be attributable in part to greater accumulated disadvantage over a range of life opportunities. But these shorter life expectancies mean that black elders represent a considerably smaller proportion of African-American citizens than do elders of other ethnic groups (He et al., 2005).

Second, there are lower proportions of married couples among older black Americans than among all other major ethnic groups. Since African-American elders have a greater incidence of disability, the relative absence of marital partners creates a more serious shortage of spousal caregivers. However, the greater tendency of older black women to live with other relatives – rather than using commercial long-term care venues – largely compensates for this shortage.

Third, older black Americans have a poverty rate nearly three times that of their white counterparts. Older African-Americans have lower median incomes for various demographic subgroupings, and household net worth among them is considerably lower (He et al., 2005). Consequently, elders in black families are, on average, less well prepared to meet exceptional medical and long-term care expenses commonly experienced by elders. Yet similar, if not even more extensive, educational and other resource deficiencies afflict black youth who represent a much larger cohort of the African-American population.

Fourth, black elders are concentrated regionally in a swath running from Texas to New Jersey across the southeastern United States (exempting Florida), plus the rust belt states of Illinois, Michigan, New York, and Ohio (He et al., 2005). Particularly, the southeastern members of this group of states, characterized by Elazar's (1966) traditionalistic culture, tend to perform poorly in terms of state-level public social programs aimed at vulnerable target populations. So competition for scarce public-sector resources resembles an intense zero-sum game.

In summary, black elders constitute a smaller proportion of the African-American population than older citizens do of the American population generally. Additionally, through likely symbiotic influences of distinctive family patterns, limited financial resources, and social discrimination, black households have developed more extensive social patterns of taking care of their elders within the extended family than have Americans generally. Moreover, although older African-Americans often experience severe deficiencies in income and other material resources, arguably even more egregious resource shortfalls afflict the much more numerous black youngsters who are near the beginning, rather than the end, of their lives (USCB, 2000). For instance, the states in which African-Americans have the greatest legislative presence also routinely have the highest rates of infant mortality (USCDC, 2002) and teenage pregnancy (USNCHS, 2002). And public-sector social program resources are routinely exceptionally skimpy in the states in which older African-Americans form the largest percentages of the population.

Accordingly, even if black legislators share the general family support orientation of women legislators, they might place a higher priority on directing limited public resources toward the support of African-American children rather than elders. Indeed, if competition for public social program resources is (or is perceived as) zero-sum, African-American legislators may view the predominantly white elders who draw on a state's public social program resources as competing with the needs of minority children.

It is the central hypothesis of this study that, for these reasons, African American legislators are not as "age friendly" as women legislators.

LEGISLATIVE INFLUENCE OF SEX AND ETHNICITY: IMPORTANT EXPLANATORY VARIABLES?

Factors that may contribute to cross-state variation in state age friendliness include the varying degrees to which women and African-Americans are represented among states' prominent public officials. In the aftermath of 1960s social changes, academic interest in women legislators rested largely on descriptive representation or how women become legislators. This concern continues into the present (e.g., Dolan, 2004, 2006; Paxton, Hughes, & Green, 2006; Rule, 1981, 1990; Sanbonmatsu, 2002, 2006b; Welch & Studlar, 1990). Since the mid-1970s, the numbers of women legislators have increased substantially. With these increases, academic interest shifted somewhat from descriptive representation to substantive representation or what differences the presence of increasing numbers of women produces on legislative substance (Barrett, 2001; Bolzendahl & Brooks, 2007; Carroll, 2001, 2008;

Diamond, 1977; Dodson, 2001; Kathlene, 2001; Orey & Smooth, 2006; Pitkin, 1967; Preuhs, 2006; Reingold, 2008; Smooth, 2008; Thomas & Welch, 2001; Tolleson-Rinehart & Stanley, 1994; Wolbrecht & Campbell, 2007).

In some legislative domains (e.g., public works), women legislators' attitudes do not differ much from those of men. However, both biological (e.g., hormones such as oxytocin and nurturing offspring during infancy) and social (e.g., imitating their mothers as children) influences likely foster inclinations among many women toward greater connectedness with others than those characteristic of many men. So, cross-sex differences are clearly evident (Dodson, 2001; Reingold, 2008), and distinctive female legislative objectives arise from physiological and socially constructed elements including institutional norms and constraints (Duerst-Lahti & Kelly, 1995; Gilligan, 1982; Kathlene, 2001; Kenney, 1996).

Women legislators exhibit different policy and legislative priorities and institutional strategies than their male counterparts. They often choose to serve on health and human services as well as education committees that deal with issues involving families and children (Burrell, 1994; Carroll, 2008; Saint-Germain, 1989; Swers, 1998; Thomas, 1994; Thomas & Welch, 1991). Women tend to retain these interests even as they rise to leadership positions in legislative chambers (Deen & Little, 1999). Women are also distinctly more interested in legislation involving women's rights (Carroll, 2008). Additionally, women's orientations toward legislation in some areas, rather than being framed by "economic man" incentives, are often more supportive and nuanced – for example, greater interest in rehabilitation and less in punishment with respect to criminality (Kathlene, 2001). Further, women, perhaps because they are, even today, less numerous than their male legislative colleagues, are more prone to organize themselves across committee assignments and even party lines on matters of common interest (Reingold, 2008).

The development of an African-American middle class since the 1960s means that public issues associated with family social and economic needs are widely shared across black and other American families (e.g., Robinson, 2010). Recent research suggests that black legislators support state-level public policies improving access to education and employment as well as a range of other public social programs targeted on families with children (e.g., Barrett, 2001; Bratton, Haynie, & Reingold, 2006; Orey & Smooth, 2006; Preuhs, 2006; Smooth, 2008).

While women and African-American legislators generally share support of education, health-care reform, unemployment, and economic development legislation, African-American legislators tend to focus on issues of interest to blacks more than white legislators of either sex (Barrett, 1995, 1997; Darcy & Hadley, 1988; Simien, 2005). Thus, black legislators may have different priorities on age-friendly legislation as a consequence of having different constituencies to support. Research also suggests, for instance, that black women legislators show ambivalence toward women's movement activities that focus on middle-class white women (Breines, 2002; Fuller, 2004; Prestage, 1977; Zajicek, 2002).

RESEARCH DESIGN AND DATA

In an earlier study, we found that the persistent presence of a significant proportion of women in a state's legislature had a positive effect on a state's age friendliness (Giles-Sims et al., 2012). In this study, we examine whether African-American legislators extend their support to families' elders as women legislators do and offer an explanation as to why they do not. Specifically, we investigate how, if we control for a range of other well-known influences on state orientation and public policy, the sex and ethnicity composition of states' legislatures affect support for older citizens finding a meaningful life, sustaining health and accessing high-quality medical care, and acquiring high-quality long-term care – our dependent variables. Thus, while three of our four dependent variables center on legislative outcomes, they do so, not in the conventional sense of whether or not a state has passed particular legislation, but rather in terms of the specific character of policy designs and delivery (e.g., a Medicaid nursing facility long-term care program's resource depth and service quality). We draw on a cross-sectional data set for the 50 states and use ordinary least squares (OLS) regression for analysis. Our study is cross-sectional by necessity since some of the dependent variable data are unique to a particular year and other data are available only once a decade. We lag the independent variables at 2000 and the dependent variables follow as soon as feasible a few years later. All of our indicators are state-level.

The literature on women's substantive representation employs three types of measures for translating representation into influence on legislative substance. Some studies use the simple percentage of women in a state's legislature on the assumption that, as this percentage grows, so too does the capacity for influencing substance. Other researchers think that women must be present in a "critical mass" (Grey, 2002; Jaquette, 1997) in order to have much influence on legislation; 15 (Kanter, 1977) to 30 (Paxton et al., 2006) percent of the seats are variously used as a criterion. Still others are concerned with how long women have had a substantial presence in a legislature and thus the degree to which their presence has become conventional or routine (Carroll, 2001; Kenney, 1996; Rosenthal, 1998; Thomas, 1994). Although we recognize that the influence cannot be inferred directly from presence, we adopt the simple percentage option here. As we explain below, we do so primarily to match the procedure necessary for black legislators.

Data and practices for measuring minority legislative influence are less well developed. We ended up limiting ourselves to African-American legislators, leaving aside Asian, Hispanic, or Native American legislators. In 2000, for instance, Hispanic members exceeded 10 percent of their state legislatures in only 4 states, whereas African-American legislators met this criterion in 15 states, so focusing on blacks provides vastly more variation on minority legislative representation than relying on other ethnic minorities. Additionally, African-Americans have a lengthier tradition of organized political action in support of selected aspects of family-friendly public policy than do other minority groups. Thus, if any single minority group is apt to be age friendly as well, blacks would appear to be a likely possibility. Since even African-American legislators reached 20 percent (a modest threshold) in only five states in 2000, and had achieved those levels only recently, using either a threshold or the length of time the blacks have had a substantial legislative presence sharply reduces variation on this independent variable. So, we employ the percentage of a state's legislature composed of black legislators in 2000 as our measure.

This procedure (and any alternative) requires a decision as to what to do with respect to black women legislators. In 2000, there were 7,424 state legislators. Of these, 1,672 were women; 571 were African-American, and 146 were black women. In our early exploratory analyses, we found that any effects of these 146 black women legislators (or slightly less than 9 percent of women legislators and just over 25 percent of black legislators), considered independently, were simply overwhelmed by the effects of the larger groups of black male and white women legislators. So, we count these women twice, once as women legislators, and again as African-American legislators. In light of our hypothesis above, this is a conservative decision. The presence of a number of persons in both groups should serve to dampen differences between the two groups, making our anticipated outcome marginally less likely.

We add to our models four state-level variables that, given our purpose here, serve as controls. Since we have limited degrees of freedom, we need to keep the total number of our independent/control variables relatively small. We draw on Karch's (2007) version of a "standard model" for explaining cross-state policy variation: state ideology, political party competition, state material (tax) capacity, and the need for the policy. We also employ an index for Elazar's (1966) conception of culture as an independent variable. It provides support for our explanation of the surprising strength of African-American legislators' influence (Table 1).

Dependent Variables

Meaning: This is a state's score on the *making meaningful contributions and finding supportive community* dimension of state age friendliness (Lockhart & Giles-Sims, 2010). It is calculated by adding a state's z-scores for (1) the state's Gini index (reversed as a measure of income equality), (2) Putnam's Comprehensive Social Capital II index for the state, (3) the percentage of a state's $65+$ residents with incomes above the federal poverty level, and (4) the percentage of a state's $65+$ residents voting in the 2004 presidential election. The first two elements of this scale focus on a state's total adult population, indicating the degree to which a state's overall socioeconomic environment supports civic involvement and community attachment. This broader social context arguably contributes to shaping the narrower one composed of older citizens in part by socializing the large proportion elders who live in the state prior to their old age. The latter two elements focus on the same factors with regard to a state's $65+$ residents. The alpha for this scale (.80) indicates the strong relations among all four components.

Health & Medical Care: This is a state's score on the *sustaining health and accessing high-quality medical care* dimension of state age friendliness (Lockhart & Giles-Sims, 2010). It is calculated by adding a state's z-scores for (1) the state's score on the Centers for Disease Control's healthy aging index, (2) a state's rank on the "best practices" conception of Medicare medical care quality (Jencks, Huff, & Cuerdon, 2003), (3) a state's rank on the "coordination of care elements" conception of Medicare medical care quality (Baicker & Chandra, 2004), and (4) the percentage of a state's Medicare decedents who are *not* admitted to an intensive care unit (ICU) or similar unit during their last six months of life (alpha $= .82$). All elements of this scale (and the two dependent variables that follow below) focus on a state's $65+$ population.

Long-Term Care (NF): This is a state's score on the *finding accessible and high-quality long-term care* dimension of state age friendliness (Lockhart & Giles-Sims, 2010). It is calculated by adding a state's z-scores for (1) state Medicaid certified nursing facility beds per one thousand $65+$ state

Table 1.   Variable Descriptions, Sources, and Dates.

Variable	Source	Date
Dependent Variables		
Meaning: Scale alpha = .80; composed of added *z*-scores of four elements: state's Gini index (reversed); state's score on Putnam's comprehensive social capital II index; % of 65 + state residents above federal poverty level; and % of 65 + state residents voting in the 2004 presidential election	From Lockhart and Giles-Sims (2010): http://census.gov/hhes/ www/incme/histince/state/ state4.html; http:// www.bowlingalone.com/ StateMeasures.xls; http:// pubdb3.census.gov/macro/ 032006/pov/ new46_100125_14.html; http:// census.gov/population/www/ socialdemo/voting.cps2004.html	1999, 2000, 2005, and 2004
Health & Medical Care: Scale alpha = .82; composed of added *z*-scores of four elements: state's score on CDC's healthy aging index; state's rank on "best practices" Medicare medical care quality; state's rank on "coordination of care" Medicare medical care quality; and % of state's Medicare decedents *not* in ICU during last six months of life	From Lockhart and Giles-Sims (2010): http://www.cdc.gov/aging/ pdf.saha_2007.pdf; Jencks et al. (2003); Baicker and Chandra (2004): http:// www.dartmouthatlas.org/data/ download/ 2005_eol_medpar_state.xls	2004, 2000– 2001, 2000– 2001, and 2005
Long-Term Care (NF): Scale alpha = .65; composed of added *z*-scores of four elements: state Medicaid nursing facility beds per one thousand 65 + state residents; % of state's Medicaid expenditures devoted to nursing facilities; state Medicaid nursing facility expenditures (adjusted for state cost of living) per one thousand 65 + state residents; and quality of state nursing facility processes scale (alpha = .74): added *z*-scores for the % of state nursing facilities *without* deficiencies with respect to preserving resident dignity, facility housekeeping, residents experiencing accidents, and food sanitation	From Lockhart and Giles-Sims (2010): Harrington et al. (2005), Table 2 & USDC (2004), Table 20; *USDHHS* (2005), Table 110; *USDHHS* (2005), Table 110 & USDC (2004), Table 20 and Berry, Fording, and Hanson (2000) updated via the ICPSR archive: http:// www.icpsr.umich.edu; Harrington et al. (2005), Tables 38, 40, 45, and 48, respectively	2003, 2003, 2003, and 2003

Table 1. (*Continued*)

Variable	Source	Date
HCBS$/MNF$: State HCBS aged/disabled long-term care expenditures/state Medicaid nursing facility long-term care expenditures	Burwell et al. (2003): http:// www.hcbs.org/, search Brian Burwell > Table 1 (PDF)	2003
Independent Variables		
Women's Legislative Influence: Percentage of state legislative representatives (both houses) who are women	Center for American Women and Politics (CAWP), Rutgers University: http:// www.cawp.rutgers.edu	2000
Blacks' Legislative Influence: Percentage of state legislative representatives (both houses) who are African-American	Joint Center for Political and Economic Studies: http:// www.jointcenter.org	2000
State Ideology: State citizen liberalism	Berry et al. (1998) updated via ICPSR archive: http:// www.icpsr.umich.edu	2000
Party Competition: Ranny (folded) state political party competition index	Bibby and Holbrook (2004)	2000
State Tax Capacity: Total state taxable resources per capita indexed to the U.S. average	National Center for State Higher Education Policymaking and Analysis: http://higheredinfo.org	2000
% State Population 65 +: Percentage of a state's population that is 65 or older	USCB (2000): http:// www.census.gov > Census 2000 > Summary File 1	2000
State Political Culture: Index for Elazar's state cultural assessments. 1 = strongly traditionalistic; 15 = strongly moralistic	Elazar (1966, p. 110)	Mid-1960s

residents, (2) the percentage of the state's Medicaid expenditures devoted to nursing facilities, (3) state Medicaid nursing facility expenditures per one thousand $65+$ state residents, and (4) Lockhart and Giles-Sims' (2010) quality of state nursing facility processes index (alpha $= .65$). As the appended (NF) suggests, this variable rests on states' Medicaid nursing facility long-term care programs, excluding HCBS alternatives. Data on HCBS programs are often inadequate for cross-state comparisons comparable to those for nursing facilities (Mollica & Johnson-Lamarche, 2005).

HCBS\$/MNF\$: Our fourth dependent variable is designed to counter the nursing facility bias of the previous variable, using the only sufficiently rigorous data available (Burwell, Sredl, & Eiken, 2003). It represents a state's (Medicaid) HCBS expenditures divided by its Medicaid nursing facility expenditures, providing an index of the degree to which states support HCBS alternatives to nursing facility care with public funds. Older citizens needing professional assistance with ADLs routinely prefer either to remain in their own homes or live in a community-based congregate setting such as an assisted-living complex rather than to enter institutional environments such as nursing facilities. Since the U.S. Supreme Court's *Olmstead v. L.C.* ruling in 1999, states have made greater efforts to employ and financially support these alternatives to nursing facility care. This ruling encouraged states to offer these options, and alternatives to nursing facilities are usually less expensive per person served.

Independent Variables

Women's Legislative Influence (Hereafter *Women's Influence*): This variable indicates the percentage of women representatives in a state's legislature (both houses together) in 2000. The literature on women's legislative representation suggests that this variable will exert strong positive effects on *meaning, health & medical care*, and *HCBS\$/MNF\$*. Because women may be more closely attuned to elder care issues than men and thus may favor HCBS over nursing facility care, we think that this variable will have a negative effect on *long-term care (NF)*.

African-Americans' Legislative Influence (Hereafter *Blacks' Influence*): This variable measures the strength of African-Americans' influence in state legislatures in terms of the proportion of seats (both houses collectively) held by blacks in 2000. As explained above, we count *all* African-American legislators, male or female. So in 2000, 146 black women legislators are included in *women's influence* and also in *blacks' influence*. This double counting increases variation on *blacks' influence*. It also portrays ambiguity (and thus may fit well with some of these legislators' ambivalence) as to whether these legislators are representing women or blacks more prominently (Barrett, 1997; Prestage, 1977; Simien, 2005). We expect that this variable will produce low and likely negative effects on all four of our dependent variables.

State Ideology: Ideology provides an index of state predisposition or inclination, the first of Karch's (2007) four general factors explaining cross-state policy differences. We use Berry, Ringquist, Fording, and Hanson's (1998) index for state citizen liberalism. We anticipate that this variable will exert low-level positive effects on all four of our dependent variables.

Party Competition: Competition among political parties is the second general factor in Karch's (2007) model. We use Ranney's (1965) folded index of state party competition that rests on how closely the major parties divide the seats of a state's legislative chambers (Bibby & Holbrook, 2004). We expect that this variable will produce low positive or negative effects on all four of our dependent variables because political party differences over supporting older citizens are more muted than those for public assistance programs for working-aged persons.

State Tax Capacity: Material resource depth is Karch's (2007) third general factor affecting states' policies and programs. A state's tax capacity or its total taxable resources per capita is commonly used as an indicator of this concept. Our measure indexes states to the national average. We anticipate that this variable will have positive effects with respect to three of our dependent variables, particularly with respect to long-term care (NF). But, because HCBS long-term care is less expensive, it may be favored by less wealthy states. Thus, *tax capacity* may exert a negative effect on HCBS$/MNF$.

Percentage of State Population 65 + (Hereafter *% State Population 65 +*): Karch's (2007) fourth criterion involves the level of need for a particular state policy. This is often measured by the size of the target population. Accordingly, we use the percentage of a state's population that is 65 +. Karch suggests that greater need often prompts greater positive state response. This might be the case here in spite of raising costs since, as Schneider and Ingram (1993) as well as Cook and Barrett (1992) argue, older persons are often held in positive regard by both public officials and ordinary citizens. So, we expect that *% state population 65 +* will produce positive, but not strong, effects on all four of our dependent variables.

Culture: This is our index for Elazar's (1966) cultural distinctions among the American states: traditionalistic, individualistic, and moralistic. We had reservations about using *culture* and *liberal* in the same analysis. But, as Table 2 shows, they correlate (positively) at only .24, and we discern no disruptive effects of including both as independent variables in the same

Table 2. Simple Pearson Correlation Coefficients Among the 11 Variables in the Analysis.

	Meaning	Health & Medical Care	Long-Term Care (NF)	HCBS$/MNF$	Women's Legislative Influence	Blacks' Legislative Influence	State Ideology	Party Competition	State Tax Capacity	% State Population 65+
Health & Medical Care	.79***									
Long-Term Care (NF)	.17	.15								
HCBS$/MNF$	.26	.22	-.11							
Women's Legislative Influence	.49***	.57***	-.06	.32*						
Blacks' Legislative Influence	-.66***	-.66***	.03	-.22	-.49***					
State Ideology	.03	.24	.32*	-.12	.23	-.02				
Party Competition	-.08	-.09	.02	.08	-.08	.13	.22			
Tax Capacity	.15	.13	.31*	.00	.35*	-.10	.34*	.23		
% State Population 65+	-.03	.10	.21	-.22	-.09	-.02	.33*	-.01	-.22	
Culture	.76***	.69***	.16	.20	.60***	-.58***	.24	-.01	.28	-.02

*Significant at <.05; **significant at <.01; ***significant at <.001. All variables are state level, and $N = 50$.

regression models. We use this variable to help explain the surprisingly strong effects that *blacks' influence* exerts on *meaning* and *health & medical care*. While Elazar's assessment of state cultures dates from the mid-1960s, these cultures are based on long-standing, basic beliefs and values that transcend contemporary opinions on issues of the day. A number of studies find that Elazar's assessments hold up well against competition with other, arguably more sophisticated measures (Johnson, 1976), as well as across time and continue into the present to usefully contribute to predicting and explaining cross-state policy differences (Fisher & Pratt, 2006; Hanson, 1991; Kincaid, 1982; Mead, 2004; Moran & Watson, 1991). Our index starts at the bottom with the most traditionalistic states (assigned a 1) and runs up along Elazar's distinct categories (1966, p. 110) through the individualistic states to the most moralistic states (assigned a 15). We expect that *culture* will exert positive effects – likely stronger for *meaning* and *health & medical care* – on all four of our dependent variables.

In addition to the independent variables listed above, we examined, but dropped from the analysis, four others. The percentage of state's population that is African-American and the percentage of state 65 + population that is minority correlate, respectively and statistically significantly, with *blacks' influence* (which was essential) at .96 and .33, so we used *blacks' influence* in place of either of the others. A dummy variable for South/not South correlates at .72 with *culture*, and we used the latter, more nuanced measure in place of the former. The percentage of a state's women legislators who are Democratic exerts no strong effects. We dropped it from the analysis in order to maintain degrees of freedom.

RESULTS

Table 2 shows the correlations among the 11 variables in the analysis. Among the four dependent variables *meaning* and *health & medical care* correlate closely (.79); otherwise these variables are independent of one another. Correlations among our independent variables are generally low and unproblematic. Unfortunately, the exceptions to this generalization involve the three independent variables of primary interest: *women's influence* with *blacks' influence* (−.49), *culture* with *women's influence* (.60), and *blacks' influence* (−.58). We did not anticipate the strength of these correlations. But the absence of a strong positive correlation between *women's influence* and *blacks' influence* fits with a literature that shows the women's movement is not always inclusive or supportive of minority

Table 3. 12 Ordinary Least Squares (OLS) Models for Four Dependent Variables.

IVs	Model 1: Meaning	Model 2: Meaning	Model 3: Meaning	Model 4: Health/ Medical Care	Model 5: Health/ Medical Care	Model 6: Health/ Medical Care	Model 7: Long-Term Care (NF)	Model 8: Long-Term Care (NF)	Model 9: Long-Term Care (NF)	Model 10: HCBS$/ MNF$	Model 11: HCBS$/ MNF$	Model 12: HCBS$/ MNF$
						DVs						
Liberal	-.025 (.037) $p=.498$	-.007 (.031) $p=.814$	-.027 (.024) $p=.277$	.022 (.035) $p=.543$	.039 (.029) $p=.190$	.026 (.027) $p=.333$	.078 (.046) $p=.097$	.081 (.046) $p=.086$	.069 (.046) $p=.137$	-.002 (.002) $p=.398$	-.002 (.002) $p=.467$	-.002 (.002) $p=.443$
Compete	-4.565 (6.112) $p=.459$	-.747 (5.802) $p=.884$	.018 (3.955) $p=.996$	-6.287 (5.802) $p=.284$	-2.658 (4.820) $p=.584$	-2.158 (4.383) $p=.625$	-6.003 (7.538) $p=.430$	-5.199 (7.685) $p=.502$	-4.720 (7.504) $p=.533$	.256 (.335) $p=.449$	.304 (.340) $p=.376$	.308 (.343) $p=.374$
Tax Capacity	1.578 (2.937) $p=.594$	1.302 (2.411) $p=.593$	.330 (1.884) $p=.862$	-.424 (2.788) $p=.880$	-.687 (2.287) $p=.765$	-1.322 (2.088) $p=.530$	10.250** (3.622) $p=.007$	10.192** (3.646) $p=.008$	9.584* (3.574) $p=.010$	-.131 (.161) $p=.317$	-.135 (.161) $p=.409$	-.140 (.164) $p=.396$
% 65+	.112 (.266) $p=.676$	-.003 (.219) $p=.990$	.029 (.171) $p=.866$	.178 (.252) $p=.483$	.070 (.208) $p=.739$	.090 (.189) $p=.635$	.385 (.328) $p=.246$	.361 (.332) $p=.282$	.381 (.324) $p=.246$	-.015 (.015) $p=.317$	-.016 (.015) $p=.277$	-.016 (.015) $p=.288$
Women's Legislative Influence	.168* (.067) $p=.015$	.040 (.061) $p=.519$	-.040 (.050) $p=.425$	.209** (.063) $p=.002$	.087 (.058) $p=.141$	.035 (.055) $p=.530$	-.228** (.082) $p=.008$	-.255** (.092) $p=.008$	-.305** (.094) $p=.002$	.008* (.004) $p=.030$	.007 (.004) $p=.115$	.006 (.004) $p=.166$
Blacks' Legislative Influence		-.271*** (.057) $p=.000$	-.141** (.051) $p=.008$		-.258*** (.054) $p=.000$	-.173** (.056) $p=.004$		-.057 (.087) $p=.514$	.024 (.096) $p=.801$		-.003 (.004) $p=.378$	-.003 (.004) $p=.552$
Culture			.471*** (.087) $p=.000$			.308** (.097) $p=.003$			.295 (.166) $p=.083$			.003 (.008) $p=.714$
Adjusted R^2	.064	.369	.618	.183	.450	.546	.236	.226	.263	.059	.055	.036

*Significant at <.05; **significant at <.01; ***significant at <.001. Standard errors are in parentheses. N for all variables = 50. DVs, dependent variables; IVs, independent variables.

movements (Bratton et al., 2006; Breines, 2002; Fuller, 2004; Zajicek, 2002).

Table 3 displays 12 OLS regression models, three models for each of four dependent variables. The first set (Models 1–3) has *meaning* as its dependent variable. Model 1 provides a "baseline" with *women's influence* and our four control variables. This model is similar to, but weaker than, one we employed previously, using a length-of-substantial-presence calculation for women's influence. *Women's influence* exerts the sole statistically significant (positive) influence, but the model explains only 6 percent of the cross-state variation of *meaning*. Adding *blacks' influence* in Model 2 reduces the effect of women's influence (eliminating its statistical significance), reveals a negative, statistically significant effect for *blacks' influence*, and raises the cross-state variation explained to about 35 percent. The addition of culture in Model 3 adds a strong, statistically significant positive effect for this variable and raises the cross-state variation explained to 60 percent.

Models 4–6, with *health & medical care* as the dependent variable, follow a very similar pattern as *blacks' influence* and *culture* are added progressively. This is not surprising considering the high correlation (.79) between *meaning* and *health & medical care*.

Models 7–9 have *long-term care (NF)* as their dependent variable. These models follow a different pattern. Across all three models *tax capacity* reveals a statistically significant, positive effect, while *women's influence* provides a statistically significant negative effect. On the basis of previous work, we predicted both these statistically significant effects. Our explanation for the seemingly surprising negative effect for *women's influence* was that women legislators strongly favor using HCBS long-term care over nursing facility care since HCBS alternatives represent the predominant preference of elders and are also less expensive per person served (Giles-Sims et al., 2012). The cross-state variation in *long-term care (NF)* explained by these three models remains roughly constant (around 25 percent).

In the previous study, this explanation was sustained when we shifted to *HCBS\$/MNF\$* as our dependent variable, as in Models 10–12 of Table 3. This explanation is sustained again in Model 10 in which *women's influence* provides the only statistically significant (positive) effect. But this effect, while having by far the lowest *p*-values across the three models, does not retain statistical significance when *blacks' influence* and *culture* are added in Models 11 and 12, respectively. The cross-state variation in *HCBS\$/MNF\$* is quite low, only around 5 percent, in these three models.

In summary, when *meaning*, *health & medical care*, and HCBS\$/MNF\$ are the dependent variables (Models 1–6 and 10–12), adding *blacks' influence* to the analysis wipes out the statistically significant, positive effect of *women's influence* in Models 1, 4, and 10. Adding culture in Models 3, 6, and 12 reduces the negative effect of *blacks' influence*, but does not eliminate its statistical significance in Models 3 and 6. Indeed, *blacks' influence's* effects on *meaning* and *health & medical care* are surprisingly strong, more robust than the generally small proportions of African-American state legislators (a mean of 7 percent, and a maximum of just under 26 percent with only five states exceeding 20 percent) could be reasonably imagined to support. Our interpretation is that *women's influence* and particularly *black's influence* are each "standing in" for rival cultures, moralistic and traditionalistic, respectively. African-American legislators are most numerous in states exhibiting Elazar's traditionalistic culture, although it is unlikely that they adhere to this culture themselves. In contrast, *women's influence* is highest in states with Elazar's moralistic culture, and many women legislators may well sympathize with this culture.

The models in Table 4 examine this explanation. They include more independent variables than can be supported by 50 cases, so we view these models heuristically. When we add interaction between *culture* and *women's influence* as well as *blacks' influence* to the analysis, the independent effects of *women's influence* and *blacks' influence* recede from statistical significance. *Culture* acquires a statistically significant positive effect on *meaning*. *Culture's* interaction with *women's influence* produces a statistically significant positive effect on *HCBS$/MNF$*, and its interaction with *blacks' influence* produces statistically significant negative effects on *meaning* and *health & medical care*. These results are less systematic than we would prefer, but they are consistent with our suggested explanation above for the surprisingly strong effects of *blacks' influence* on *meaning* and *health & medical care*.

Because *culture* and particularly *meaning* are arguably endogenous, we ran two-stage-least-squares (2SLS) regression counterparts for Models 1–3 in Table 3 and Model 1 in Table 4. We do not display these models because their results are quite similar to those of the OLS models, albeit slightly weaker. Thus, there is little sign, at least at this level of aggregation, of endogeneity.

DISCUSSION

Implications

Aside from the effects of our independent variables of primary interest – *women's influence*, *blacks' influence*, and *culture* – only one variable attains

Table 4. Four Ordinary Least Squares (OLS) Models for Four Dependent Variables.

IVs	DVs			
	Model 1: Meaning	Model 2: Health/Medical Care	Model 3: Long-Term Care (NF)	Model 4: HCBS$/ MNF$
Liberal	−.025	.040	.071	−.001
	(.023)	(.024)	(.048)	(.002)
	$p = .287$	$p = .101$	$p = .145$	$p = .678$
Compete	3.205	−.526	−4.646	.065
	(3.934)	(4.049)	(8.202)	(.355)
	$p = .420$	$p = .897$	$p = .574$	$p = .855$
Tax Capacity	.885	.521	9.817*	−.073
	(1.833)	(1.866)	(3.822)	(.166)
	$p = .632$	$p = .784$	$p = .014$	$p = .662$
% 65+	.056	.169	.391	−.014
	(.161)	(.165)	(.335)	(.014)
	$p = .727$	$p = .313$	$p = .250$	$p = .356$
Women's Legislative	.152	.057	−312	−.014
Influence	(.114)	(.118)	(.239)	(.010)
	$p = .191$	$p = .663$	$p = .199$	$p = .184$
Blacks' Legislative	.067	.082	.050	−.008
Influence	(.086)	(.089)	(.180)	(.008)
	$p = .433$	$p = .363$	$p = .782$	$p = .308$
Culture	1.096**	.568	.301	−.049
	(.296)	(.305)	(.618)	(.027)
	$p = .001$	$p = .070$	$p = .629$	$p = .074$
Culture × Women's	−.021	−.002	.001	.002*
Influence	(.011)	(.012)	(.024)	(.001)
	$p = .074$	$p = .846$	$p = .976$	$p = .040$
Culture × Blacks'	−.032**	−.044**	−.005	.000
Influence	(.012)	(.012)	(.024)	(.001)
	$p = .008$	$p = .001$	$p = .847$	$p = .639$
Adjusted R^2	.669	.660	.227	.094

*Significant at <.05; **significant at <.01; ***significant at <.001. Standard errors are in parentheses. N for all variables = 50.
DVs, dependent variables; IVs, independent variables.

statistically significant effects in Table 2: *tax capacity* in Models 7–9 with *long-term care (NF)* as the dependent variable. These results show that our independent variables of primary interest exert their effects under controls that are well recognized (Karch, 2007) as influential in explaining cross-state policy differences. We explained above why several of these variables might be less influential in the instance of policies targeted on older citizens.

With respect to our three primary independent variables, we had previously found that *women's influence* exerted a strong positive effect on three of the dependent variables also in this study and a strong negative effect on *long-term care (NF)* (Giles-Sims et al., 2012). For reasons that we introduced above, it seemed sensible that the persistent presence of a significant proportion of women delegates in a state's legislature would be influential in fostering age-friendly orientations and policies.

We expected that we would find African-American legislators did not actively support and likely offered some resistance to the influence of women representatives in this regard. We imagined that this would be the case because particularly in the states in which African-American legislators hold higher proportions of the seats – states in which public social program resources are generally quite limited – they might find it necessary to develop priorities distinct from women legislators. Many black children are "at risk" in a variety of ways, and it is reasonable to imagine that the problems these youngsters face at the outset of their lives would take precedence, among black legislators, over those of older and predominantly white citizens who draw heavily on state pubic social program resources.

Accordingly, we expected that *blacks' influence* would exert modest, likely negative, effects on all our dependent variables (Bratton et al., 2006; Breines, 2002; Fuller, 2004; Zajicek, 2002). These expectations are consistent with our results for the two dependent variables involving long-term care (*long-term care (NF)* and *HCBS\$/MNF\$*) but stand at odds with those for *meaning* and *health & medical care*. In this latter pair of instances, *blacks' influence* exerts statistically significant negative influences, effects much stronger than those which *women's influence* exerts in a positive direction.

Given that the proportions of black legislators are so small, exceeding 20 percent in only five states and averaging 7 percent, it seems a stretch to imagine that such a generally small coterie of representatives would be capable of producing such sharply negative consequences for *meaning* and *health & medical care*. It is likely then that the proportion of a state's legislators who are black is closely (but not necessarily causally) associated with some other factor, such as states' political culture, that is more central to the source of these negative effects. Thus, we think that a state's political culture is at least partially responsible for the state's age friendliness with respect to *meaning* and *health & medical care*, and that in varying degree what we are picking up through *blacks' influence* and *women's influence* when *culture* is excluded from the analysis are the effects of *culture* as registered through these other variables.

For instance, Elazar's moralistic culture is influential in states in which public policies benefitting the public broadly, and particularly its most vulnerable members, are widely supported. States in which this culture is prominent also have larger proportions of women legislators (see Table 2.) So, while these women legislators make a contribution to state age friendliness independent of that fostered by culture, *culture* exerts a powerful effect of its own on *women's influence, meaning,* and *health & medical care.*

The instance of *blacks' influence* is more complicated. States in which Elazar's traditionalistic culture is influential are generally states in which a range of public social programs benefitting vulnerable citizens are notoriously skimpy, so it makes sense that the traditionalistic culture exerts a strong negative effect in these states that depresses support for age-friendly social policies. Additionally, most of these states have relatively large proportions of African-American representatives (see Table 2). So, institutional change (i.e., the personnel of the legislature) has occurred more rapidly than aspects of these states' cultures. But when black legislators, who are predominantly members of the political party that is usually more supportive of public policies benefitting vulnerable groups, are faced with stark zero-sum alternatives, some may perceive age-friendly public social programs as relatively low priorities in the competition for scarce public social program resources; their hesitancy to support age-friendly programs contributes an increment to explaining poor state performance on some dimensions of state age friendliness. This suggestion is illustrated by *blacks' influence* retaining its statistically significant effect in interaction with *culture* in the models having *meaning* and *health & medical care* as the dependent variables.

Limitations

Our study has three prominent limitations and is thus exploratory and suggestive rather than definitive. First, the N is relatively small (50). Second, the three independent variables of primary interest exhibit fairly high intercorrelations. Third, the study is cross-sectional rather than longitudinal.

Future Research

Against the influences of all women legislators and all male African-American legislators, the influence of 146 black women legislators, considered independently, exerts little effect in our national study. We expect to design a regional study in which we can determine the character of their independent influence on age-friendly state policies. Further, as the population in the United States continues to age, having a better understanding of the dynamics influencing the relative support of elders will be increasingly important. So a related study with a larger N, acquired through longitudinal data, on how race, ethnicity, and sex interact would be extremely valuable.

REFERENCES

Baicker, K., & Chandra, A. (2004). Medicare spending, the physician workforce and beneficiaries' quality of care. *Health Affairs* (web version) W4-184 (April 7).

Barrett, E. J. (1995). The policy priorities of African American women in state legislatures. *Legislative Studies Quarterly, 20*(2), 223–247.

Barrett, E. J. (1997). Gender and race in the state house: The legislative power. *Social Science Journal, 34*(2), 131–144.

Barrett, E. J. (2001). Black women in state legislatures: The relationship of race and gender to legislative experience. In S. J. Carroll (Ed.), *The impact of women in public office* (pp. 185–204). Bloomington, IN: Indiana University Press.

Berry, W. D., Fording, R. C., & Hanson, R. L. (2000). An annual cost of living index for the American states, 1960-1995. *Journal of Politics, 62*(2), 550–567.

Berry, W. D., Ringquist, E., Fording, R. C., & Hanson, R. L. (1998). Measuring citizen and government ideology in the American states, 1960-1993. *American Journal of Political Science, 42*(1), 327–348.

Bibby, J. F., & Holbrook, T. M. (2004). Parties and elections. In V. Gray & R. L. Hanson (Eds.), *Politics in the American states* (pp. 62–99). Washington, DC: CQ Press.

Bolzendahl, C., & Brooks, C. (2007). Women's political resources and welfare state spending in 12 capitalist democracies. *Social Forces, 85*(4), 1509–1534.

Bratton, K. A., Haynie, K. L., & Reingold, B. (2006). Agenda setting and African American women in state legislatures. *Journal of Women, Politics & Policy, 28*(3/4), 71–96.

Breines, W. (2002). What's love got to do with it? White women, black women and feminism in the movement years. *Signs: Journal of Women in Culture & Society, 27*(4), 1095–1134.

Burrell, B. (1994). *A woman's place is in the House: Campaigning for Congress in the feminist era.* Ann Arbor, MI: University of Michigan Press.

Burwell, B., Sredl, K., & Eiken, S. (2003). *Medicaid long term care expenditures* (And related tables can be retrieved from http://www.hcs.org/; search Brian Burwell > Table 1 (PDF)). Cambridge, MA: Thomson Medstatt.

Carroll, S. J. (2001). Representing women: Women state legislators as agents of policy-related change. In S. J. Carroll (Ed.), *The impact of women in public office* (pp. 3–21). Bloomington, IN: Indiana University Press.

Carroll, S. J. (2008). Committee assignments: Discrimination or choice? In B. Reingold (Ed.), *Legislative women: Getting elected, getting ahead* (pp. 135–156). Boulder, CO: Lynne Rienner Publishers.

Cook, F. L., & Barrett, E. (1992). *Support for the American welfare state.* New York, NY: Columbia University Press.

Darcy, R., & Hadley, C. D. (1988). Black women in politics: The puzzle of success. *Social Science Quarterly, 69*(3), 629–645.

Deen, R. E., & Little, T. H. (1999). Getting to the top: Factors influencing the selection of women to positions of leadership in state legislatures. *State and Local Government Review, 31*(2), 123–134.

Diamond, I. (1977). *Sex roles in the state house.* New Haven, CT: Yale University Press.

Dodson, D. L. (2001). Acting for women: Is what legislators say, what they do? In S. J. Carroll (Ed.), *The impact of women in public office* (pp. 225–242). Bloomington, IN: Indiana University Press.

Dolan, K. (2004). *Voting for women: How the public evaluates women candidates.* Boulder, CO: Westview Press.

Dolan, K. (2006). Symbolic mobilization? The impact of candidate sex in American elections. *American Politics Research, 34*(6), 687–704.

Duerst-Lahti, G., & Kelly, R. M. (Eds.). (1995). *Gender power, leadership and governance.* Ann Arbor, MI: University of Michigan Press.

Elazar, D. J. (1966). *American federalism: A view from the states.* New York, NY: Thomas Y. Crowell.

Fisher, P., & Pratt, T. (2006). Political culture and the death penalty. *Criminal Justice Policy Review, 17*(1), 48–60.

Folbre, N., Reimers, C., & Yoon, J. (2009). Making do and getting by: Non-market work and elderly women's standard of living. *Journal of Women, Politics and Policy, 30*(2/3), 198–221.

Fuller, A. A. (2004). What difference does difference make? Women, race-ethnicity, social class and social change. *Gender, Race and Class, 11*(4), 8–29.

Giles-Sims, J., Green, J., & Lockhart, C. (2012). Do women legislators have a positive effect on the supportiveness of states toward older citizens? *Journal of Women, Politics and Policy, 33*(1), 38–64.

Gilligan, C. (1982). *In a different voice: Psychological theory and women's development.* Cambridge: Harvard University Press.

Grey, S. (2002). Does size matter? Critical mass and New Zealand's women MP's. *Parliamentary Affairs, 55*(1), 19–29.

Hanson, R. L. (1991). Political culture variations in state economic development policy. *Publius, 21*(2), 63–81.

Harrington, C., Carrillo, H., & Mercado-Scott, C. (2005). *Nursing facilities, staffing, residents, and facility deficiencies, 1998 through 2004.* San Francisco, CA: Department of Social and Behavioral Sciences, University of California.

Hartmann, H., & English, A. (2009). Older women's retirement security: A primer. *Journal of Women, Politics and Policy, 30*(2/3), 109–140.

He, W., Sengupta, M., Verkoff, V. A., & DeBarros, K. A. (2005). *65+ in the United States: 2005.* Washington, DC: Census Bureau, U.S. Department of Commerce & National Institutes of Health, U.S. Department of Health and Human Services.

Howes, C. (2009). Who will care for the women? *Journal of Women, Politics and Policy, 30*(2/3), 248–271.

Jaquette, J. S. (1997). Women's power: From Tokenism to critical mass. *Foreign Policy, 108*, 23–37.

Jencks, S. F., Huff, E. D., & Cuerdon, T. (2003). Change in the quality of care delivered to Medicare beneficiaries, 1998-2000-01. *Journal of the American Medical Association, 289*(3/January 15), 305–312.

Johnson, C. A. (1976). Political culture in the American states: Elazar's formulation examined. *American Journal of Political Science, 20*(3), 491–499.

Kanter, R. M. (1977). Some effects of proportions on group life: Skewed sex ratios and responses to token women. *American Journal of Sociology, 82*(5), 965–990.

Karch, A. (2007). Emerging issues and future directions in state policy diffusion research. *State Politics and Policy Quarterly, 71*(1), 54–80.

Kathlene, L. (2001). Words that matter: Women's voice and institutional bias in public policy formation. In S. J. Carroll (Ed.), *The impact of women in public office* (pp. 22–48). Bloomington, IN: Indiana University Press.

Kenney, S. J. (1996). Field essay: New research on gendered political institutions. *Political Research Quarterly, 49*(2), 445–466.

Kincaid, J. (1982). Introduction. In J. Kincaid (Ed.), *Political culture, public policy and the American states* (pp. 2–15). Philadelphia, PA: Institute for the Study of Human Issues.

Lockhart, C., & Giles-Sims, J. (2010). *Aging across the United States: Matching needs to states' differing opportunities and services.* University Park, PA: Penn State University Press.

Mead, L. M. (2004). State political culture and welfare reform. *Policy Studies Journal, 32*(2), 271–296.

Mollica, R., & Johnson-Lamarche, H. (2005). *State residential care and assisted living: 2004.* Washington, DC: Department of Health and Human Services.

Moran, D. R., & Watson, S. S. (1991). Political culture, political system characteristics and public policies among the American states. *Publius, 21*(2), 32–48.

Orey, B. D., & Smooth, W. (2006). Race *and* gender matter: Refining models of policy making in state legislatures. *Journal of Women, Politics and Policy, 28*(3/4), 97–119.

Paxton, P., Hughes, M. M., & Green, J. L. (2006). The international women's movement and women's political representation, 1893–2003. *American Sociological Review, 71*(6), 898–920.

Pitkin, H. F. (1967). *The concept of representation.* Berkeley, CA: University of California Press.

Prestage, J. (1977). Black women state legislators. In M. Githens & J. Prestage (Eds.), *A portrait of marginality: The political behavior of the American woman.* New York, NY: David McKay.

Preuhs, R. R. (2006). The conditional effects of minority descriptive representation: Black legislators and policy influence in American states. *Journal of Politics, 68*(3), 585–599.

Ranney, A. (1965). Parties in state politics. In H. Jacob & K. Vines (Eds.), *Politics in the American states: A comparative analysis* (pp. 61–99). Boston, MA: Little, Brown and Co.

Reingold, B. (2008). Women as officeholders: Linking descriptive and substantive representation. In C. Wolbrecht, K. Beckwith & L. Baldez (Eds.), *Political women and American democracy* (pp. 128–147). New York, NY: Cambridge University Press.

Robinson, E. (2010). *Disintegration: The splintering of black America.* New York, NY: Doubleday.

Rosenthal, C. S. (1998). *When women lead: Integrative leadership in state legislatures.* New York, NY: Oxford University Press.

Rule, W. (1981). Why women don't run: The critical contextual factors in women's legislative recruitment. *Western Political Quarterly, 34*(1), 66–77.

Rule, W. (1990). Why more women are state legislators. *Western Political Quarterly, 43*(2), 437–448.

Saint-Germain, M. A. (1989). Does their difference make a difference? The impact of women on public policy in the Arizona legislature. *Social Science Quarterly, 70*(4), 956–968.

Salganicoff, A., Cubanski, J., Ranju, U., & Newman, T. (2009). Health coverage and expenses: Impact on older women's well-being. *Journal of Women, Politics and Policy, 30*(2-3), 222–247.

Sanbonmatsu, K. (2002). Political parties and the recruitment of women to state legislatures. *Journal of Politics, 64*(3), 791–809.

Sanbonmatsu, K. (2006). *Where women run: Gender and party in the American states.* Ann Arbor, MI: University of Michigan Press.

Schneider, A., & Ingram, H. (1993). Social construction of target populations: Implications for politics and policy. *American Political Science Review, 87*(2), 334–348.

Simien, E. (2005). Race, gender and linked fate. *Journal of Black Studies, 35*(5), 529–550.

Smooth, W. G. (2008). Gender, race, and the exercise of power and influence. In B. Reingold (Ed.), *Legislative women: Getting elected, getting ahead* (pp. 175–196). Boulder, CO: Lynne Rienner Publishers.

Swers, M. L. (1998). Are women more likely to vote for women's issue bills than their male colleagues? *Legislative Studies Quarterly, 23*(3), 435–448.

Thomas, S. (1994). *How women legislate.* New York, NY: Oxford University Press.

Thomas, S., & Welch, S. (1991). The impact of gender on activities and priorities of state legislators. *Western Political Quarterly, 44*(2), 445–456.

Thomas, S., & Welch, S. (2001). The impact of women in state legislatures: Numerical and organizational strength. In S. J. Carroll (Ed.), *The impact of women in public office* (pp. 166–181). Bloomington, IN: Indiana University Press.

Tolleson-Rinehart, S., & Stanley, J. R. (1994). *Claytie and the Lady: Ann Richards, Gender and Politics in Texas.* Austin: University of Texas Press.

U.S. Census Bureau (USCB). (2000). *State population by age and race.* Retrieved from http://www.census.gov > Census 2000 > Detailed Tables > United States + Table P12B.

U.S. Centers for Disease Control (USCDC). (2002). *Infant death records.* Retrieved from http://wonder.cdc.gov/lbd-v2002.html

U.S. Department of Commerce (USDC). (2004). *Statistical abstract of the United States.* Washington, DC: USDC. Retrieved from http://www.census.gov

U.S. Department of Health and Human Services (USDHHS). (2005). *Healthcare finance review: Medicare and Medicaid statistical supplement.* Washington, DC: USDHHS.

U.S. National Center for Health Statistics (USNCHS). (2002). *Teenage births in the United States: Trends 1991-2000.* Retrieved from http://www.cdc.gov/nchs/data/nvsr/nvsr50/nvsr50_09.pdf

Welch, S., & Studlar, D. T. (1990). Multi-member districts and the representation of women: Evidence from Britain and the United States. *Journal of Politics, 52*(2), 392–412.

Wolbrecht, C., & Campbell, D. E. (2007). Leading by example: Female members of parliament as political role models. *American Journal of Political Science, 51*(4), 233–247.

Zajicek, A. M. (2002). Race discourses and antiracist practices in a local women's movement. *Gender and Society, 16*(2), 155–174.

INTERSECTIONAL IDENTITIES AND WORKER EXPERIENCES IN HOME HEALTH CARE: THE NATIONAL HOME HEALTH AIDE SURVEY

Carter Rakovski and Kim Price-Glynn

ABSTRACT

As the population ages in the United States and globally, health-care demands are rising and varied, including the growth of home health care. Small, regional, qualitative studies indicate both satisfaction and exploitation in home health-care work. These intimate, caring relationships with clients may be especially challenging for minorities due to client prejudice and structural marginalization. This study broadens the scope of current research by addressing issues facing home health-care workers using large-scale, nationwide data.

Using nationally representative data of home health aides in the US, the National Home Health Aide Survey (NHHAS), we evaluate which features of work are related to overall satisfaction. The prevalence and sources of discrimination and working conditions are examined according to workers' intersectional gender, race, ethnicity, and class identities.

Issues in Health and Health Care Related to Race/Ethnicity, Immigration, SES and Gender
Research in the Sociology of Health Care, Volume 30, 261–280
ISSN: 0275-4959/doi:10.1108/S0275-4959(2012)0000030014

Satisfaction was highest for those who were extremely satisfied with challenging work, learning new skills, and were most supported in their caring labor. Salary was the area with the most frequent dissatisfaction. Support for reproductive and caring labor was often inadequate. Black women and men reported the highest levels of discrimination (about 28.0%), followed by Hispanic women and men (16.5% and 10%, respectively). The largest source of discrimination was patients (80.4%). There were differences in job outcomes according to intersectional identities of race, class, and gender.

Discrimination, low wages, and not having enough support for both reproductive and caring labor are problems for home health aides. Improving home health aide work is also likely to improve patient outcomes.

Keywords: Direct care workers; home health care; home health aides; intersectionality; caring labor.

INTRODUCTION

The changing organization of work within the long-term care industry needs to be examined with respect to its effect on workers. In particular, there has been a shift away from long-term stays in hospitals and skilled nursing facilities (SNFs) toward community-based home health care (Decker, 2005). This change of context from institutional health-care settings to private homes has had corresponding changes for health-care workers who now provide care with fewer resources like extensive medical equipment, ergonomic settings, and colleagues. In 2004, there were 624,000 home health aides (HHAs) and 701,000 paid care attendants in private homes in the United States and these numbers are increasing (National Occupational Research Agenda (NORA), 2009). HHAs are forecast to grow the fastest among all US health-care occupations (974,000 and 988,000 workers projected in 2014, respectively) (NORA, 2009).

HHAs are a diverse group of direct care workers (DCWs) that work for home health agencies. In this study, DCWs includes the following job titles: HHA, home care aide, personal care attendant, hospice aide, certified hospice and palliative nursing assistant, and certified nursing assistant. DCWs are involved in hands-on patient care, excluding housekeepers and those with higher degrees such as registered nurses or specialists like nutritionists.

DCWs working in hospitals and SNFs help clients with activities of daily living (ADLs), such as dressing, bathing, eating, transferring, and toileting. HHAs assist with ADLs too, but they also help with instrumental ADLs, such as meal preparation, cleaning, and shopping. As an HHA described it, "We're maids plus" (Stacey, 1995, p. 839). They often drive to more than one home and are sent by supervisors to fill in at other homes (Aronson & Neysmith, 1996).

While HHAs care for the frailest and most dependent people in our society, HHAs themselves are a vulnerable population. HHAs are often women (91.8%), ethnic/racial minorities (49.7%), and immigrants (23.7%), who have completed less than a high school education (30.9%) (Montgomery, Holley, Deichert, & Kosloski, 2005). HHAs are on average older (mean = 42.8) than DCWs in SNFs (mean = 36.4) and hospitals (mean = 38.0) and less likely to be US citizens (16.2% non citizens, compared to 8.2% and 6.4% in SNFs and hospitals, respectively) (Yamada, 2002). Women HHAs are more likely to be minorities (51%), single mothers (22%) and foreign born (22%) than all women in the US workplace (30%, 14%, and 13%, respectively) (Smith & Baughman, 2007). Their training ranges between on-the-job experiences to specific credentials and certification that is dependent on the type of employment and the state in which the DCW is working. According to the National Home Health Aide Survey (NHHAS), the majority (83.9%) of HHAs received training prior to beginning work.

HHAs also face greater economic inequalities compared to other health-care workers; their poverty rates are higher and the average wages are lower for DCWs in home care than in SNFs and hospitals (Yamada, 2002). The low wages of home care workers are historically tied to race, class, and gender (RCG) among caring laborers (Duffy, 2007). Research suggests that between 19% and 22% live below the poverty line (compared to 13% of the general population) and an additional 25–28% live near the poverty line (Montgomery et al., 2005; Yamada, 2002). HHAs have lower average wages than facility-based workers (Kemper et al., 2008; Yamada, 2002). When asked about factors most critical to improving their jobs, HHAs cite increased wages rather than other factors (Kemper et al., 2008). Compared with facility-based jobs, home care jobs offer fewer opportunities for advancement.

In addition to discrimination based on race/ethnicity, immigrant status, class, gender, citizenship and educational background, DCWs face various injuries and hazards in their workplace. DCWs experience musculoskeletal pain and injuries, exposure to hazardous drugs and other chemicals, exposure to infectious diseases, traumatic situations, deaths of clients, and physical/verbal assaults from clients (Institute of Medicine [IOM], 2008; Miranda, Punnett, Gore, & Boyer, 2011; NORA, 2009; Zhang, et al. 2011).

HHAs suffer injuries from lifting and transferring patients, human and animal bites, assaults, and scratches (Bercovitz et al., 2011). Miranda et al. found 56% of DCWs in SNFs had been physically assaulted in the past three months, and those DCWs who experienced multiple assaults were more likely to report widespread musculoskeletal pain (2011). Tak, Sweeney, Alterman, Baron, and Calvert reported that one third of DCWs in SNFs had sustained injuries in the past year due to client aggression (2010). Zhang et al. conducted interviews and focus groups with both DCWs and supervisors in SNFs (2011). Their research uncovered numerous DCW risks, specifically, ergonomic issues, trip hazards, needle sticks, combative residents, and infectious diseases, many of which were not recognized by supervisors (Zhang et al., 2011). Sophie, Belza, and Young described similar risks from interviews with DCWs working in SNFs with the addition of burdens of responsibility and emotional stress (2003).

The workplace risks encountered by HHAs are not as well documented as DCWs in SNFs but are likely different (Aronson & Neysmith, 1996; Yamada, 2002). Hasson and Arnetz compared DCWs working in two settings (SNFs and home care) in Sweden (2007). DCWs in home care reported less sufficient knowledge but also less mental and emotional exhaustion than their facility-based counterparts. Home care workers were more influenced by feeling their job was "dead-end" in their intention to leave than workers in SNFs (Brannon, Zinn, Mor, & Davis, 2002).

Context and Content of Home Care Work

DCWs find satisfaction with their work because of their commitment to clients, caring for others, and challenging work (Nishikawa, 2011; Rakovski & Price-Glynn, 2010; Stacey, 2005). In the National Nursing Assistant Study, 98% of respondents reported "caring for others" as one of the reasons they continued in their jobs, and 50% reported it as the main reason (Rakovski & Price-Glynn, 2010). In a study of consumer-directed home care workers, 66% listed commitment to their clients as one of the top three reasons they took and remained in their jobs (Howes, 2008). This reason was listed far more frequently than any other reason, especially wages (9%) and health insurance (18%). Home care workers who report caring for clients as an important reward are less likely to intend to leave the job (Brannon, Barry, Kemper, Schreiner, & Vasey, 2007).

The literature on caring labor emphasizes the gendered devaluation of caring labor (England, 2005). Since caring labor is seen as women's responsibility and something women accomplish *naturally* as opposed to jobs that require *work*, similar to the expectations around motherhood, caring labor is normatively devalued as not amounting to work at all or rendered invisible (Cancian, 1986; Chodorow, 1978; Hochschild, 1983). Context also matters. As Hondagneu-Sotelo argues, domestic labor is "distinctive not in being the worst job of all but in being regarded as something other than employment" (2007, p. 9). Since HHAs' labor is influenced by its location in clients' homes, HHAs working conditions vary considerably by the type of setting under study, but are usually described as problematic. Stacey describes the more than thirty HHAs she studied from California as "overworked" (2005). The overwork stems, in part, from a chronic shortage of workers, high turnover, and organizational policies regarding adequate staffing levels (Harrington et al., 2000).

The overwhelming responsibility that home care workers feel toward clients can lead to exploitation. As a worker in a study by Aronson and Neysmith explained, "Some things I do because there's nobody else to do them. So it's either me or it doesn't get done" (1996, p. 70). In addition to the isolation that can exacerbate feelings of responsibility, DCWs use a family metaphor to understand their relationships (Berdes & Eckert, 2007), and administrators encourage DCWs to think of their clients "like family" (Dodson & Zincavage, 2007). These intimate, caring relationships can lead to worker abuse and exploitation, particularly in home health care (Aronson & Neysmith, 1996; Stacey, 2005).

The literature suggests that race, immigrant status, culture, and religion continue to matter for DCWs. In a study of DCWs in SNFs in Massachusetts, Allensworth-Davies et al. reported that nonwhite DCWs perceived their organizations to be less culturally competent and their coworkers as more negative to their race than white DCWs (2007). The overrepresentation of minorities among DCWs and their underrepresentation among supervisors and clients may exacerbate problems, including a lack of attention and sensitivity to issues like racism (Dodson & Zincavage, 2007). DCWs who experience on-the-job racism may be less likely to come forward to address prejudice. Similar findings for immigrant status, culture, and religion persist. Sloane, Williams, and Zimmerman argued immigrant status had an independent negative effect on job satisfaction and increased intention to leave for DCWs in SNFs (2010). Solaris found that cultural and religious background was more important than gender in determining the way HHAs understood their work in a small, qualitative study among Russian immigrants (2006). Jewish HHAs constructed themselves and their work in a narrative of professionalism, while Orthodox Christian

HHAs used a model of sainthood and fictive kinships that framed their work as personal (Solaris, 2006).

Caring labor relationships are complex. HHAs' family references are a proxy for their intimate bonds with patients, reflecting the kind of care HHAs seek to provide, and the similarities between these work relationships and those HHAs have had with their own aging parents (Berdes & Eckert, 2007). By contrast to the family metaphors used by DCWs, clients often characterize workers through invisibility and distancing. Lynn May Rivas, in her work on personal care assistants, argues the best care looks "effortless" by making DCWs and their labor invisible, then the relationship is commodified and cheap (Rivas, 2003, p. 78). Moreover, due to clients' desires for independence and the purchase of that independence through the labor of HHAs, it becomes apparent that HHA visibility may run counter to clients' notions of self-determination. For clients to preserve feelings of independence, it is better to see the HHA as an object they purchased, not as an equal or recognizable contributor. Clients accomplish distancing through the use of medical terms and acronyms used to describe these workers, like HHA or PCA, instead of caring terms. Clients' use of this language professionalizes and distances them from being the one who needs help or care in a position of weakness or subservience and elevates them into a position of power, as a supervisor.

Contradictions

Despite many potential hazards, home health-care work is not a zero sum game. As Kemper et al. (2008) point out, some of the differences in home-based direct care jobs compared with those in nursing homes and assisted living facilities may actually produce better outcomes for HHAs. Since the location of work is in client homes, HHAs have more autonomy about how their work is organized than other DCWs (Kemper et al., 2008; Stacey, 2005). For example, home care workers generally have greater autonomy and control over their schedules. HHAs also tend to have more responsibility for and control over patient care and may be able to build deeper and more meaningful relationships with clients and families than other DCWs (Howes, 2008; Stacey, 2005; Kemper et al., 2008). HHAs may also be less hurried than facility-based workers. Over 90% of HHAs stated they had enough or more than enough time to help clients with ADLs (Bercovitz et al., 2011). These job attributes may foster HHA's willingness to accept lower wages and fewer benefits for more autonomous and relaxed working conditions. HHA independence, however, is a double-edged sword. DCWs who work independently in homes of clients may become more isolated and experience greater levels of job stress than other DCWs (Morris, 2009). Home care jobs also usually involve considerable travel and less consistent hours (Howes, 2008; Kemper et al., 2008).

Research Questions

The present study uses the NHHAS to address the risks and rewards of home care work and whether these are distributed equally among groups of workers by the intersectional identity characteristics of gender, race, and socioeconomic status. Specifically, this study addresses the following questions:

1. How satisfied are HHAs with aspects of their work?
2. Which aspects of HHA work are related to overall job satisfaction?
3. Is there evidence of prejudice and discrimination toward HHAs, and if so, what are the sources?
4. Do aspects of home health-care jobs, including satisfaction and discrimination, differ by intersectional group identities?

METHODS

Intersectionality

Scholars have proposed a variety of techniques for analyzing diverse characteristics of selfhood, like RCG (Collins, 1993; King, 1988). Feminist and critical race scholars have favored multidimensional approaches that see identities as "interconnected" in their influence over power and inequality (Browne & Misra, 2003; Collins, 1993). Intersectional RCG research seeks to uncover the ways in which multiple facets of identity influence life and work (and vice versa) in overlapping and interactive ways (Landry, 2007). Despite strong theoretical support, intersectionality has not been widely studied within different occupations (Browne & Misra, 2003). Further, highly skilled and paid professional workers have been the primary focus of social identity research in the workplace, especially treatment by supervisors, coworkers, and clients (Browne & Misra, 2003; Correll, Bernard, & Paik, 2007). The present study attempts to address these gaps in the literature by looking at the affects of RCG on organizational measures of inequality among low-wage, home health-care workers. Drawing on Leslie McCall's "categorical approach," we use the existing available analytical categories – gender, race, education, and income – to strategically examine relationships and inequalities within and between social groups (McCall, 2005). We also situate these identity characteristics within organizational, economic, and contextual workplace issues.

Data Source

Data are from the NHHAS, the first nationally representative sample survey of HHAs in the United States (Bercovitz et al., 2011). The survey was sponsored by the Department of Health and Human Services' Office of the Assistant Secretary for Planning and Evaluation (ASPE) in order to understand issues related to worker satisfaction and retention. NHHAS, a two-stage probability sample survey, was a supplement to the 2007 National Home and Hospice Care Survey (NHHCS) conducted by the Centers for Disease Control and Prevention's National Center for Health Statistics in conjunction with ASPE. Aides who worked in agencies that participated in the NHHCS were sampled for the NHHAS. Aides who directly involved in providing ADL assistance were eligible and were interviewed using computer-assisted telephone interviewing. Further details of the sampling and data collection can be found at http://www.cdc.gov/nchs/nhhas.htm.

Despite the strengths of the sampling method and data collection, the NHHAS does not include some variables in the public-release data file. Citizenship status was not released and its exclusion is a weakness of the present study. Few intersectional identities could be studied using the NHHAS. Race was limited to three categories: white, black, and other. Because the other category was ambiguous and small, especially for men, we excluded it from this analysis. We created a separate category for those who identified as Hispanic. Age and wages were also limited at the upper ends (65 and $25.00, respectively). Aides working at agencies not included in the NHHCS were also not eligible for inclusion.

Sample Characteristics

Of the 3,377 HHAs interviewed, 96.9% were women (Table 1). The average age was 45.6 years. The majority self-identified as white (67.2%) with 20.9%

Table 1. Sample Description $(n = 3377)^a$.

	%	Mean (SD)
HHA characteristics		
Gender, Age and Race:		
Female	96.9	
Age		45.6 (11.7)[b]
Hispanic, Latino/Latina	7.0	
African American	20.9	
White	67.2	
Other racial group	4.9	
Marital status:		
Married/living with partner	62.0	
Separated/Divorced	20.3	
Widowed	5.2	
Never married	11.6	
Education:		
Less than high school graduate	12.7	
Holds high school degree or GED	50.6	
Some college or college graduate	36.7	
Total annual household income:		
Less than 10 K	3.1	
10 K – under 20 K	15.8	
20 K – under 30 K	27.9	
30 K – under 40 K	19.8	
40 K-under 50 K	13.2	
50 K or more	20.2	
Work-related characteristics		
Hours worked per week		33.3 (10.7)
Hourly pay		11.4 (2.6)
Months worked at current job		76.5 (73.2)
Works more than one job	15.9	
Time worked as a home health aide:		
Less than two years	8.3	
Two to five years	19.5	
Six to ten years	19.3	
Eleven to twenty years	36.7	
More than twenty years	16.1	
Location of work:		
Inpatient facility	5.6	
Patient homes	64.5	
Both homes and inpatient facilities	29.9	
If patient homes, multiple patients	89.2	
Agency characteristics		
Location:		
Metropolitan	38.7	
Micropolitan	35.6	
Neither	25.7	

Table 1. (*Continued*)

	%	Mean (SD)
Ownership:		
Chain	23.1	
Independent (not chain)	76.9	
Profit status:		
For profit agency	31.1	
Not for profit	68.9	
Agency type:		
Home health	28.6	
Hospice	35.6	
Mixed	35.8	

[a]Some survey items have smaller sample sizes due to missing data.
[b]Age was coded as 65 when age was 65 or greater.

African American, and 7.0% Hispanic or Latino/a. The majority of HHAs were married or living with a partner (62.0%) and have at least a high school degree (87.3%). Household incomes reflect the low wages of caring labor. The average hourly rate was $11.40, despite working at their current job on average 76.5 months (or more than 6 years). Most worked in multiple patient homes and were distributed fairly evenly between urban and rural areas. Unlike DCWs in SNFs, HHAs were mostly working in independently owned agencies (76.9%) that were not-for-profit (68.9%).

Composite Measures and Analytic Strategy

All NHHAS survey questions were examined to find the appropriate questions to measure worker satisfaction. Five survey items were chosen to create a measure of *job satisfaction*. The first question was, "How satisfied are you with your current job," which had the following responses: extremely dissatisfied (0), somewhat dissatisfied (1), somewhat satisfied (2), and extremely satisfied (3). The second question, "If HHA had to decide whether to take current job again, would HHA take it," included responses ranging from: definitely not take it (0), probably not take it (1), probably take it (2), and definitely take it (3). The third question, "Would HHA recommend friend or family work as HHA," provided responses including: definitely not recommend (0), probably not recommend (1), probably recommend (2), and definitely recommend (3). The fourth and fifth items were about the respect HHAs feel given to them by their supervisors and the agency. The responses were as follows: a great deal (2), somewhat (1), and not at all (0). These five items had good reliability (Cronbach's $\alpha = 0.80$). The scale was made by averaging the scores across the five items (in order to make a scale with all of the non missing items). This scale was converted into a z-score by subtracting the mean and dividing by the standard deviation. This results in a *job satisfaction* scale with a mean of 0 and standard deviation of 1. Positive scores represent above-average satisfaction, and negative scores represent below-average satisfaction.

The NHHAS reported satisfaction with aspects of the current job, specifically, salary, benefits, learning new skills, and challenging work. Satisfaction was indicated by four responses: extremely dissatisfied, somewhat dissatisfied, somewhat satisfied, and extremely satisfied. In addition, two other aspects of the job, *reproductive labor* and *caring labor*, were measured by combining survey items. *Reproductive* measures the amount of time they feel they have for the reproductive labor aspects of their job, and *caring labor* measures the amount of space allowed by the facility for the caring aspects of their job (Duffy, 2007; Lopez, 2006). *Reproductive labor* is the sum of two variables: "During a typical workweek, how much time do you have to give individual attention to residents who need activities of daily living (ADL) assistance?" and "During a typical work week, how much time do you have to complete other duties not directly related to residents?" Each item was scored 0 (not enough time), 1 (enough time), or 2 (more than enough time). *Reproductive labor* ranges from 0 (least time) to 4 (most time).

Caring labor is a composite score from four survey items. The survey items and their responses are as follows: "To what degree do you feel your supervisor respects you as part of the health care team?" not at all (0), somewhat (1), or a great deal (2); "Are you assigned to care for the same clients on most days that you work?" clients change (0) or are the same or a combination (1); "In general, does supervisor encourage you to discuss the care and well-being of clients with their families?" no (0) or yes (1); and "My supervisor listens to me when I am worried about a client's care" somewhat disagree or strongly disagree (0), somewhat agree (1), or strongly agree (2). These responses were summed to create a score ranging from 0 to 6, where 0 indicates the job is least supportive of caring labor and 6 indicates the job is the most supportive of caring labor.

Hourly wages were self-reported by HHAs with an upper limit of \$25.00 or more. We created a *benefits summary score* by summing nine dummy items, where a one indicates that a benefit was available to the respondent. The following nine benefits were used: retirement, health insurance for family, health insurance for self, time off for good work, bonuses, sick leave, personal days, paid vacation days, and supplemental pay for transportation. For our measurement of *socioeconomic status*, we drew on the work of Oakes and Rossi (2003). They conceptualize socioeconomic status as a function of material capital (i.e., income), human capital (i.e., education), and social capital (i.e., social networks and support). Since we could not measure social capital with these data, we created a scale that equally weighted education and total family income. Then, we split the sample into the top quartile and the lower three quartiles for comparison of gender and race by socioeconomic status on job outcomes. All other variables were taken directly from NHHAS survey items.

Mean job satisfaction scores were calculated across various aspects of the job. The prevalence of reported discrimination was calculated by the percent of respondents indicating they experienced discrimination overall and within six race/ethnic and gender groups. Chi-square tests were calculated for each discrimination outcome (yes/no) across the six groups. Finally, the averages for aspects of the job (i.e., injuries, wages, benefits, and satisfaction) were calculated across all six race/ethnic and gender groups. Four of the six groups were further differentiated by social class. Latino men and black men were not compared by class due to small sample sizes.

FINDINGS

In accordance with previous research, the majority of HHAs remained at their jobs because of the value they place on caring for clients (71.7%) and reported above-average job satisfaction ($M = 0.10$) (Table 2). Satisfaction was highest for those who were extremely satisfied with challenging work ($M = 0.27$), learning new skills ($M = 0.29$), salary ($M = 0.53$), benefits ($M = 0.39$), and were most supported in their caring labor ($M = 0.38$). Those who reported the lowest levels of satisfaction were extremely dissatisfied with having challenging work ($M = -2.30$), learning new skills ($M = -1.92$), had little support for caring labor ($M = -2.42$), and were not trusted to make patient care decisions ($M = -1.35$). Over 30% reported one or more injuries in the last year, and they also reported low levels of job satisfaction. Salary was the area with the most dissatisfaction (11.7% were extremely dissatisfied). Time and support for reproductive and caring labor also were areas in need of improvement for theses workers.

Discrimination due to race or ethnicity was reported by 10.8% of HHAs (Table 3). The largest source of discrimination was patients (80.4%). However, 91.2% of all HHAs also reported feeling respected by patients "a

Table 2. Sources of Satisfaction and Dissatisfaction with Current HHA Work $(N = 3359)$[a].

	N	Mean Satisfaction[b]		n	Mean Satisfaction
Values caring			*Discrimination*		
Stay at job to care for others	2403	0.10	(due to race/ ethnicity)	362	−0.41
Challenging work			*Salary*		
Extremely satisfied	2049	0.27	Extremely satisfied	836	0.53
Somewhat satisfied	1239	−0.37	Somewhat satisfied	1603	0.12
Somewhat dissatisfied	49	−1.13	Somewhat dissatisfied	526	−0.39
Extremely dissatisfied	9	−2.30	Extremely dissatisfied	394	−1.09
Learning new skills			*Benefits*		
Extremely satisfied	1950	0.29	Extremely satisfied	1304	0.39
Somewhat satisfied	1212	−0.30	Somewhat satisfied	1211	−0.04
Somewhat dissatisfied	139	−0.78	Somewhat dissatisfied	358	−0.42
Extremely dissatisfied	50	−1.92	Extremely dissatisfied	325	−0.98
Trusted to make patient care decisions			*Feel respected by the agency*		
Strongly agree	2826	0.08	Strongly agree	2864	0.09
Somewhat agree	434	−0.30	Somewhat agree	406	−0.41
Somewhat disagree	58	−0.87	Somewhat disagree	61	−0.77
Strongly disagree	34	−1.35	Strongly disagree	23	−1.09
Reproductive labor			*Caring labor*		
4 Most supportive	579	0.16	6 Most supportive	1120	0.38
3	768	0.06	5	1132	0.21
2	1649	0.01	4	576	−0.16
1	249	−0.33	3	273	−0.88
0 Least supportive	96	−0.82	2	118	−1.35
Number of injuries			1	62	−2.42
0	2751	0.06	0 Least supportive	5	−2.04
1–2	573	−0.20			
3 or more	651	−0.89			

[a]Some survey items have smaller sample sizes due to missing data.
[b]Mean satisfaction is the satisfaction with their current job scale, standardized as a z-score with a mean of 0 and standard deviation of 1. Positive scores represent higher than average satisfaction, while negative scores represent lower than average satisfaction.

Table 3. Prevalence of Discrimination in Current Job by Source and Intersectional Identity ($N = 3350$).

	N	Experienced Discrimination (%)	Source: Patients (%)	Patients' Family (%)	Agency Management (%)	Coworkers (%)	Respected by Patients (%)
Overall	*3350*	*10.8*	*80.4*	*55.0*	*17.5*	*16.3*	*91.2*
Latina women	224	16.5	75.7	59.5	21.6	10.8	89.7
White women	2188	4.5	72.7	42.4	14.1	14.1	93.1
Black women	678	28.0	84.2	62.1	18.0	18.4	90.6
Latino men	10	10.0	100.0	100.0	0	0	60.0
White men	64	0	0	0	0	0	90.8
Black men	21	28.6	100.0	33.3	0	0	95.5
p-value		**		*			**

p-values from Chi-square tests. **p < 0.001, *p < 0.05.

great deal" (Table 3). Black women and men reported the highest levels of discrimination (28.0% and 28.6%, respectively). Latina and Latino HHAs reported the next highest levels of discrimination (16.5% and 10%, respectively). Latino HHAs also reported the least amount of respect by clients (only 60.0% reported a great deal), although the sample size was small ($n = 10$). A small, minority of white women reported discrimination (4.5%), and no white men reported discrimination. For those HHAs reporting discrimination, the majority cited patient family members as a source (55.5%). Less than 20% reported management or coworkers as a source of discrimination.

There were differences in job outcomes among workers according to their intersectional identities of RCG (Table 4). White men and women of the upper SES (top quartile) were the most likely to report injuries ($M = 0.25$ and 0.30, respectively). Wages and benefits differed by social class for all groups with the upper class group receiving higher wages and benefits. White men and women on average received the highest number of benefits ($M > 6.0$). Black men ($M = 4.10$) and Latino men ($M = 5.10$) on average received the lowest number of benefits. However, for the other aspects of the job, race and gender mattered more than social class. White men reported the most support and time for caring labor and had the highest job satisfaction scores. Black men, black women, and Latino men had lower than average job satisfaction scores. Latina and white women were about average. Reproductive labor scores did not vary significantly across groups, ranging between 2.13 and 2.80.

Table 4. Job Satisfaction and Working Conditions by Race, Class, and Gender.

Social Class		n	Injuries	Caring Labor[a]	Reproductive Labor[a]	Job Satisfaction[b]	Hourly Wage	Number of Benefits[c]
Latina women	Lower quartiles	180	0.19	4.72	2.20	0.01	11.31	5.23
	Top quartile	31	0.19	4.68	2.39	−0.08	12.17	5.38
White women	Lower quartiles	1725	0.26	4.81	2.49	0.05	11.35	6.32
	Top quartile	399	0.30	4.81	2.38	0.07	11.80	6.35
Black women	Lower quartiles	588	0.20	4.73	2.47	−0.17	10.90	5.87
	Top quartile	65	0.12	4.97	2.38	−0.05	13.36	6.22
Latino men[d]		10	0.10	4.90	2.80	−0.57	12.80	5.10
White men	Lower quartiles	47	0.17	5.33	2.68	0.26	11.39	6.05
	Top quartile	16	0.25	5.47	2.27	0.11	12.14	6.50
Black men		23	0.04	4.83	2.13	−0.06	11.60	4.10

[a]Caring and reproductive labor are coded such that higher numbers represent more support and time for this work.
[b]Job satisfaction is coded as a z-score where positive values are above-average satisfaction and negative values are below-average satisfaction.
[c]Number of benefits ranges from 0 benefits to 9 benefits offered.
[d]Latino men and Black men were not shown by class due to small sample sizes.

DISCUSSION

This study presented characteristics of HHAs, their satisfaction with aspects of their work, estimates for the prevalence of discrimination, and how these vary by the race/ethnicity, gender, and social class of the workers. These findings support previous research that HHAs are overwhelmingly women, about one third are minorities, and they have low wages and incomes. Sources of dissatisfaction include wages, benefits, and discrimination, mostly from patients and their families. By contrast, HHAs did not find significant institutional discrimination. HHAs are satisfied with being trusted to make patient care decisions, feeling respected by their agencies, having challenging work, and learning new skills. These findings reflect the importance of context for HHAs. Work in private homes seems to expose HHAs to clients' and their families' prejudice in ways that might be mitigated by a more open institutional setting.

Caring labor is of great importance to DCWs (Rakovski & Price-Glynn 2010). DCWs compensate for the negative aspects of their profession by the pleasure of caregiving through daily intimate contact with their clients. They also gain status by being recognized informally as the "true caregivers" by clients, other health-care professionals, and sometimes client family members (Bullock & Waugh, 2004). HHAs reported needing more time for both caring and reproductive labor. Not surprisingly, job satisfaction was low for those who did not feel supported in their caring labor. Like other DCWs, HHAs struggle to provide a nurturing setting and just care despite pressures to complete tasks quickly.

In terms of our intersectional analysis, race and gender emerged as important variables. Social class did not have an effect on the content of the work, but was associated with higher wages and benefits. However, it is reasonable that wages and social class are related, since household income, along with education, was used to create the social class variable. White men and women were the most satisfied with their work. White men had the most time and support for caring labor. These outcomes are likely due, at least in part, to both the race and gender politics of their clients. In particular for white men HHAs, clients may be reluctant to push for speedups the way they will for women of color. It is also possible that context plays a role. These findings stand in contrast to white male and female DCWs working in institutions who report less support for caring and reproductive labor (Price-Glynn & Rakovski, 2012). Perhaps the work setting – private homes – is shaping these outcomes. Despite these advantages, white men and women also had the highest number of injuries.

During the rise of medicine at the turn of the last century, nurses were less successful than doctors in creating a high-wage, high-status profession, and medical professions became increasingly gender-stratified (Duffy, 2011). Home health-care workers are at the nexus of the lowest levels of nursing and domestic work, both of which have suffered economically by their association with women, immigrants, and minorities (Duffy, 2011). However, it still needs to be examined whether, within low-wage workers, there is stratification by race, immigrant status, and gender. Our findings did not reveal substantial or clear hierarchies in terms of benefits and wages by intersectional identities of workers.

Differences in discrimination were evident. Black men and women reported the most discrimination. However, using quantitative, survey data may underestimate instances of mistrust or miscommunication due to race or ethnic differences or biases. Workers may not wish to disclose negative events due to social desirability bias. HHAs may also downplay some aggressive, patient behavior as an expected part of the job. The lower levels of discrimination with coworkers and agencies as sources is something that can be addressed at agencies, perhaps more easily than discrimination at the patient level. Agency supervisors have little control over a work environment that includes patients' private homes. Lopez (2006) found that organizations who promote honest, open dialogues between DCWs and clients increase worker satisfaction, compared to organizations that stress a customer service model for DCW/client interactions. Agencies can support HHAs when they challenge bad behavior from clients and create space for more authentic, balanced relationships. This is in contrast to the common practice of promoting fictive kin ties where all of the obligation and duties are one-sided.

Turnover is notoriously high among HHAs, likely driven by low wages. Among a large sample of home care workers in Maine, low wages and lack of affordable, employer-provided health care were more significant drivers for both intent to leave and actual turnover than other job characteristics (Morris, 2009). DCWs economic struggles remain persistent over the last several decades. Yamada (2002) examined the characteristics of DCWs across settings and how they changed between 1987–1989 and 1997–1999. While health insurance benefits improved, wages declined (Yamada, 2002). Our study also found more dissatisfaction with wages and benefits, compared to other aspects of the job. Wages continue to be vital to improving HHAs' working conditions and job satisfaction.

Despite the strengths of this study, there were also weaknesses. Using a secondary data analysis research method, we were limited by the survey items in the NHHS public-release files. The NHHS did not release citizenship information and only contained three racial categories (white, black, and other) and one ethnicity (Hispanic). We also had small sample sizes for men, especially black and Latino men. Open-ended responses to survey items were not released to the public. Those responses may reveal issues not anticipated by the survey design. However, the NHHS was modeled after the National Nursing Assistant Survey and allows comparisons of DCWs across settings (Bercovitz et al., 2011).

Future research is needed to explore interventions to improve the working conditions and job satisfaction of HHAs. Interventions and programs are needed to support HHAs who feel discriminated against by clients and their families. There is also a need for more space, time, and recognition of both reproductive or "dirty" work and emotional labor or caring work. The majority of HHAs were satisfied with feeling respected by their agencies and trusted to make care decisions. Caring for others is one of the main reasons DCWs continue despite low wages, rushed schedules, and injuries. Efforts must be ongoing to create a safe working environment for the increasing number of people who will work in home health care in the near future.

REFERENCES

Allensworth-Davies, D., Leigh, J., Pukstas, K., Geron, S. M., Hardt, E., Brandeis, G., ... Parker, V. A. (2007). Country of origin and racio-ethnicity: Are there differences in perceived organizational cultural competency and job satisfaction among nursing assistants in long-term care? *Health Care Management Review*, *32*(4), 321–329.

Aronson, J., & Neysmith, S. M. (1996). You're not just in there to do the work: Depersonalizing policies and the exploitation of home care workers' labor. *Gender & Society*, *10*, 59–77.

Bercovitz, A., Moss, A., Sengupta, M., Park-Lee, E. Y., Jones, A., Harris-Kojetin, L. D., & Squillace, M. R. (2011). An overview of home health aides 2007. *National health statistics reports*. US Department of Health and Human Services: Centers for Disease Control and Prevention National Center for Health Statistics.

Berdes, C., & Eckert, J. M. (2007). The language of caring: Nurse aides' use of family metaphors conveys affective care. *The Gerontologist*, *47*, 340–349.

Brannon, D., Barry, T., Kemper, P., Schreiner, A., & Vasey, J. (2007). Job perceptions and intent to leave among direct care workers: Evidence from the better jobs better care demonstrations. *The Gerontologist*, *47*(6), 820–829.

Brannon, D., Zinn, J., Mor, V., & Davis, J. (2002). An exploration of job, organizational, and environmental factors associated with high and low nursing assistant turnover. *The Gerontologist*, *42*(2), 159–168.

Browne, I., & Misra, J. (2003). The intersection of gender and race in the labor market. *Annual Review of Sociology*, *29*, 487–513.

Bullock, H. E., & Waugh, I. M. (2004). Caregiving around the clock: how women in nursing manage career and family demands. *Journal of Social Issues, 60,* 767–786.

Cancian, F. M. (1986). The feminization of love. *Signs, 11,* 692–709.

Chodorow, N. J. (1978). *The reproduction of mothering: Psychoanalysis and the sociology of gender.* Berkeley, CA: University of California Press.

Collins, P. H. (1993). Toward a new vision: Race, class, and gender as categories of analysis and connection. *Race, Sex and Class, 1,* 25–46.

Correll, S., Bernard, S., & Paik, I. (2007). Getting a job: Is there a motherhood penalty? *American Journal of Sociology, 112*(5), 1297–1338.

Decker, F. H. (2005). *Nursing homes 1977–99: What has changed, what has not?* Hyattsville, MD: National Center for Health Statistics.

Dodson, L., & Zincavage, R. (2007). It's like a family: Caring labor, exploitation, and race in nursing homes. *Gender & Society, 21,* 905–928.

Duffy, M. (2011). *Making care count: A century of gender, race, and paid care work.* New Brunswick, NJ: Rutgers University Press.

Duffy, M. (2007). Doing the dirty work: Gender, race, and reproductive labor in historical perspective. *Gender & Society, 21*(3), 313–336.

England, P. (2005). Emerging theories of care work. *Annual Review of Sociology, 31,* 381–399.

Harrington, C., Kovner, C., Mezey, M., Kayser-Jones, J., Burger, S., Mohler, M., ... Zimmerman, D. (2000). Experts recommend minimum nurse staffing standards for nursing facilities in the United States. *The Gerontologist, 40*(1), 5–16.

Hasson, H., & Arnetz, J. E. (2007). Nursing staff competence, work strain, stress and satisfaction in elderly care: A comparison of home-based care and nursing homes. *Journal of Clinical Nursing, 17,* 468–481.

Hochschild, A. R. (1983). *The managed heart : Commercialization of human feeling.* Berkeley, CA: University of California Press.

Hondagneu-Sotelo, P. (2007). *Domestica: Immigrant workers cleaning and caring in the shadows of affluence.* Berkeley, CA: University of California Press.

Howes, C. (2008). Love, money, or flexibility: What motivates people to work in consumer-directed home care? *The Gerontologist, 41,* 46–59.

Institute of Medicine. (2008). *Retooling for an aging America: Building the health care workforce.* Washington, DC: National Academy of Sciences.

Kemper, P., Heier, B., Barry, T., Brannon, D. B., Angelelli, J., Vasey, J., & Anderson-Knott, M. (2008). What do direct care workers say would improve their jobs: Differences across settings. *The Gerontologist, 48,* 17–25.

King, D. K. (1988). Multiple jeopardy, multiple consciousness: The context of a black feminist ideology. *Signs: Journal of Women in Society, 14,* 42–72.

Landry, B. (2007). *Race, class and gender: Theory and methods of analysis.* Upper Saddle River, NJ: Pearson Prentice Hall.

Lopez, S. H. (2006). Emotional labor and organized emotional care: Conceptualizing nursing home care work. *Work and Occupations, 33,* 133–160. doi:10.1177/0730888405284567

McCall, L. (2005). The complexity of intersectionality. *Signs: Journal of Women in Society, 30,* 1771–1800.

Miranda, H., Punnet, L., Gore, R., & Boyer, J. (2011). Violence at the workplace increases the risk of musculoskeletal pain among nursing home workers. *Occupational and Environmental Medicine, 68,* 52–57.

Morris, L. (2009). Quits and job changes among home care workers in maine: The role of wages, hours, and benefits. *The Gerontologist, 49*(5), 635–650.

Montgomery, R. J., Holley, L., Deichert, J., & Kosloski, K. (2005). A profile of home care workers from the 2000 Census: How it changes what we know. *The Gerontologist, 45*(5), 593–600.

Nishikawa, M. (2011). Redefining care workers as knowledge workers. *Gender, Work, and Organization, 18*(1), 113–136.

National Occupational Research Agenda (NORA). (2009). Occupational Safety and Health Research and Practice in the U.S. Healthcare and Social Assistance (HCSA) Sector. *Developed by the NORA Healthcare and Social Assistance Sector Council*, Retrieved from http://www.cdc.gov/niosh/nora/comment/agendas/hlthcaresocassist/

Oakes, J. M., & Rossi, P. H. (2003). The measurement of SES in health research: Current practice and steps toward a new approach. *Social Science & Medicine, 56*, 769–784.

Price-Glynn, K., & Rakovski, C. (2012). Who rides the glass escalator? Gender, race and nationality in the national nursing assistant study. *Work, Employment and Society, 26*(5), 830–856.

Rakovski, C., & Price-Glynn, K. (2010). Caring labour, intersectionality, and worker satisfaction: An analysis of the national nursing assistant study (NNAS). *Sociology of Health & Illness, 32*, 400–414.

Rivas, L. M. (2003). Invisible labours: Caring for the independent person. In B. Ehrenreich, A. R. Hochschild & A. Russell (Eds.), *Global woman: Nannies, maids and sex workers in the new economy* (pp. 70–84). London: Granta Books.

Sloane, P. D., Williams, C. S., & Zimmerman, S. (2010). Immigrant status and intention to leave of nursing assistants in U.S. nursing homes. *Journal of the American Geriatric Society, 58*, 731–737.

Smith, K., & Baughman, R. (2007). Caring for America's aging population: A profile of the direct-care workforce. *Monthly Labor Review, 130*(9), 20–26.

Solaris, C. (2006). Professionals and Saints: How immigrant careworkers negotiate gender identities at work. *Gender & Society, 20*(3), 301–331.

Sophie, J., Belza, B., & Young, Y. (2003). Health and safety risk at a skilled nursing facility: Nursing assistants' perceptions. *Journal of Gerontological Nursing, 29*(2), 13–21.

Stacey, C. L. (2005). Finding dignity in dirty work: The constraints and rewards of low-wage home care labour. *Sociology of Health & Illness, 27*, 831–854.

Tak, S., Sweeney, M. H., Alterman, T., Baron, B., & Calvert, G. M. (2010). Workplace assaults on nursing assistants in U.S. nursing homes: A multilevel analysis. *American Journal of Public Health, 100*(10), 1938–1945.

Yamada, Y. (2002). Profile of home care aids, nursing home aids, and hospital aides: Historical changes and data recommendations. *The Gerontologist, 42*, 199–206.

Zhang, Y., Flum, M., Nobrega, S., Blais, L., Qamili, S., & Punnet, L. (2011). Work organization and health issues in long-term care centers: Comparison of perceptions between caregivers and management. *Journal of Gerontological Nursing, 37*, 32–40.